PSYCHOTHERAPY
A Practical Introduction

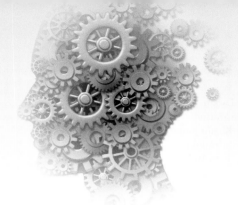

PSYCHOTHERAPY
A Practical Introduction

Adam M. Brenner, MD

Vice Chair for Education
Department of Psychiatry
University of Texas Southwestern Medical Center

Laura S. Howe-Martin, PhD

Associate Professor
Department of Psychiatry
University of Texas Southwestern Medical Center

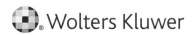. Wolters Kluwer

Philadelphia • Baltimore • New York • London
Buenos Aires • Hong Kong • Sydney • Tokyo

Acquisitions Editor: Chris Teja
Development Editor: Ariel S. Winter
Editorial Coordinator: John Larkin
Marketing Manager: Kirsten Watrud
Production Project Manager: Kirstin Johnson
Design Coordinator: Stephen Druding
Manufacturing Coordinator: Beth Welsh
Prepress Vendor: TNQ Technologies

9 8 7 6 5 4 3 2 1

Printed in China

Library of Congress Cataloging-in-Publication Data

ISBN-13: 978-1-975126-78-0

Cataloging in Publication data available on request from publisher

lww.com

The editors wish to acknowledge the additional editing contribution of Amy S. Brenner MSW, LCSW.

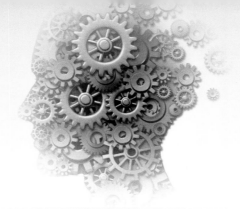

Contributors

Amy S. Brenner, MSW, LCSW
Volunteer Clinical Faculty
Department of Psychiatry
University of Texas Southwestern Medical Center
Dallas, Texas

Deborah L. Cabaniss, MD
Professor of Clinical Psychiatry
Department of Psychiatry
Columbia University
New York, New York

Erin M. Crocker, MD
Clinical Associate Professor
Department of Psychiatry
University of Iowa
Iowa City, Iowa

Sallie G. De Golia, MD, MPH
Clinical Professor
Department of Psychiatry and Behavioral Sciences
Stanford University School of Medicine
Stanford, California

Prasad R. Joshi, MD, PhD
Psychiatrist
Scranton Counseling Center
Scranton, Pennsylvania
Assistant Professor
Department of Psychiatry
Cornell University
New York, New York

Alexander S. Kane, MD
Assistant Professor
Department of Psychiatry
Cornell University
New York, New York

Heidi Koehler, PhD, ABPP
Assistant Professor
Department of Psychiatry
University of Texas Southwestern Medical Center
Dallas, Texas
Fort Worth VA Outpatient Clinic
VA North Texas Healthcare System
Fort Worth, Texas

Alison E. Lenet, MD
Assistant Clinical Professor
Department of Psychiatry
Columbia University Vagelos College of Physicians and Surgeons
New York, New York

Ben Lippe, PhD
Assistant Professor
Department of Psychiatry
University of Texas Southwestern Medical Center
Dallas, Texas

Shirali Patel, MD, MPhil
Assistant Professor
Department of Psychiatry and Behavioral Sciences
Baylor College of Medicine
Houston, Texas

Lindsey Pershern, MD
Associate Professor
Department of Psychiatry
University of Texas Southwestern Medical Center
Dallas, Texas

Mona A. Robbins, PhD
Assistant Professor
Department of Psychiatry
University of Texas Southwestern Medical Center
Dallas, Texas

Donna M. Sudak, MD
Professor of Psychiatry
Vice Chair for Education
Drexel University
General Psychiatry Residency Program Director
Tower Health-Brandywine Hospital Psychiatry
Philadelphia, Pennsylvania

Larry Thornton, MD
Professor
Department of Psychiatry
University of Texas Southwestern Medical Center
Dallas, Texas

Megan E. Tan, MD, MS
Clinical Assistant Professor
Department of Psychiatry and Behavioral Sciences
Stanford University
Palo Alto, California

Randon S. Welton, MD
Professor of Psychiatry
The Margaret Clark Morgan Chair of Psychiatry
Northeast Ohio Medical University
Rootstown, Ohio

Matan White, MD
Clinical Assistant Professor
Department of Psychiatry
University of Texas Southwestern Medical Center
Dallas, Texas

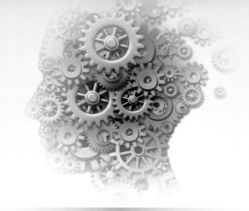

Contents

SECTION 3

Psychotherapy in Nontraditional Settings

SECTION 4

Further Directions in Learning Psychotherapy

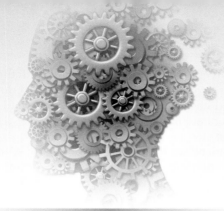

Introduction—How to Read This Book

This is the book we would have liked to have read when we were beginning our own clinical training in psychotherapy. We hope it will be similarly valuable to today's psychiatry residents, psychology graduate students, social work interns, and other trainees in mental health. Psychotherapy can be daunting to learn for the first time—there is a long, complex history, a lot of professional terminology, disagreement among experts, numerous schools of thought etc. Fortunately, you do not need to master the whole literature of psychotherapy to begin working effectively with your patients. Understanding the principles common to all therapies, appreciating the essential concepts of the major approaches to therapy, and knowing how to adapt these principles and concepts to different settings will allow you to be of great help to the people who entrust their care to you. That is the purpose of this book.

We have written this book so that it can be read straight through as a whole, or by selecting specific chapters that speak to your current training situation. Perhaps you are reading this as part of a course or didactic series, or perhaps you have just started in your first psychotherapy clinic and are needing a useful (brief) reference to help you feel more oriented. We hope this text can serve both purposes, while also sparking your interest in more in-depth learning.

Case studies are used frequently, to help illustrate the material in a more concrete manner, and each chapter includes a list of questions to help you check your own learning and provides references for further learning. Of note, the case studies in this book are the creation of each author or coauthors and are fictional in nature. Each of these case studies has been informed and shaped by our actual accumulated clinical experiences. Nonetheless, any resemblance to an actual person within the cases is coincidental. However, any self-disclosure made by our authors throughout their chapters is genuine.

Throughout the chapters you will find additional information in **text boxes.** These are meant to expose you to valuable ideas and topics that are not covered in the main text of the chapter. They can be read in the order they appear as part of the chapter, or they can be revisited by the reader when useful. Similarly, at the end of each chapter, we have included **resources for further learning**. It is our hope that these additional resources will inspire you to begin a lifetime of learning psycho-therapy. All our authors would agree that psychotherapy education during training at best provides "a good start"—an entire career of growth in expertise and deepening your understanding lies ahead.

Also, you may have noticed we have chosen to use "Mr. A" or "Ms. A" throughout each case study, even when discussing patients who are minors. We recognize this approach represents a binary approach to gender and note that the case studies did not include an example of the inclusive alternative "Mx. A" terminology. In addition, we recognize that the use of such titles as "Mr./Ms./Mx." reflects a formality that is not required or encouraged in all training environments, or across all cultures. Our practice as supervisors is to encourage what we view as a sense of formality and respect in this manner, for both the patient and the clinician, while also recognizing the use of these titles is a specific professional and cultural practice.

Now, onto how the book is outlined. **Section 1** provides a backdrop on the **fundamentals of psychotherapy** and the necessary **common elements** that span psycho-therapy methods and are crucial to beginning any therapy. We also hope it causes you to feel intrigued and excited at the prospect of working with patients of your own through psychotherapy. This section provides guidance on creating a **thoughtful psychotherapy case conceptualization** and also direction with regard to **choosing a therapy that will match your patient.**

Section 2 dives into four fundamental areas of psychotherapy that are considered **core competencies** for most psychotherapy training programs, including psychiatry residency. Chapters are specifically devoted to describing and applying **Supportive Psychotherapy, Cognitive-Behavioral Therapy,** and **Psychodynamic Therapy.** In addition, there is a chapter on the importance of considering **Culture and Systems.** Each of these chapters uses clear definitions of core concepts and illustrative case studies to apply beginner-level concepts. None of these therapeutic approaches can be covered entirely in a single chapter, but we have worked with our expert authors to provide you with a solid foundation.

Section 3 explores some of the unique settings in which psychotherapy is used. Many of these will mirror the settings in which you are or will be receiving psycho-therapy training. Special considerations exist for applying psychotherapy (of any kind) to **community mental health settings, consultation-liaison/medical settings, ER and crisis environments,** and **inpatient psychiatric units.** While we often stereotype psychotherapy as a 50-minute outpatient office visit, we know psychotherapy has a role and can be used effectively in every setting where treatment for mental illness and behavioral health is provided.

Section 4 addresses some key issues of the next steps of your development as therapists, in particular collaboration and supervision. The authors will orient you to the subject of **integrating psychotherapy and medication treatments**, the pros and cons of doing so in a single session, and ways for nonprescribers to collaborate more clearly with prescribers to boost their patients' care. In addition, there is a **specific chapter on psychotherapy supervision**. We strongly recommend reading this chapter prior to initiating supervision, as it contains several helpful (and practical) tips for making the most of your supervisory learning relationship.

We are enthusiastic to share this book with you and hope it prompts a keen interest in the art and science of psychotherapy!

Adam M. Brenner, MD
Laura S. Howe-Martin, PhD
UT Southwestern Medical Center, Dallas, Texas

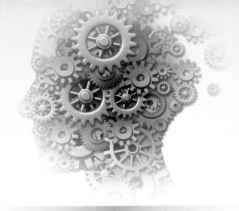

Section 1

BEGINNING PSYCHOTHERAPY

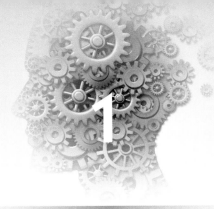

The Lay of the Land

ADAM M. BRENNER, MD

Learning to do psychotherapy can be daunting. There are many different kinds of therapy, and some of them have elaborate theoretical underpinnings, along with quite a bit of unnecessary jargon. Many of us struggled as beginning therapists to see the forest among all the intimidating trees. This first chapter will help you get the "lay of the land." In other words, what do you need to know about the "forest" of psychotherapies to not feel lost as you begin studying and doing therapy? In this chapter we will discuss:

1. What is psychotherapy?

2. What are the challenges (and rewards) unique to learning psychotherapy?

3. What are the core features of most psychotherapies?

4. How does psychotherapy work?

5. Does psychotherapy affect the mind or the brain?

6. What are the advantages and disadvantages of psychotherapy, compared with other kinds of treatments?

WHAT IS PSYCHOTHERAPY?

I remember being a beginning therapist and trying to explain to my new patients what psychotherapy was, while feeling unsure I could answer this question for myself. One of the reasons why it is so challenging to learn psychotherapy is that there is no universally accepted definition of "psychotherapy." It is an umbrella term used to encompass a wide range of different treatments. In that regard, Merriam-Webster[17] defines psychotherapy in an understandably broad and inclusive way: "Treatment of mental or emotional disorder or of related bodily ills by psychological means." In other words, psychotherapy is a treatment for a wide range of presentations (physical, mental, emotional) and that it is psychological—as opposed to physical, nutritional, pharmaceutical, etc. This definition is certainly true, but it leaves us with many questions. What are the "psychological means" through which therapy works? How are these "psychological means" created in the relationship between a therapist and a patient? And how is this relationship both like and unlike other important and helpful relationships in a patient's life?

Every student in a mental health training program has brought some preconceptions about psychotherapy. Sometimes those preconceptions are based on your own prior experience in psychotherapy. If so, you may have had a vivid experience of what a particular type of therapy looks like in the hands of one clinician. One of the learning goals in this book is to help you put that specific experience into the larger context of psychotherapy. However, for other trainees, your only prior exposure to psychotherapy may have been through depictions in popular culture. And depending on whether this has been through *The Sopranos* or *Frazier* or any of hundreds of other movie, TV, or literary therapists, you may have dramatically different ideas of what psychotherapy will look like. Sometimes, the picture is of a generally silent and reserved figure who listens, says very little, and yet somehow peers into the dark depths of the soul. In other instances, the therapist appears as a wise and warm sage who provides guidance—spiritual, moral, practical—that will finally set the patient on the right path. And unfortunately, sometimes the image is of a charismatic but unbalanced healer who uses electrifying interventions, but whose work is always balanced on the razor's edge and where boundaries exist just to be dramatically broken. We assume that you come to this subject with a similar task of sorting out an array of inspiring, confusing, disturbing, and contradictory depictions of psychotherapy.

Our patients are no different in that they also bring their own preconceptions into therapy. Sometimes, they have already been in psychotherapy and expect their new treatment to be like the previous one. Sometimes, they have absorbed the same stereotypes from pop culture described previously. Other patients expect that psychotherapy will be like their other physician visits—a description of the problem, a diagnosis, and then instructions. They will need you, as their new therapist, to help them understand what they are actually signing up for.

In some ways, defining "psychotherapy" will take this entire book. But, here are some ideas I have found useful to organize my own explorations of therapy that may be helpful to get you started. *In psychotherapy, we try to help a patient with some problem that matters a great deal to them, is often difficult to talk about initially, and has already failed to be helped by their usual resources. We create a unique kind of relationship, so that we can use listening, talking, and being together to purposefully initiate relief, change, and growth.*

CHALLENGES AND REWARDS UNIQUE TO LEARNING PSYCHOTHERAPY

Most of us who have been doing therapy for a while can still vividly remember how anxious we were with our first patients. Part of this anxiety was uncertainty about our own competence, but we were also unsure what "good psychotherapy" was supposed to look like! In most areas of health care, a provider will watch someone else perform a procedure—generally at least several times—before attempting to provide the treatment themselves. For example, a physical therapist treating you has previously watched someone else conduct this same type of therapy from start to finish, and this would be a fair expectation. In other areas of health care, training in simulation laboratories has become essential—the trainee will often have watched and practiced the treatment procedure on a mannequin or a simulated patient before they try with a real patient.

But, neither multiple observations nor simulations are likely to occur before your first psychotherapy session with a patient. Why is that? Part of the reason is practicality. A very short course of psychotherapy might be 10 to 20 sessions, and these will be spread out over many weeks. That is a lot of time to devote to observation or simulation. In fact, a training program may arrange for a therapy to be observed behind a one-way mirror, or for a therapy to have been filmed so that the trainees can watch. There is a great deal to be learned this way, but even that approach has innate limitations. One of the strange things about psychotherapy as a treatment process is that the therapy that is observed or filmed is never exactly the same as it would have been without the observers or the cameras. The patient will behave differently, and the therapist will also. Sometimes people are more inhibited, sometimes they become more performative, but either way, you are not going to see what would have happened if the therapy had been conducted in the usual cocoon of therapeutic privacy.

Another difficulty is psychotherapy is an incredibly complex process. Although you can be taught theoretical principles, rules of thumb, techniques, and specific interventions, each moment in psychotherapy has too many possible meanings and too many possible helpful responses for a trainee to successfully "script out" what should happen. This has important implications for learning therapy. Watching one therapy session—or even several—will not fully prepare you for conducting your own psychotherapies because the combination of your own personality, your specific patients, and your therapeutic approach will all differ. This is one of the wonderful paradoxes of psychotherapy. While there are many profound commonalities to all human beings, each person is still absolutely distinct and has a story no one else has ever told. This is part of why many therapists still find their work fascinating, even after decades of practice.

Both sides of this tension turn out to be great sources of personal growth and fulfillment for therapists. On the one hand, therapists find truth in the old saying by Terence, "Nothing human is alien to me."[18] All of us share longings to be loved and to love, to have a valued identity, and to be appreciated for our work. All of us need to feel we belong—to a family, a community, a congregation, or a political party, etc. All of us feel frightened when vulnerable or threatened, and all of us become angry when hurt or attacked. All of us feel regret and guilt when our actions fall short of our standards, and all of us feel shame when we are faced with something about ourselves that seems unacceptable, defective, or disgusting. When we meet with patients, we come in touch with the things that make us all human. *It is a moving and humbling privilege.*

And yet, no individual can be reduced to any schematic or equation defined by these needs and feelings, because the story of each person is always irreducibly unique. And, that story is critical to each person's understanding of themselves. Sometimes, the patient's story that they convey in psychotherapy sounds more like a myth or fairy tale. Other patients may tell you a story that fits the kinds of fiction and movie genres that we are all familiar with—they tell their life as if it were a tragedy, or a heroic quest, or a romantic comedy. And yet other patients will tell a story that defies genre, because it is complex and nuanced, or because it is fragmented and confusing. What all of these stories have in common is that they attempt to answer fundamental questions of existence and cause—"Why am I who I am?" and "How did I get to be where I am in life?"

Another difficulty in learning psychotherapy is it can resemble many other experiences people have outside of treatment. Psychotherapy is surely not the only way in which people engage with each other with the goal to help, to learn, to grow, and to comfort. This occurs within parent–child relationships, friendships, romantic relationships, teaching, mentoring, and many other ways of relating. In all those instances, two (or more) people are talking and the goal is to help and be helped. In fact, many learners find themselves in psychotherapy training programs because they have in the past shown some particular aptitude for listening and helping in these spontaneous and less formal relationships. Often, someone has told the student or resident, "You should think about being a therapist!"

Patients will often, quite understandably, expect therapy to proceed like those other spontaneous and natural helping relationships. That would mean, for example, that there would be the degree of reciprocity and mutuality found in a friendship. Or that there would be a strong emphasis on advice-giving, like a parent or a mentor or executive coach would provide. It helps to remember that patients usually come to therapy already having tried to address their problems through these other, more typical channels. It is only when these other approaches are not sufficient that a patient seeks out a mental health professional. So, an important part of the task in learning psychotherapy is to understand how it will be actually different from all those other helping encounters and relationships. What is it that we will offer that goes beyond the help found in all those other arenas? Or to put a sharper point on it, what is that we are being paid for?

MAKING SENSE OF THE VARIETIES OF THERAPY

So, if we are not providing advice about important decisions, and we are not forming the usual kinds of reciprocal social relationships that people enjoy or lean on, what in fact are we doing for our patients? What happens in psychotherapy that actually helps the patient? Let us imagine a person who comes to therapy looking for help with some kind of distressing thought, or mood problem, or troubling behavior. Our new patient is probably not only suffering from the direct impact of their symptom or behavior. They often feel ashamed of their situation, alone and isolated by it, and afraid that nothing can be done. I am going to suggest that we will help this new patient in two very different ways. There is risk that this will oversimplify a complex topic and, like with any rules of thumb, there will be exceptions. Nonetheless, it is helpful when approaching a new and intimidating field of study to have a basic scaffolding to hold onto and on which to place the many details.

First, we help our patients by *providing comfort, safety, and support*. As a result, they feel more hopeful and less alone. These effects are often referred to as some of the "common elements" of psychotherapy[1-3] (there will be much more on these common elements later). Second, we *help our patients learn something new*, something that they would not be able to learn in any other relationship or setting. The specifics of what is learned and how can vary enormously from one therapy to the next. Some

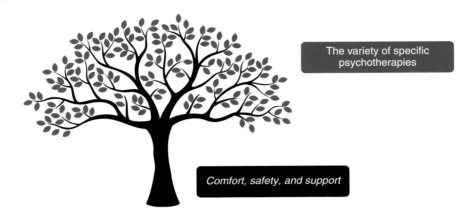

FIGURE 1.1 The tree of psychotherapies.

authors have suggested the metaphor of a "tree" of psychotherapies, with the common elements of comfort and support being the trunk of the tree, and the specific therapies with their different kinds of learning the branches (*Figure 1.1*). A similar metaphor is the "Y model," where the stem of the "Y" is the common elements/ supportive therapy and the two upper branches are the two major approaches of psychodynamic and cognitive behavioral therapy[4] (these specific therapies will be discussed in later chapters) (*Figure 1.2*).

For example, in cognitive behavioral therapy (CBT), the therapist teaches the patient quite directly.[5] The therapist may teach the patient to identify distorted patterns of thinking and how to correct them. Or, the therapist may teach the patient techniques for modulating emotions, desensitizing themselves to anxious situations, or changing maladaptive behaviors. The learning may continue between appointments as well if the therapist assigns an "action plan" or "homework" to the patient. In contrast, a psychodynamic therapist tends to help the patient learn in a more indirect way. The therapist believes the patient needs to learn about aspects of their own mind that are under the surface, and typically inaccessible to conscious introspection, perhaps because they are too disturbing for the patient to be fully aware of.[6] In that case, the therapist creates a process where unconscious material can be discovered and learned about together. In the process, the therapist and patient will also learn about the patient's ways of being with another person, patterns that the

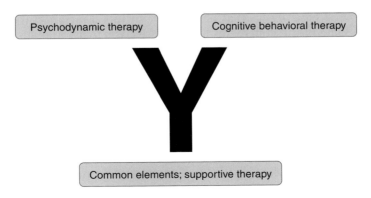

FIGURE 1.2 The Y model of psychotherapy.

patient may also have been unaware of, and the possibility of learning different ways of relating begins to open. Regardless, both rely heavily on a solid trunk of common factors and a comforting, safe, and supportive psychotherapeutic relationship.

As you can see from these two examples, the kinds of teaching and learning that happen in different approaches to psychotherapy can be very distinct, and you will learn much more about these in the chapters on psychodynamic therapy, cognitive behavioral therapy, supportive therapy, and social systems approaches to psychotherapy. It is our hope that this book will provide a solid platform from which you can also learn about and explore many other psychotherapy approaches, which are beyond the scope of this introductory book.

THE IMPORTANCE OF COMMON FACTORS OF PSYCHOTHERAPY

It is useful to understand the vital importance of common elements of therapy when thinking of the very first meeting between the patient and their prospective therapist. As new therapists, it is very common to feel preoccupied with what we do not know how to do and thereby feel that what we have to offer is inadequate. The good news is that this is not true. What you bring to the patient even at the beginning of your training is already quite powerful. New therapists are often surprised when a patient returns for the second session and reports that they felt much better after that first encounter. *How can the patient feel better when I, the therapist, felt overwhelmed and inept?* The fact is we actually do not have to do anything fancy or brilliant for the patient to get some real relief at that first meeting.

Those of us who come to therapy through medical school can usually remember experiences as beginning medical students where we met with patients for the first time to "take a history." Often we felt guilty for intruding or for wasting the patient's time, as we were not able to offer the patient a diagnosis or treatment plan. And yet, we were surprised when the patient later thanked us, or told the attending physician how helpful we had been. Similarly, psychotherapy researchers described a wonderful study where college professors with no training in counseling or therapy met with distressed students and, lo and behold, the students felt better.[6] Why is it that patients can feel helped by a well-intentioned—but still untrained—student or college professor?

There are several basic things that help make our initial meetings with a patient therapeutic. Some of these elements can seem so basic that you might easily overlook them. One is that the patient told you what is troubling them. You then proceeded to take them seriously and showed that their concerns matter to you. This is known in the psychotherapy research literature as the Hawthorne effect: being seen as worth another person's careful attention is powerful.[1] Another fundamental element is that you did not recoil in shock or horror when the patient talked about the material they find disturbing or shameful. You might take for granted that you would not think of responding that way, but your response to the patient may make a profound impression. In fact, you probably even asked them to tell you more about the things that they feel are most terrible and off-putting. The last fundamental element is that you seemed to have at least some (even if vague) idea about how psychotherapy is going to be helpful to the patient and conveyed some confidence in the process. Notice these fundamental elements do not include great insights about the unconscious meanings of their problems, or the ability to describe an explanatory model of their symptoms, or that you made a profound connection between their distress and their early developmental experiences. None of that is necessary to lay the groundwork for successful therapy during the first meeting.

If the initial meeting has included some of these fundamental elements, the patient is likely to leave the meeting in a very different state than they were in at the beginning. First, the patient may have been feeling alone with their distress, and now they feel that you are in this with them. The two of you are together in bearing this problem, whatever it turns out to be. Second, they may have been feeling that their experience or symptoms make no sense, or as people often put it, that they are "crazy." At the end of the meeting they feel you actually could understand something of what they are going through. Third, they may have felt ashamed, or freakish, because of what they are experiencing. At the end of the meeting, however, they feel you were able to accept them as they are. And finally, at the beginning of the session they may have felt desperate and hopeless, having tried everything they could think of to cope and having it fail. But at the end of the meeting, they feel hopeful and tentatively expectant of some kind of change.

Those four effects—(1) Together (not alone); (2) Understood (not incomprehensible); (3) Accepted (not rejected); (4) Hopeful (not demoralized)—are of course not limited to the initial meeting. They will be repeatedly reinforced throughout the entire treatment. One of the most important research findings about psychotherapy is not only that all therapies have these elements in common, but these elements also account for much of the beneficial impact of any specific therapy.[2] That is worth repeating, because it is counterintuitive. Even though you will be spending a great deal of time and effort to learn the theory and technique of specific psychotherapies, *most of the benefit is actually going to be generated by careful attention to promoting these common elements.*

Now here is a strong caveat to what was just stated—this does *not* mean that the effort to learn and apply a specific therapy is not time well spent. First, specific therapeutic techniques do account for a substantial part of the effect, and you and your patient will want to be making use of every kind of treatment advantage available. But just as important, it is not possible to optimize the full extent of the common effects of therapy unless you are also providing a specific therapy. Your capacity to help the patient feel understood will draw on your understanding of some theory of what has gone wrong. Similarly, I described the crucial importance of the patient feeling hopeful about the plan. This can only come about because you convey that the specific psychotherapy you will be using has a specific method of some kind and that you will be applying this method together, in the service of alleviating the patient's suffering.

Jerome Frank's classic text, *Persuasion and Healing*, emphasized the importance of the specific theory and method, or what he called "myth" and "ritual."[7] Frank found that when he looked at psychotherapies of different kinds they shared certain characteristics with therapeutic relationships that occur in spiritual or cultural traditions of helping around the world. These characteristics are as follows: (1) A conceptual scheme (or myth) that provides a plausible meaning or explanation for the problems. This results in a possibility of mastery and decreasing helplessness. (2) A ritual or procedure that is believed to be effective. This ritual provides both a direct source of hopefulness, and an opportunity to work together on shared tasks that generate incremental gains.

To review, a patient may come away from their initial psychotherapy sessions feeling better in some predictable ways—less alone, less ashamed, and more hopeful. Taken together, common factors theories and research serve as a solid "trunk of the psychotherapy tree" that can further be developed by learning specific therapies (or "branches") to improve outcomes. However, what is it about human beings that creates the conditions for these common elements to have such profound effects, and for psychotherapy to therefore "work"?

THE IMPORTANCE OF ATTACHMENT IN PSYCHOTHERAPY

One of the reasons the unique relationships within psychotherapy produce change lies in the fact that we are primates, and primates are born with an attachment system. Thinking about attachment is very helpful for understanding how the common elements are rooted in our deepest nature. Psychotherapy schools in the 20th century were slow to appreciate the importance of attachment. Some early schools of therapy (such as psychoanalysis) emphasized how people were driven by the biological urges of hunger, sex, and aggression, while other early schools of therapy (such as behaviorism) were more focused on the ways reward and punishment could be used to modify behaviors. The idea that every human being was built to seek out a secure attachment during development was not on their radar. John Bowlby and Mary Ainsworth were pivotal figures in influencing the field of mental health and behavior toward the centrality of attachment.[8]

Bowlby drew on clinical experience as a therapist, on naturalistic observation of children, and on laboratory studies of primates.[9] Especially important were observations of children who had suffered from deprivation of parental care or from disruptive separations. Acutely, such children could seem listless, needy, and anxious, while over the long term they might have problems with depression, aggression, or antisocial behavior. These observations were also completely consistent with Harlow's famous studies of infant monkeys. In response to separation from their mothers, films showed the baby monkeys clinging desperately to the most minimal available substitutes, such as a wire frame covered with a thin towel. In both human and other primate young, separation resulted in a common set of reactions—first the baby would cry or call out in protest, then seem sad and despairing, and finally become detached from the caregiver, but with significant emotional and behavioral scars.

After demonstrating that this early connection was critical, Bowlby described how attachment happens, and Ainsworth later provided empirical evidence for this theory through designing experiments (the Strange Situation Classification) to assess the various attachment styles that exist between children and their caregivers. Per Bowlby's theory, both the baby and the parent had built-in behavioral systems designed to foster these connections. This is absolutely crucial, because primate babies are quite helpless when born and will not survive very long at all without a caregiver hovering nearby. When babies experience a separation, they cry. Parents find this such a disturbing sound that they immediately want to find the cause and stop it (and not just parents, as anyone who has sat near a crying baby on an airplane can attest). When the parent returns and picks the child up, the comfort, relief, and then even joy of the child is clear.

Babies also provide positive signals, such as smiling or babbling, that draw their parents (and others) to engage them and hold them. Once the baby and the parent are mutually engaged, they immediately start mimicking and responding to each other's faces. This generally happens quite automatically, but is a wonderful early experience of learning how to be attuned to another person and how to modulate each other's emotional state.

Our point here is that patients are not a "blank slate" when they present for therapy. As primates, they have an attachment system that is built to reach out for a protective other, and as primates we have reciprocal instincts to comfort in response. Of course, the patient's early attachment experiences will have a profound influence on the shape of how they seek attachment as an adult. Some will have had an experience of relatively tuned-in and reliable caregivers. These fortunate patients had a "secure attachment" and even in the face of their symptoms and distress, they will approach the therapist in a spirit of optimistic expectation. Ainsworth demonstrated through the Strange Situation research that when a secure attachment has not been possible the toddler will modify their own behaviors to cope as best they can with the pain of separation or neglect, even if these new behaviors are maladaptive later in life. Some patients who had inconsistent or unresponsive caregivers will come to their new therapist under the shadow of these "insecure attachments." They might have learned to adopt a stance of not needing anyone, although deep down there are still great yearnings to connect. Or, they might have learned to demand and grab hold tightly to any available caregiver. This is a fairly reasonable response if you could not count on your caregivers to be attuned and responsive to your needs. In our chapter on beginning a therapy (Chapter 4), we will have more to say about patients who had serious trauma as a child and how this shapes their initial experience of therapy. However, just being aware of these possibilities can help us to tolerate our patient's maladaptive ways of seeking and avoiding attachment, and help the patient use psychotherapy to learn healthy new ways of being connected.

DOES PSYCHOTHERAPY AFFECT THE MIND OR THE BRAIN?

Is psychotherapy affecting the "mind" or the "brain"? This is an area of significant and lively discussion within mental health care and research. In the past, mental health clinicians often thought of treatments as either biologic or psychosocial. This fed into a tendency to think of medications, as a clearly biologic treatment, acting on the brain, whereas psychotherapies, as psychosocial treatment, were seen as acting on the mind. Today, we should all recognize that this is a false and misleading dichotomy. Several decades of functional imaging research have made it clear that psychotherapy results in changes in brain function.[10,11] For example, functional imaging allows researchers to see whether specific regions or circuits are either overactive or underactive compared to healthy controls, by looking at the degree of blood flow or metabolism throughout the brain. Numerous studies in patients with conditions such as social phobia, obsessive compulsive disorder, post-traumatic stress disorder, and depression provide compelling demonstrations that we are generating measurable changes in brain function by talking to our patients. Clearly everything that we experience as our "self," all of our mental life, is rooted in the brain.

However, the relationship of the mind and the brain has been puzzling and vexing our greatest thinkers throughout human history. And it *still* remains a largely unresolved question! We have only the most tentative ideas about how neuronal activity, subjective feeling, and thoughts actually relate to one another. Fortunately, we do not have to resolve this question to be effective psychotherapists. It is enough if we understand from neuroscience research that all mental life is rooted in the brain.[12,13] Injuries to the brain result in changes in a person's thoughts, feelings, behaviors, personality, and even identity. And as you just read, making changes in thoughts and feelings results in physiological changes in the brain.

This can further be illustrated through the neurobiology of both attachment and learning. Attachment and "social pain" is an area of research that clearly demonstrates the connection between mind and brain. It turns out that experiences of social pain—the humiliation, anxiety, and confusion that accompany feeling rejected or excluded—have a remarkable overlap with the distress of physical pain.[14] The brain uses opioid receptors to signal the distress of both a physical injury and an interpersonal one, and then uses endogenous opiates to relieve the distress. In experiments that involve isolating puppies and causing separation distress, administering a low dose of morphine is as effective on distress as it would be if the puppies were in physical pain. And, reuniting mothers and puppies increases endogenous opiate levels in both mother and puppy. The same part of the brain that regulates and represents the experience of physical wounds—the anterior cingulate cortex—also regulates and represents our patients' experiences of the pain of rejection and isolation. Given how absolutely essential attachment is for baby primates—and therefore how extreme the danger of separation—it makes sense that the brain would call into service these older mechanisms for protection from physical pain. These same brain mechanisms for monitoring and soothing social pain are ready for the therapist and patient to activate when they meet, even for the initial encounter.

As we discussed earlier, all psychotherapies involve new learning of one kind or another, and research on learning also shows the convergence of mind and brain. Eric Kandel and others were able to demonstrate how the brain changes when animals learn, a process known as "plasticity."[12,13] These changes can involve growth of new synapses (connections between neurons), pruning of existing synapses (reduction in the number of connections between neurons), or changes in the strength of specific synaptic connections. Kandel eventually received the Nobel Prize in Medicine for this work. Furthermore, Kandel himself thought this was directly relevant to psychotherapy: "Insofar as psychotherapy or counseling is effective and produces long term changes in behavior it presumably does so through learning, by producing changes in gene expression that alter the strength of synaptic connections and structural changes that alter the anatomical pattern of interconnections between nerve cells in the brain."[12]

However, what is learned is encoded into memory through two very distinct neurobiological systems.[13,15] Both of these memory systems are important to our work in psychotherapy and need to be highlighted. First, some memory is called "declarative" or "explicit." This is the memory of specific facts or events that we can consciously bring to mind. The hippocampus and the neocortex are particularly crucial to this kind of memory and learning. The second kind of memory is called "procedural" or "implicit." This kind of memory is used for learning how to do something or encoding relational patterns and generally operates without conscious awareness. For example, attachment patterns and expectations are held as procedural or implicit memory.

To use a simple analogy, when I drive to work on my usual route I am using implicit memory for both the task of driving itself and for following the route. I do not have to think about either operating the car or finding my way, leaving me consciously free to talk to a companion, listen to a news story on the radio, or reflect on a challenging situation at work. However, if my usual route is blocked by an accident, I may need to think very explicitly and consciously about how to find a new route and how to do it safely.

Many patients come to therapy because, for whatever reason, their established and automatic ways of relating or being in the world are no longer working. When they discover those "routes" are blocked, they need to learn new options. One of the very exciting things about therapy is that sometimes this learning occurs very explicitly, with the patient and the therapist talking about obstacles to trust (for example) in their relationship and resolving them together. However, much of the time the patient may also be learning implicitly.[15] You as the therapist may not feel that much is happening and you may wonder whether you are really having an impact. But the patient, through the repeated experience of your reliability and steady interest, might be having a very profound experience of implicit learning about what might be possible within healthy attachment relationships. Fortunately, therapy clearly utilizes both the brain structures and circuits that manage procedural/implicit memory as well as those that support conscious/explicit memory.

THE ADVANTAGES OF PSYCHOTHERAPY

Some patients seek psychotherapy as the intervention of choice because they wish to avoid the risks or side effects of other treatment modalities. Other patients, however, are reluctant to consider psychotherapy, perhaps because they hoped for a treatment that will be faster or more focused than "just talking." Where does psychotherapy fit among the array of possible treatments aimed at alleviating mental suffering? There are, after all, other ways to have a therapeutic impact on the mind and the brain. Psychotherapy is not without real risks and costs, but it also has some very distinct advantages that include its capacity for highly focused intervention.

Although there are many medications that produce crucial and sometimes life-saving changes in patients, it is important to realize that medications are the bluntest possible instrument. When a patient is given a medication that works on dopamine or serotonin or GABA receptors, that medication will be administered to every circuit and neuron throughout the entire brain that uses that neurotransmitter. In addition, most medications also have lesser effects on other, nontargeted neurotransmitters and receptors, often resulting in side effects. Some are nagging and minor, but others can be quite profound. The loss of sexual function in a young person trying to recover from depression is no small thing. The subjective dulling of creativity or aliveness that some patients with bipolar disorder report from mood stabilizers or antipsychotic medications can feel like a great loss. In this context, the capacity to use some of the newer neuromodulation interventions such as transcranial magnetic stimulation to target a specific structure or circuit in the brain could be a great advantage.

For example, let us consider a patient who presents with all the classic signs of a major depressive episode after suffering a humiliating loss in his career. We can give him a serotonin reuptake inhibitor that will work throughout every area of the brain where serotonin is involved in circuits, which is very extensive. Or, we can consider a targeted neuromodulation such as a transcranial magnetic stimulation to activate or quiet a specific brain structure or circuit.

However, it is important to remember that there already is a procedure that is more specific than either neuromodulation or psychotropic medications. It is a procedure that evolved alongside the brain itself, over millennia of evolution, as the primary means of affecting highly specific and crucial change in the brain. In the face of life's greatest pains and losses, relationships and talking are how our brain was "designed" to be comforted, repaired, and healed.

One of the things that may have drawn you to mental health was appreciating that even though losses can lead to depression, and depressions can have similar symptoms from one patient to the next, no two depressed or grieving patients are ever the same. The details of their stories and therefore the specific meaning of the loss are unique. This meaning is encoded in the brain at the level of organization of synaptic networks that can only be selectively reached through the use of language and behavior.[16] When we ask the patient in psychotherapy to talk about their subjective experience of a recent loss, we can activate that highly specific synaptic network. We will be able to impact just those neurons associated with each other through the memory of the specific events, their association to past events that magnify or mitigate the impact, and their association to specific implicit ideas about his identity, value in the world, and value to other people he cares about. This is one of the ways that psychotherapy can do things that no other biologic intervention can do.

THE RISKS OF PSYCHOTHERAPY

While it is true that psychotherapy has the advantages of specificity and avoiding many of the side effects of other treatments, it also has disadvantages or risks of its own. These are important to recognize, because when we invite a patient to begin therapy, we are also asking them to take on these costs. First, psychotherapy as it is traditionally provided is expensive to patients and requires significant resources. Even if we offer the lowest fees we can, it is still a very time-consuming process. And time is a "zero sum game"—the time spent commuting to and from and attending therapy is time that cannot be used for work, studying, caring for children or the elderly, in hobbies, in community, etc. Second, therapy is almost always painful, at least at some point in the process. If the patient is addressing the truly painful parts of their story, they may leave the session still hurting emotionally for some time. Third, therapy is not always successful in alleviating suffering, nor is it always the best treatment approach. At times, we choose a therapy approach that is the "best" treatment available per the current research, only to see it fail because it does not fit with the patient's values or expectations. Psychotherapy is not a cure-all, nor is it appropriate for all patients at all times.

Finally, the same mechanisms that underlie the impressive power of the common elements of therapy—trust, hope, attachment—also make the patient vulnerable. Although we make use of the power of attachment to support and to heal, that experience is confined to the therapy hour. They may experience the pain of disappointment as they face the limits of the therapy relationship. Although patients can "internalize" this experience, and carry the mental image of the therapist with them throughout the rest of the week, this is still a far cry from having you actually there when they are in pain. In the chapter on starting therapies (Chapter 4), we will discuss why it is necessary to have these limits and boundaries—they make it possible for therapy to happen. When those limits are not maintained by the therapist, we can cause great harm to the patient, including experiences of exploitation, abuse, and exacerbation of the presenting illness. These "boundary violations" are perhaps the greatest potential risk of psychotherapy and should be taken very seriously by the new therapist.

Conclusion

In this chapter, we have seen that psychotherapy is a general term that covers an array of approaches, but that all psychotherapies all involve one person trying to help and heal another person through talking about important, distressing matters. Psychotherapy can be challenging to learn because both the therapist and the patient will bring preconceptions (and misconceptions) to the process, based on media and cultural depictions of therapy, and based on analogies to other helping relationships. Psychotherapy can also be difficult to learn because we need to embrace both our common humanity and each patient's profound uniqueness. We then saw that we can begin to orient ourselves by thinking about how therapy works. There are some beneficial effects that all therapies share, including reducing aloneness, shame, and hopelessness. These "common effects" are partly rooted in a universal human capacity to seek out and to provide attachment. We also saw that there are therapeutic benefits specific to each kind of therapy rooted in learning. Learning is a crucial part of therapy but what kinds of things we want the patient to learn can be very different. Because attachment and learning are both well-described neurobiological processes, we found it makes little sense to confine the work of psychotherapy to either the brain or the mind, or divide treatments into "biological" or "psychosocial." All mental life is mediated through brain function, and psychotherapy generates clear changes in the brain. Finally, we looked at the significant advantages that psychotherapy offers as a treatment modality, especially the capacity for a degree of specificity and focus unmatched by any other intervention. We also noted, however, that psychotherapy is a powerful process, and there are real costs and risks that must be respected as well.

Self-Study Questions

1. How do we define psychotherapy? How is it similar to and different from other important relationships in a patient's life?

2. List and describe at least two "common factors" of psychotherapy.

3. Describe why the concept of attachment is important in psychotherapy.

4. List at least two risks and two benefits of psychotherapy as a treatment approach.

RESOURCES FOR FURTHER LEARNING

Etkin A, Pittenger C, Polan HJ, Kandel ER. Toward a neurobiology of psychotherapy: basic science and clinical applications. *J Neuropsychiatry Clin Neurosci.* 2005;17:145-158.

Feinstein R, Heiman N, Yager J. Common factors affecting psychotherapy outcomes: some implications for teaching psychotherapy. *J Psychiatr Pract.* 2015;21:180-189.

Fonagy P. *Attachment Theory and Psychoanalysis.* New York, NY: Other Press LLC; 2001.

Frank JD, Frank JB. *Persuasion and Healing: A Comparative Study of Psychotherapy.* 3rd ed. Baltimore, MD: Johns Hopkins University Press; 1991.

Lieberman MD. *Social: Why Our Brains Are Wired to Connect.* New York, NY: Broadway Books; 2013.

Plakun EM, Sudak DM, Goldberg D. The Y model: an integrated, evidence-based approach to teaching psychotherapy competencies. *J Psychiatr Pract.* 2009;15:5-11.

REFERENCES

1. Feinstein R, Heiman N, Yager J. Common factors affecting psychotherapy outcomes: some implications for teaching psychotherapy. *J Psychiatr Pract.* 2015;21:180-189.

2. Wampold BE. How important are the common factors in psychotherapy? An update. *World Psychiatry.* 2015;14(3):270-277.

3. Nahum D, Alfonso CA, Sönmez E. Common factors in psychotherapy. In: Javed A, Fountoulakis K, eds. *Advances in Psychiatry.* Cham: Springer; 2019.

4. Plakun EM, Sudak DM, Goldberg D. The Y model: an integrated, evidence-based approach to teaching psychotherapy competencies. *J Psychiatr Pract.* 2009;15:5-11.

5. Beck JS. *Cognitive Behavior Therapy: Basics and Beyond.* 2nd ed. New York, NY: The Guilford Press; 2011.

6. Cabaniss DL. *Psychodynamic Psychotherapy: A Clinical Manual.* 2nd ed. Chichester, England: Wiley Blackwell; 2016.

7. Frank JD, Frank JB. *Persuasion and Healing: A Comparative Study of Psychotherapy.* 3rd ed. Baltimore, MD: Johns Hopkins University Press; 1991.

8. Fonagy P. *Attachment Theory and Psychoanalysis.* New York, NY: Other Press LLC; 2001.

9. Bowlby J. *A Secure Base: Parent-Child Attachment and Healthy Human Development.* New York, NY: Basic Books; 1988.

10. Etkin A, Pittenger C, Polan HJ, Kandel ER. Toward a neurobiology of psychotherapy: basic science and clinical applications. *J Neuropsychiatry Clin Neurosci.* 2005;17:145-158.

11. Schore AN. "*Toward a new paradigm of psychotherapy*". In: *The Science of the Art of Psychotherapy.* New York, London: WW Norton and Company; 2012.

12. Kandel E. A new intellectual framework for psychiatry. *Am J Psychiatry.* 1988;155:457-469.

13. Kandel ER. Neurobiology and the future of psychoanalysis: a new intellectual framework for psychiatry revisited. *Am J Psychiatry.* 1999;156:505-524.

14. Lieberman MD. *Social: Why Our Brains Are Wired to Connect.* New York, NY: Broadway Books; 2013.

15. Fuchs T. Neurobiology and psychotherapy: an emerging dialogue. *Curr Opin Psychiatry.* 2004;17:479-485.

16. Kendler KS. Explanatory models for psychiatric illness. *Am J Psychiatry.* 2008;165(6):695-702. doi:10.1176/appi.ajp.2008.07071061.

17. Merriam-Webster. *Psychotherapy.* In: *Merriam-Webster.com Dictionary.* n.d. Available at https://www.merriam-webster.com/dictionary/psychotherapy. Accessed March 1, 2020.

18. Williams R. *Latin Quips at Your Fingertips.* Barnes and Noble Books; 2001.

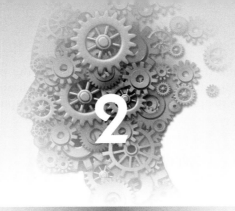

Case Conceptualization and Psychological Assessment in Psychotherapy

LAURA S. HOWE-MARTIN, PhD

Case Study

Trainee X has been treating a 34-year-old Korean-American, cisgender, able-bodied female (Ms. M) for the past several weeks. The initial therapy intake reflected long-standing difficulties with social anxiety and poor self-esteem, resulting in a provisional diagnosis of persistent depressive disorder and social anxiety disorder. However, during the third and fourth sessions, the patient became agitated with Trainee X for "being too hung up on goals" and "expecting too much." Throughout the next several sessions, Ms. M continued to report additional symptoms, including obsessive-type ruminations that cause insomnia, a distant history of hair-pulling behaviors, and transient paranoia. At that point, Trainee X consulted their supervisor and an advanced peer about this case and is now perplexed regarding diagnosis and treatment planning. Trainee X begins to work with the patient on the "problem of the week" during each therapy session, but becomes increasingly frustrated with the lack of treatment progress and Ms. M recently commented that therapy is "maybe a waste of time."

PART I: CASE CONCEPTUALIZATION
(ALSO KNOWN AS "CASE FORMULATION")

The purpose of this chapter is to explain why case conceptualization (sometimes referred to as *case formulation*) is a vital part of treatment, and to review several ways this process can become more straightforward for beginning therapists. Case conceptualization is *not* solely a lengthy recount of a patient's history or symptom presentation, although this information is valuable to the process of building the conceptualization. Instead, the process of case conceptualization results in a working hypothesis about why the patient is experiencing these symptoms or challenges now.

WHY CONCEPTUALIZE?

Gardening is a useful metaphor for illustrating the importance of case conceptualization for psychotherapy. Imagine having a handful of seeds, soil, and a generally pleasant climate. If you simply fling these seeds toward the soil and tamp them down with your foot, *something* will happen. It is quite possible *many* plants will grow. But—and here is the challenge—you will never quite understand *what* will grow or *why*. In addition, you will not know *which* plants will pop up, until many weeks or months pass. At that point, you will have to scramble to change your gardening methods and even transplant a few of these plants to a more appropriate growing environment. This is not an ideal way to grow a truly flourishing garden that develops from one season to the next.

In addition, you ideally learn about the science and art of gardening through gathering research and gaining real-world experience over time. The garden is also impacted by the environment, realistic expectations, and your goals as a gardener. Further, season after season, year after year, you would tend to your garden. Sometimes it would lie fallow, and at other times, there would be intense activity of tilling and preparation.

In the same way, therapy requires case conceptualization that is based on experience, impacted by goals, and tended routinely. The best case conceptualizations involve ongoing revision that incorporates new information, so as to revise or confirm hypotheses.

At this point, you may be thinking, "Is it realistic to do a thorough case conceptualization *for all patients all the time*?" The answer is: perhaps not. Or, at least not in an extremely detailed manner. However, it *is* possible to cultivate a habit of creating a thoughtful case conceptualization at the beginning of each new therapy case, and then working deliberately to continue revising it as treatment progresses, so as to tailor interventions appropriately.

INTRODUCING A TRANSTHEORETICAL CASE CONCEPTUALIZATION

What I will emphasize throughout this chapter is the importance of building a solid foundation for your chosen therapy intervention plan. To return to the gardening metaphor, the process of case conceptualization requires you to thoughtfully use research, education, and clinical experience (along with your supervisor's guidance) to select the seeds, timing, and environment for your garden. This process will help you better predict and replicate useful interventions, tailored to your patients' needs and preferences, as well as help you maintain a consistent direction in therapy.

2

We will revisit the details of this transtheoretical case conceptualization framework later in the chapter, but I will go ahead and introduce the idea here, so that you have a clear understanding of what I mean by a "case conceptualization" (again, also referred to as a "case formulation"). There are many ways to conceptualize patients, most of which are based on specific theoretical treatment approaches, professional training environments, cultural influences, and personal preference/experience of the therapist. This chapter will not try to cover all the factors that impact our understanding of patient behaviors. Instead, please see the list of references at the end of this chapter for helpful readings on case conceptualization and subsequent chapters in this book on theory-specific approaches to therapy.

There are three basic questions that can serve as a foundation for a transtheoretical case conceptualization framework and can be used to help you form hypotheses, regardless of your theoretical orientation. These ideas are not new and have been introduced by others in the field, using different formats, languages, and steps (see examples by Eells,[1] Liese and Esterline,[2] and Ridley and Jeffrey[3]). In fact, the works by Eells,[1,4] Johnston and Dallos,[5] and Frank and Davidson[6] are a few very helpful resources to help you deepen your understanding of case conceptualization, far beyond what is introduced in this chapter.

Figure 2.1 outlines three basic questions that will help you shape an initial hypothesis. Regardless of the patient's presentation, situation of the therapy encounter, or your theoretical orientation, you should be able to tentatively answer each of these three questions, at *any* point in the treatment process.

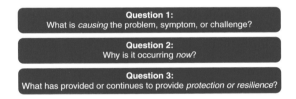

Question 1:
What is *causing* the problem, symptom, or challenge?

Question 2:
Why is it occurring *now*?

Question 3:
What has provided or continues to provide *protection or resilience*?

FIGURE 2.1 Three basic conceptualization questions.

Articulating consistent responses to these three questions can be challenging, even with a lot of experience. However, addressing these questions about each new patient will continue to develop and inform your work as a therapist. If you continue to struggle to articulate answers to these questions, or find yourself providing very inconsistent responses from session to session, the interventions you are using in each therapy session will likely be undeveloped and/or highly variable. Again, much like flinging seeds into the soil in different patterns or times, you will find that "things will grow" in treatment, but you will not really know why.

Case Study: Initial Case Conceptualization Sketch

After meeting with Ms. M for the initial therapy intake session, Trainee X briefly jots down a few additional notes for later documentation and their upcoming supervision session the next day.

Chief complaint: relationship problems, poor self-esteem, anxiety; Provisional diagnoses: persistent depressive disorder + social anxiety disorder

Question 1: *What is causing the problem, symptom, or challenge?* Social anxiety may have preceded depression symptoms. Need more info on family mental health history, early relationships, cultural background, and substance use history.

Question 2: *Why is it occurring now?* Patient mentioned very recent breakup and some ongoing "family problems" but did not elaborate. Has been in group therapy but not individual therapy for past 3 years with good symptom response per patient, until recently.

Question 3: *What has or continues to provide protection or resilience?* Patient has stable employment and housing, college degree, access to health care. Need to further assess additional strengths.

WHAT IS THE LITERATURE ON CASE CONCEPTUALIZATION?

A review of case conceptualization in the empirical literature can help us understand why conceptualization is considered essential to the practice of psychotherapy, while remaining inconsistent in actual practice.

The process of case conceptualization is consistent with evidence-based practice psychotherapy guidelines adopted by the American Psychological Association[7] and considered a core skill or competency by the American Board of Psychiatry and Neurology.[8] A brief literature review will reflect multiple publications on this topic, although most are focused on a specific theory and are not necessarily transtheoretical.

In addition, while limited research indicates a positive impact of conceptualization on patient care and provider understanding of patients,[9,10] other studies reflect ambivalence about the impact of case conceptualization on patient care.[11,12] This may be because even the terms "conceptualization" and "formulation" are not used uniformly, and there are no specific guidelines for what composes a "good" case conceptualization. This leads to difficulties with both reliability and validity of the process, within and among clinicians (for more in-depth details, see Ref. 13). In addition, specific theoretical approaches use the term "conceptualization" in a different manner than is proposed in this chapter. For example, a cognitive case conceptualization, which is a core feature of cognitive behavioral therapy, is acknowledged as being nonholistic and focused primarily on cognitions that are prompting and sustaining patient symptoms,[14,15] instead of the patient's life story.

In sum, although case conceptualization is highly encouraged and considered a core feature of quality psychotherapy practice, there is no consistent, reliable approach to conceptualization within the broad field of psychotherapy. Regardless of the contradictory results within the literature, I would continue to argue that there are several practical benefits as a beginning therapist to creating a habit of building case conceptualizations, which are reviewed in the next section.

WHAT ARE THE PRACTICAL BENEFITS OF CASE CONCEPTUALIZATION?

Case Conceptualization Helps You Know Your Patient

The sorts of background information that are useful for case conceptualization are covered further below in an example and diagram. For now, let us just say that the process of gathering this information with a patient and from collateral sources (and even being aware of the information you do not know) is a wonderful way to begin to really get to know your patient. Most patients who come to see you for psychotherapy struggle to feel heard, and to have their thoughts and feelings given weight by those around them. By asking your patients key information about their current struggles, their history, their culture, and their important relationships, you will succeed in making the patient feel heard and will start the process of honoring their experiences. You will also learn how your patient views the world and others in it, and gain insight into what may provide hope amid the suffering. So while data gathering can seem overwhelming during that first session, or at times extremely mundane, this process in and of itself allows you to demonstrate a striking interest in your patient's story that is likely a unique experience for them. Make the most of it!

Case Conceptualization Incorporates and Goes Beyond Differential Diagnosis

Case conceptualization is *not* the same as a differential diagnosis. The process of differential diagnosis cannot really tell us what to do in psychotherapy, nor does it give us enough information to formulate useful hypotheses about a patient's behavior. However, careful differential diagnosis can often provide part of the answer to the first question—what is causing the problem, symptom, or challenge? You should think of differential diagnosis as an important component to the process of conceptualization, but only one part. In contrast, it is the entire process of a case conceptualization that helps us put together an understanding of why *these* symptoms or problems are occurring at *this* point in time.

You are likely familiar with differential diagnosis from your introduction to psychopathology course and/or rotations within a clinical setting, and likely have used diagnostic systems such as the DSM-5[16] or ICD-11.[17] Differential diagnosis involves considering inclusion, exclusion, and outcome criteria to label a cluster of known symptoms using an established diagnostic system—for example, major depressive disorder, single episode, moderate, or panic disorder without agoraphobia, if you use a diagnostic system such as the DSM-5.[16] Careful differential diagnosis can be helpful for identifying potential treatments of choice, communicating clearly with patients or other professionals, and filing claims for third-party payers. In addition, a careful differential diagnosis can be helpful for identifying potential empirically supported interventions that may (or may not) be applicable.

Some clinicians use a patient's current diagnosis as the sole basis for treatment (eg, "The primary diagnosis is a substance use disorder; therefore, I am going to use motivational interviewing"). While the treatment-per-diagnosis approach is not entirely inaccurate, if you base treatment solely on a single DSM-5 or ICD-11 diagnosis, your treatment will inevitably lack the complexity and specificity needed to treat a vast majority of patients seated in front of you. In addition, a diagnostic label generally does not address the questions of "why." As a result, you will often be left with more questions than answers if you base treatment solely on a diagnosis.

Case Conceptualization Can Help Understand Behaviors Inside (and Outside) of the Session

Case conceptualization provides the therapist a hypothetical framework or "lens" through which to interpret and understand a patient's behavior, within the context of a therapeutic approach. Three specific therapeutic approaches (supportive psychotherapy, cognitive behavioral therapy, and psychodynamic psychotherapy) are explored in detail in later chapters of this book. However, this is a good opportunity to give a brief example of how each of these therapies might use their own theoretical case conceptualization or "lens" to understand Ms. M's behavior.

When Ms. M stated therapy may be "a waste of time," a therapist using *supportive psychotherapy* may conceptualize this behavior as an expression of frustration due to the circumstances overwhelming her typically sufficient ability to cope. In comparison, a therapist using *cognitive behavioral therapy* may conceptualize this behavior as one possible example of an underlying core belief (eg, worthlessness). A therapist using *psychodynamic therapy* may conceptualize this behavior as a parallel of how this patient interacts with important others in their life. Similarly, if Ms. M did not show for the next session and did not call to cancel the appointment, each of these therapeutic approaches would conceptualize the no-show behavior differently as well. Yet all provide some explanation of "why this is happening" and "why now."

As you can see, one part of conceptualization allows the therapist to create a hypothetical lens through which to understand a patient's behavior. However, as noted in the next sections, the chosen theoretical orientation is not the sole driver of a quality, holistic case conceptualization.

Case Conceptualization Helps Direct Intervention(s)

Case conceptualization should strive to identify and match the patient's needs with the appropriate interventions. As will be described further in the chapter, this process involves assessment of prior psychotherapy treatment outcomes, as well as assessment of current strengths/areas of resilience. In addition, completing this process thoughtfully may result in implementing a different type of therapy than was initially proposed, or even referring a patient for an entirely different form of treatment (see guidance on managing psychotherapy fails by Markowitz and Milrod[18]). It also means recognizing that *your* preferred interventions as a therapist are not *the* interventions that may be most helpful to a patient at any given time. It cannot be emphasized enough that although therapy can be an effective treatment that takes many forms, it is not a salve for all presenting problems.

In that regard, the type of history-taking that helps form a solid case conceptualization works to identify treatment needs *beyond the scope of psychotherapy*, and therefore adds to this more holistic approach. For example, Ms. M. may have a history of chronic pain, for which she is seeking care from both a chiropractor and a pain management physician. Or she may have a history of immigration challenges that requires re-referral to a lawyer and intermittent attention to the stress associated with threatened deportation. It will be important to continuously recognize the other treatment needs and the importance of other types of healing, over and above psychotherapy.

Case Conceptualization Provides a Foundation

At some point during the therapy treatment process, you will find yourself confused and unsure with regard to the direction of therapy. Sometimes this is due to lack of experience. However, even with years of experience, you will intermittently ask yourself, in the midst of session, "*What exactly am I supposed to be doing with this patient and why?*"

Think of your case conceptualization as providing a useful plan that you can return to, particularly during times of confusion. If you have completed a carefully written or verbalized case conceptualization, you can more easily become oriented during session. You will be able to use new or seemingly inconsistent information provided in session to mentally "fill in" the gaps in your case conceptualization. You can also move ahead with treatment during that very session and avoid relapsing into therapy habits that are neither helpful nor consistent with the treatment plan.

In addition, creating a thoughtful case conceptualization will provide you with the practice and routine necessary to think through each patient's treatment plan. This includes the practice of *revising* your case conceptualization when new information arises or when you face a roadblock in treatment. Again, if we return to the gardening metaphor, it is very difficult to make the next plan or step if you have been flinging seeds into the soil without purpose or a guide. However, your case conceptualization will provide an idea of the hypotheses you have considered, before you choose to shift directions.

GATHERING INFORMATION FOR A TRANSTHEORETICAL CASE CONCEPTUALIZATION

Taking a good history is a necessary foundation for creating a case conceptualization. You must continue to revise the history as new or contradictory information comes to light. Therefore, a therapist must work to obtain good background information from an initial interview, collateral informants, and/or prior treatment records, in order to be able to sufficiently conceptualize a patient. But remember, *having a complete patient history is not the same as creating a case conceptualization*. Instead, a case conceptualization *uses* the patient history to consistently answer and revise answers to the three broad questions involving identifying causes, timing, and protective factors.

So, what should be included in this history-taking process? Ideally, you will consider and include all of the information in the gray arrows located in *Figure 2.2*, for each and every patient. Notice I used the word "consider." This is because not all of this information will be readily available to you during the case conceptualization process, nor will this information always be entirely accurate (as patients will bring to therapy only what they wish to share, and what you make them comfortable to share). However, the available information and the potential gaps in that information should always be considered as important, and filled in as the treatment progresses and new information emerges.

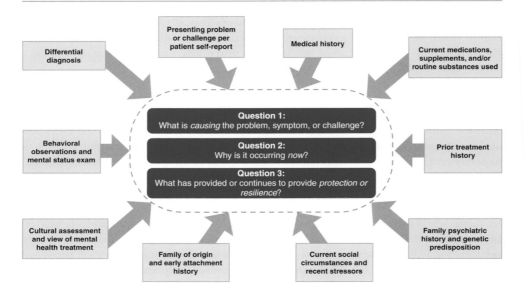

FIGURE 2.2 Case conceptualization with history.

Figure 2.3 provides an example of this information as it specifically pertains to Ms. M.

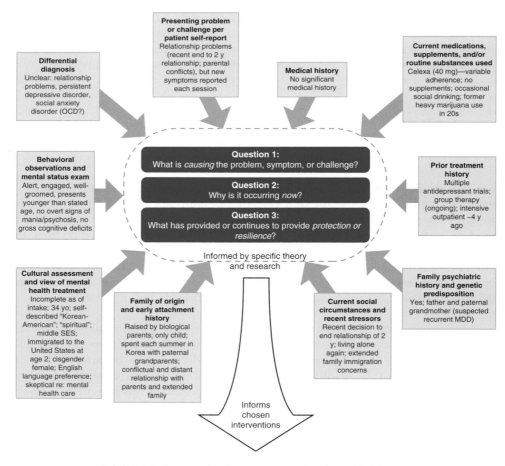

FIGURE 2.3 Case study: Case conceptualization with history.

APPLYING A TRANSTHEORETICAL CASE CONCEPTUALIZATION TO THE CASE STUDY

Case Study—Question 1: What Is Causing the Problem, Symptom, or Challenge?

Trainees often struggle to try to answer this question, amid the vast amount of information available that could explain the problem expressed by the patient in front of them. However, it is not necessary that you understand and/or incorporate *all* possible causes of *all* presenting problems to create a helpful case conceptualization. Instead, it is simply necessary for you to begin thinking through the potential causes, and incorporate these into a consistent approach to treatment that you can articulate in supervision.

Let us return to the case study of Ms. M and the information gathered earlier. We can see Ms. M is presenting for therapy because her primary care physician referred her, as antidepressants do not appear effective in managing symptoms of depression. However, by gathering information and combining this with our ability to conceptualize, we can recognize the presenting problems are not solely due to a clear-cut major depressive episode within a long-standing persistent depressive disorder. Further historical information reflects a family history of recurrent major depression (and a potential genetic predisposition for mood disorders) and chronic self-esteem problems beginning in childhood. She also views mental health care (eg, psychotherapy) with some level of skepticism. Her family does not know she has sought mental health care treatment, and she reported they would be ashamed of her because she did so. As a result, she has "done what some friends do" and sought treatment from a physician and a therapist, but is not entirely certain these approaches have been helpful. Ms. M also reported a very negative experience with a structured, intensive outpatient program in the past, and a review of collateral medical records indicates Ms. M has tried different antidepressant and mood stabilizing combinations in the past.

At this point, you would use this information to carefully consider the *potential hypotheses* for Ms. M's long-standing difficulties. What is potentially *causing* this presentation for Ms. M at this point? And what explains the multitude of changing symptoms and the expressions of frustration in therapy? These ongoing hypotheses will be shaped by your own developing therapy expertise and your supervisor's treatment preferences, as well as information from the relevant research literature. However, by using a broad history to build your hypotheses, you can avoid falling into narrow causal explanations that ignore important patient factors and empirical research.

For example, one reasonable hypothesis in Ms. M's case is that she has a genetic predisposition for depressive illness, which has waxed and waned in the form of persistent depressive disorder with significant major depressive episodes. Estrangement and conflict within her family of origin have contributed to feelings of poor self-esteem, loneliness, and isolation. These early relationship patterns have also contributed to insecure attachment patterns in adulthood that now show up in relationships (including with the therapist). Finally, Ms. M's worldview and cultural background continue to impact skepticism of mental health care and her subsequent behaviors in traditionally Western forms of therapy.

Case Study—Question 2: Why Is the Problem Occurring Now?

Sometimes, a patient's problems or challenges have persisted for years, and what you are seeing in therapy is merely a snapshot. Often, however, patients present for therapy when their current coping strategies are no longer working. They describe themselves as feeling "stuck" or overwhelmed in some way and are seeking therapy as one form of healing.

Let us consider Ms. M's presentation. Although she presented for therapy at the request of her primary care physician, many patients do not follow through with psychotherapy referrals. She clearly also viewed herself as in need of help at this particular point in her life. In this case, you would pay attention to the precipitating factors that led her to your office at this specific time. For example, you find out during the intake she has recently chosen to end a relationship after 2 years and is now living alone for the first time in over a year. In addition, her parents have reached out about their own recurrent immigration difficulties, about which Ms. M is feeling conflicted.

Ms. M is presenting in therapy with a multitude of symptoms, difficulties, and frustrations in a shifting pattern. You can then hypothesize that these recent strains (ie, the very recent loss of the relationship, the loneliness, and/or the increased and conflicted contact with her family) have caused difficulties to surface. This will help us better understand Ms. M's behaviors in therapy if, for example, we find out she experiences another loss or threatened loss, or becomes overwhelmed at a government office when she is asked to redo immigration paperwork on behalf of her parents. It will also help us understand triggers that could predict future relapses.

Regardless of your theoretical orientation, all psychotherapies are consistent in their tendency to eventually link patterns of the "there-and-then," with the "here-and-now." The more you understand the patterns of what cause your patient to feel "stuck" enough to seek therapy (and/or to avoid it or drop out of treatment), the better you will be able to create useful hypotheses.

Case Study—Question 3: What Has Provided or Continues to Provide Protection or Resilience?

Protective factors and areas of resiliency are often overlooked, particularly if you are trained in a program that is very problem- or pathology-oriented, versus one that is more strength-focused and emphasizes patient resilience. Regardless, it can become easy to overlook important areas of resiliency that contribute to this patient's ability to function day in and day out, with relatively minimal support from you as a therapist. Protective factors and areas of resiliency are vital areas to identify and reinforce through treatment.

Returning to the case study, Ms. M has used many coping strategies up to this point, and she continues to employ them to help her function on a daily basis. She is being treated as an outpatient, has developed relationships with others, and lives on her own, which indicates she has several strengths in place to help her function at a relatively high level. These strengths include motivation, consistency, creativity, social connections, and spirituality. Despite Ms. M's complaints about treatment in general, and some of the difficulties that have arisen with getting thorough symptom information, she is consistent with seeking care. She repeatedly states that she "really needs treatment," although she is unsure what kind and is skeptical, and she consistently attends appointments with you. She has held a stable job for many years, and also runs her own small business that allows her to be creative and engage socially with others, even when she is feeling poorly. She also lets you know, when asked, that she has a strong spiritual faith in "something bigger." All of these factors are important to consider in the conceptualization of Ms. M's case, in that these factors can help tailor future treatment approaches and interventions.

WHAT ABOUT SPECIFIC THEORIES AND RESEARCH?

As noted, this is a proposed *transtheoretical* approach to case conceptualization that represents simplified building blocks. The purpose of providing these in a relatively simple form is to get you in the habit of thinking through these three basic questions as vital for treatment, and then learning how to integrate various theories and interventions as you learn them. As a result, the response to your three questions will always be informed by various parts of historical information about the patient, and then informed by a specific theory and related research.

For example, a *supportive therapist* may view the primary cause of Ms. M's problems as due to a recent life event or stressor that has caused Ms. M's typically adequate coping strategies to crumble, resulting in a sense of confusion. A *cognitive behavior therapist* may view the cause of Ms. M's problems as due, in part, to maladaptive thinking patterns that reflect underlying core beliefs of worthlessness, and a history of learning that structured approaches (including pharmacotherapy) feel awkward and ineffective. A *psychodynamic psychotherapist* may view the cause of Ms. M's problems as due to early relationship patterns (into which she may or may not have insight), which gave rise to immature defense mechanisms that lead to behaviors such as hair-pulling and dissociation.

However, *all of these orientations* would incorporate the research on genetic predisposition into understanding of Ms. M's mood lability, as well as the impact of recent relationship stressors. Also, *all orientations* would consider the impact of Ms. M's cultural identities and worldview, particularly regarding mental health care practices on treatment. Finally, *all therapists* should take into account current treatment literature supporting the use of specific treatment approaches with presenting problems (eg, what the current research says about the empirically supported treatment of persistent depressive disorder and if this research literature is applicable to Ms. M).

If you look back at *Figure 2.3*, you will note that the "Informed by specific theory" line is represented by a dotted line, and is therefore porous. You may be wed to a specific therapy approach, either because your supervisor prefers that approach or it is literally the only type of therapy you are comfortable attempting initially. However, every treatment intervention and theoretical perspective must be porous and open to incorporating multiple parts of a patient's history.

In addition, your theoretical approach should not be carved in stone. In other words, your hypotheses should not be clung to in the face of contradictory information from the patient or in the face of emerging research. Sometimes, you will need to change this dotted line and the chosen interventions due to patient preferences, partial or no symptom response, emerging research, or even a change in supervisor. And that is entirely fine, as long as it is accompanied by an updated conceptualization that involves updated hypotheses.

WHAT IF I SIMPLY DO NOT KNOW YET HOW TO CONCEPTUALIZE THIS PATIENT'S CASE?

Here is one of the most challenging issues with case conceptualization—*there is not one single way to complete one.* Studies have demonstrated a lack of general consistency (or reliability) with regard to case conceptualizations, even among practitioners with a similar theoretical orientation.[13,19,20] Furthermore, the transtheoretical model mapped out in this chapter will be influenced by a therapist's theoretical and educational underpinnings. This can certainly be frustrating, and is one reason simplified treatment planning workbooks are often purchased by therapists in training.

Treatment environments do not always lend themselves to creating detailed and deeply explored case conceptualizations that unfold over the course of long-term treatment. Consultation-liaison hospital and emergency rooms are two settings that come to mind, as well as certain outpatient clinics that focus on very brief triage and intervention. In fact, the most common number of sessions for patients in outpatient practice in some settings is 1.[21] We are often constricted by limited information and limited time. However, this does not require that we abandon case conceptualization as a useful tool. Even a partially completed sketch of a case provides a good springboard for hypothesis formation regarding diagnosis and treatment, in part because it helps highlight what remains *unknown* and therefore areas for *further information gathering.*

Often, there are assumptions we know far more about our patients than we actually do. We are therefore prompted to make rapid judgments regarding diagnosis, cause, treatment recommendations, and appropriateness for treatment. Case conceptualization practice allows us to be more thoughtful about our patients' care and to integrate broader pieces of knowledge into our understanding, *as well as* help continue to highlight and consider what remains unknown and unexplained.

Perhaps you are thinking, "But I have to know! My job is to be the expert in the room!" Hopefully, your relationship with this type of thinking will change over time and with experience. This will result in becoming better at promoting expertise when you actually have it (eg, explaining common causes of mental illness, recommending specific interventions, discouraging unhelpful or dangerous therapies), while acknowledging there is quite a bit you cannot fully comprehend. To borrow from the cultural humility literature, there is great value in *knowing what you do not know* and building expertise from there.[22] Or to borrow from John Archibald Wheeler, "as our island of knowledge grows, so does the shore of our ignorance."

PART II: PSYCHOLOGICAL ASSESSMENT FOR CASE CONCEPTUALIZATION AND TREATMENT PLANNING

The topic of psychological assessment is far too broad to cover in one section of a single chapter in an introductory text. For example, psychological assessment is often used to assess if a patient is competent to stand trial, to detect likely signs of Alzheimer disease, or to assess the needs of a couple or family as part of family therapy. Instead, in this section, we are going to focus on explaining the utility of psychological assessment *for the purpose of psychotherapy*. Additional resources will be provided at the end of this chapter for those of you who want to learn more about psychological assessment.

It is important to realize most outpatient psychotherapists do not consistently use psychological testing batteries as a routine part of their psychotherapy conceptualization. This is not due to lack of test availability—there are many valid and reliable psychological tests that are available to assess a wide variety of psychological concerns. However, psychological assessment batteries are time-consuming and therefore costly. Instead, most therapists rely heavily on a combination of a clinical interview, clinical experience, and collateral information.

Also, many of the more extensive psychological tests require specific, supervised training before they can be competently and responsibly administered and interpreted. For example, some trainees are surprised when they discover they cannot learn how to administer and interpret a personality test or a neuropsychological measure during an hour-long didactic. In fact, these specific types of assessment tools are often taught as part of semester-long courses during psychology graduate training programs and later reinforced during internship and specialized postdoctoral training.

This section will focus on ways you could make use of psychological assessment tools in therapy, regardless of your current level of training. This could range from utilizing brief self-report measures more routinely or carefully curating a relationship with a professional who completes psychological assessment for more complex cases. In addition, for those of you who are trained in psychological testing, keep in mind that psychological assessment is a useful part of your psychotherapy arsenal and should not be limited to areas such as disability or neuropsychology evaluations.

WHAT SHOULD I CONSIDER WHEN CHOOSING AN ASSESSMENT TOOL?

Use Reliable and Valid Assessment Methods

The concepts of "reliability" and "validity" are very important for any assessment tool you choose to use. *Reliability* refers to a test's ability to provide similar results for the same patient over time, barring a significant change in circumstances, or similar results when administered by different providers. For example, an intelligence test should not provide wildly variable results for the same patient, unless there has been a significant neurological change.

Validity refers to a test's ability to measure what it proposes to measure. For example, if a test indicates that it is useful for specifically identifying depression, it should not also inadvertently detect panic disorder or dementia. Validity is also dependent on the *process of administration.* For example, the Montreal Cognitive Assessment (MoCA)[23-25] has a specific, standardized administration process that is required for correct interpretation of the findings. A primary care physician knows that a fasting blood draw is necessary to accurately interpret blood glucose level; without preliminary fasting or with the use of a contaminated sample, the results can inaccurately point to a problem. This is the same with valid and reliable psychological tests.

Finally, it is important to ensure the test has been validated on the *population* with which you are using it. For example, just because a test has been translated into another language, this does not mean its underlying questions or concepts are appropriate for use in that language. Translation of tests requires careful language translation methods and field testing, and almost always requires test results to be interpreted with caution. So before you use just any psychological test or tool, consult the peer-reviewed literature and confirm that the test is reliable *and* valid for use with the patient seated in front of you.

Screening Tools Are NOT Diagnostic Tools

Screening measures are brief questionnaires that are administered in writing or orally and are used to screen for the potential existence of a specific condition or concern. Most of these yield a high number of "false positives" (ie, when the test falsely indicates the presence of a condition), as screening measures need to capture all possible instances of a condition or concern, and need to have a low risk of missing the true positives (ie, individuals who have that condition or concern). However, it is important to not confuse a screening measure with a diagnostic assessment. For example, the PHQ-9[26] is used routinely in medical settings to screen for depression. However, it does not screen out other explanations for "positive" depression results, such as underlying medical conditions, treatment or drug side effects, bipolar disorder, or a myriad of other conditions that could explain high scores on a PHQ-9. This takes place during a follow-up diagnostic assessment, conducted by a trained professional who is able to take into account other potential causes of the "positive depression" results. Screening measures should never be used as diagnostic tools, no matter how fast-paced your environment may be.

Assess Your Competency

It is important to ensure that you have completed the training necessary to appropriately administer *and* interpret the measure. Some assessment measures are extremely brief and require little training to understand, administer, and interpret the results (see PHQ-9 mentioned earlier). However, others require extensive training and even proof of specific qualifications to purchase them from the publisher (eg, the MMPI-2-RF).[27] Still others fall somewhere in-between. For example, there are specific qualifications and recommendations required for appropriate training to administer specific mental status exams or specific types of structured interviews, but these trainings can be obtained either online or through careful supervision. In addition, as a trainee, it is important to discuss your *supervisor's* level of competency in supervising the administration and interpretation of any measures you incorporate into therapy. While some of your supervisors may have had strong training in a prior version of an assessment tool, they may require an updated refresher to be able to competently supervise you on the newer version.

INITIAL INTAKE ASSESSMENT TOOLS

Some therapists routinely use pretherapy assessment tools to inform the treatment plan. In many cases, this consists of a semi-structured clinical interview. Other therapists find that an unstructured clinical interview can be informative enough as to the appropriateness of a patient for group versus individual therapy, or can reflect that the patient needs a higher level of care than a trainee can provide. Check with your supervisor to get input on their preferred initial therapy intake style or format, and ask them why they choose specific methods over others.

Clinical Interviews, Semi-structured Interviews, and Structured Interviews

Clinical interviews are considered the standard in the mental health field for gathering patient information. However, the nature and quality of these initial interviews vary widely, and there are many risks inherent to relying entirely on an unstructured therapy intake interview. If an unstructured or therapist-created interview is what is used routinely in your setting, it is recommended that the same or similar interview is used with all patients, to avoid diagnostic bias or drift.

One interview approach you should familiarize yourself with is the Cultural Formulation Interview (CF).[16] This is an interview approach that can provide a good foundation for understanding the patient's perspective on their difficulties, strengths, and preferred treatment approaches. As a result, it can provide a much better understanding of your patient's worldview, before you dive into other areas of the intake (see Chapter 8 for further information on this approach).

There are also semi-structured diagnostic interviews, such as the SCID (now in its fifth version)[28] or K-SADS,[29,30] that provide specific prompts and allow for prewritten follow-up questions as needed. These interviews are very comprehensive and consistent, but are typically limited to psychiatric diagnosis and can result in a robotic process if not practiced thoughtfully.

Finally, structured interviews are typically used for research purposes, as these are interviews without any follow-up questions or flexibility for the interviewer. Entirely structured interviews (vs. semi-structured ones) are not recommended for use as part of the therapeutic process, as this complete lack of flexibility does not encourage clinical judgment and the building of quality therapeutic rapport.

Brief Symptom Measures

It is also a good idea to incorporate more structured, validated assessment methods into your therapy practice. Not only can these be time-saving, but sometimes patients will report issues or difficulties on a self-report measure that they may not report when asked directly during an intake interview or in front of other people. In addition, this creates structure and standardization to your practice. Available assessment tools are as numerous and varied as your needs might be. For example, you can use brief, self-report symptom measures (eg, the GAD-7 to assess anxiety)[31] or tools that assess acculturation stress (eg, HSI2)[32] or even assess levels of thought suppression if that is going to be a target for treatment (eg, WBSI).[33] Of course, the tools that are used will vary widely in terms of their length and focus, depending on the treatment setting, patient population, and theoretical orientation of the therapist.

Genograms

A genogram is another assessment tool that can be helpful during the intake interview. Genograms emerged from the family systems literature and can range from simple to fairly complex visual representations of the relationships involved in an extended family. In their simplest form, genograms provide a quick "family tree" or "map" of the patient's family of origin and current family relationships (as defined by the patient) through a series of circles, squares, symbols, and line types. If you are unfamiliar with the concept of genograms, it is recommended you learn more about these family maps or tools, and even complete one for yourself. Genograms are particularly helpful during an intake interview, as these help you create a brief, visual shorthand of complex relationships while asking about a patient's relationship history.[34]

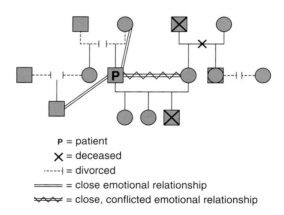

P = patient
✗ = deceased
·····┤ = divorced
═══ = close emotional relationship
∿∿∿ = close, conflicted emotional relationship

Genogram Example.

ONGOING ASSESSMENT TOOLS IN THERAPY

Routine Symptom Assessment

Some therapists systematically use validated baseline assessment measures (eg, a symptom assessment such as the HADS),[35] followed by careful implementation of a specifically chosen treatment, and then reassessment at specific intervals to assess progress. This approach, often referred to as *measurement-based care* (MBC), is similar to how other metrics are used to assess treatment progress through subjective symptom reporting. Instead of relying solely on your own perception (and related biases) to assess if a patient is improving in therapy, this approach allows you to be consistent in how you track symptoms or other targets of treatment. As a result, you can routinely reassess progress in treatment and perhaps see changes or patterns you might otherwise miss.

This approach can also be implemented with other valid and reliable measures that address other areas of importance to therapy. For example, if reducing avoidance is an important treatment target, repeated administration of a valid and reliable measure of avoidance at appropriate intervals would be useful. Another example might be the repeated use of a perceived pain scale if the target is to increase use of healthier pain management strategies.

Cognitive/Neuropsychological Assessment

In addition, psychological assessment of underlying cognitive/neuropsychological abilities can be helpful in ruling in (or ruling out) comorbid cognitive issues that are impacting progress in psychotherapy. Because neuropsychological assessment is a separate and vast topic, the following example will narrowly focus on the use of cognitive assessment as it applies to the process of psychotherapy.

For example, your patient attends therapy weekly for treatment of depression, but appears to have difficulty retaining information from session to session, although the patient presents as grossly cognitively intact. You also know there is a history of heavy alcohol use. These subtle challenges with information retention are interfering with therapy, and it is unclear if these are due to unremitting depressive symptoms or underlying cognitive impairment. A psychological assessment in the form of a brief cognitive or more thorough neuropsychological assessment would help to delineate these two diagnoses and would also provide information about patient strengths and weaknesses. These strengths could be incorporated into treatment. For example, if the patient has difficulty with both immediate and delayed recall of verbal information, but not visual information, therapy could be adapted to include more visual exercises, pictures, and visual reminders of therapy content, to bolster retention from session to session.

Personality Assessment

Psychological testing that specifically looks more in depth at symptoms, worldview, and personality style can help add to your conceptualization by providing valuable information in a rapid manner. For example, you may learn things about your patient's personality that might take a very long time to become clear in therapy.

Some personality assessments can be beneficial if we want to know more about the relationship of persisting symptoms to underlying core personality style. These include tools such as the Minnesota Multiphasic Personality Inventory (MMPI-2 and MMPI-2-RF),[27,36,37] the various Millon tests (such as the MCMI-IV),[38] the Personality Assessment Inventory (PAI),[39] the Rorschach inkblot test (and associated interpretation system),[40] and the Thematic Apperception Test (TAT).[41] Personality tests are administered by individuals with specific training in administration and interpretation, typically psychologists, as training in these is part of graduate-level clinical training programs. Training on and even ownership of these tests is also limited to individuals with specific qualifications and credentials, due to their potential for misuse.

These tests can provide valuable information about ongoing problematic symptoms, core personality traits, level of reality testing (eg, psychotic tendencies), relationship styles, underlying suicide risk, and risks for certain types of psychopathology, among other features specific to each test. These results can then be incorporated into the conceptualization and treatment approach. For example, if projective testing indicates the patient is very quietly psychotic, then the therapy approach should take this into account by incorporating reality testing and avoiding interventions that are contraindicated for psychosis.

Some of your supervisors will consider projective tests a useful and valid tool, while others will be skeptical about their place in clinical work. It is important for you to know these and similar tests contain validity indicators, which means it is more difficult for a patient to try to present in an exaggerated or dishonest manner on these tests. In addition, these tests can be reliable and valid when administered and interpreted appropriately by trained professionals, who take into account the context surrounding the patient throughout interpretation. My caution would be this—read the literature and limit use of these tests to those who have the training and qualifications to help you use them appropriately in therapy.

APPLYING PSYCHOLOGICAL ASSESSMENT TO THE CASE STUDY

Ms. M's case at the beginning of this chapter is a good example of a situation that would benefit from a psychological assessment, such as a combined personality and symptom assessment. Psychological testing provides another way of getting different types of data, which could help with understanding the patient's underlying symptoms and perspective of their world. As a result, testing could enrich our answers to the three questions from our transtheoretical case conceptualization: (1) What is causing the problem, symptom, or challenge? (2) Why is it occurring now? and (3) What has provided or continues to provide protection or resilience?

First, it is clear the initial diagnostic interview did not yield a complete picture of the treatment needs, as Ms. M continued to provide additional and sometimes contradictory information about her symptoms and history as therapy progressed. In addition, the therapeutic alliance appears to be getting tenuous. Perhaps the therapist could simply wait until the picture becomes clear. Another option is to use psychological assessment to gather additional perspectives that can be used to inform the course of treatment and potentially avoid premature termination.

Case Study: Testing Referral Process

In the case of Ms. M, the therapist decides to refer the patient for a psychological assessment in the psychology graduate program training clinic. The therapist gathers informed consent from Ms. M prior to doing so, telling her that additional data gathered from a psychological assessment will help create a more tailored therapy treatment plan. Ms. M agrees to do the assessment, and written results are provided to her therapist within 3 weeks. The therapist reviews these results with both the graduate student who completed the testing and their supervisor, so as to get an accurate understanding of the meaning of these results and how they could be used to shape treatment. The results are then reviewed with Ms. M.

Case Study: Cultural Formulation Interview

The graduate student used this opportunity to apply the CFI,[16] a brief interview taught during a graduate-level cultural diversity class. During this interview, Ms. M described the problem as "always feeling miserable and empty" and "never being good enough for [her] parents." She attributed this problem to a "flaw in [her] character" and noted that if she could just "have more willpower" she could have found a way to help herself. Ms. M expressed significant self-stigma around having any "mental problems" and noted she had not discussed any of these concerns with her family at all, only her American friends who recommended psychiatry. Ms. M noted her mother was particularly critical of any emotional expression, describing neighbors who "fall apart" and "get too angry" when difficult things occur. While Ms. M noted a willingness to "continue to try" psychiatry and psychotherapy, she described this as a "last resort." In addition, she expressed some confusion as to why her therapist always wanted to "be so collaborative about everything—she is the expert, so she should know what to do."

Case Study: Brief Assessment Results

A basic, broad symptom assessment (via the Brief Symptom Inventory [BSI])[42] reflected what has been observed in therapy, in that Ms. M reported a broad array of symptoms across this self-report measure. A very brief assessment of cognitive functioning (via the MoCA)[24] reflected no gross cognitive deficits, other than slightly poorer attention than would be expected for her age and educational background, consistent with individuals struggling with depression.

Case Study: Personality Assessment Results

Lengthier personality testing results (via the MMPI-2-RF and the Rorschach, scored with the R-PAS scoring system)[27,40] suggested that Ms. M is overreporting symptoms that reflect distress, and simultaneously understating her ability to cope with distress. Test results reflect there is no evidence of a frank psychotic disorder, although she is often distrustful of others and their intentions. These results also indicate she can and does experience very strong emotions, and has a tendency toward anger and impulsivity, although these are often not expressed. Findings also reflect that although she does experience very strong reactions, she can be interpersonally passive with others. Testing also reflected a heightened risk for suicidal ideation and alcohol use problems, when compared to normative data. These last two points are important to take into consideration for the future, as Ms. M is not currently experiencing any suicidal ideation or substance use problems. In addition, a subsequent review of the empirical literature would be helpful to this point, to evaluate what is known of suicide and substance use risk for young Korean-American women who are coping with mental health concerns.

Case Study: Applying Testing Results to Case Conceptualization

In the case of Ms. M, she began to express a variety of significant symptoms across multiple sessions, which resulted in feelings of frustration on the part of the therapist, as well as comments from Ms. M that therapy "feels like a waste of time." After receiving these test results, the trainee was better able to work with their supervisor to broaden the initial conceptualization.

1. *What is causing the problem, symptom, or challenge?*
   Psychological assessment results suggest Ms. M struggles with strong emotional experiences that are difficult for her to express in ways that are culturally acceptable. This is compounded by ongoing suspicion of others' intentions and a generally passive interpersonal style, which certainly can cause problems in social situations. Although Ms. M does not currently report any suicidal ideation or substance use problems, testing reflects an increased risk of developing these in reaction to stressors. In addition, we now have a better idea of Ms. M's own description of her problems, expectations for treatment, and cultural factors that may shape behaviors (eg, interpretations of passive interpersonal style, approved coping strategies, role expectations for the therapist). These results help contextualize and make sense of Ms. M's behaviors each week within therapy, over and above the original view of Ms. M as experiencing primarily a persistent depressive illness and social anxiety disorder. These findings do not negate the genetic disposition or the impact of insecure attachment, but instead add to the broader picture.

2. *Why is it occurring now?*
   Results reflect Ms. M may be more prone to reporting symptoms as one way to cry out for help, particularly in situations in which she believes help may not be made available to her. This helps explain why Ms. M is describing many symptoms and disorders, session after session. This new information can be incorporated with what we already know about Ms. M's ongoing skepticism of mental health care and the heightened distress due to both the recent relationship breakup and family stressors. We also now know Ms. M may be entirely unable to discuss her mental health concerns with close family members or others due to family stigma and self-stigma, resulting in therapy perhaps being the only outlet. As a result, the therapist may need to consistently reiterate to Ms. M that her concerns are going to be attended to in treatment, as Ms. M's passive interpersonal style (due to personality and/or cultural expectations) may keep her from bringing up this concern directly. Simultaneously, however, the therapist can stop trying to "chase down" specific diagnoses from the variable symptom self-reports each week, and instead focus on rebuilding the therapeutic alliance with a renewed understanding. The therapist might also need to be more directive in treatment, to align with Ms. M's expectations of the therapist.

3. *What has provided or continues to provide protection or resilience?*

There are currently no indications that Ms. M is struggling with a formal thought disorder or psychosis, nor does she have any significant cognitive problems that would create a barrier for specific types of therapy. This is helpful, as there were some concerns about a potential underlying psychosis when Ms. M reported transient symptoms of paranoia. In addition, although Ms. M may be prone to substance use problems, she has opted to pursue different coping strategies (eg, through work, social support, treatment) to assist with feelings of distress.

Conclusion

This chapter reviewed several ways to create practical "building blocks" for therapy in the service of creating a strong foundation. It reviewed the importance of thinking through a case conceptualization, the differences between patient history, differential diagnosis, and case conceptualization, and the basic questions that can form the basis of any case conceptualization. Example diagrams and several references were provided for further practice and self-directed learning.

In addition, the value of psychological assessment tools and methods for psychotherapy was also discussed. This is helpful knowledge, even if you may not yet have the background to incorporate all of these methods. The two broad tools of case conceptualization and psychological assessment can certainly be incorporated early into treatment, but also can (and should) be used intermittently as treatment progresses to improve the treatment plan and quality of care. While both take time, practice, and effort, these two approaches are also designed to help us find and maintain a path in treatment that is comprehensive, patient-centered, and empirically supported.

Self-Study Questions

1. Think of the last patient you saw in therapy (or pick up a book of case vignettes and choose from one of these). Then, sketch out a three-item case conceptualization for that patient. What is causing the symptoms or challenges? Why now? What is protective?

2. Reviewing your responses to question 1, did you incorporate relevant research into your conceptualization? Complete a brief literature review on an aspect of this case and see what you can integrate to help enhance your conceptualization.

3. What are meant by "reliability" and "validity"? And why are they important in psychological assessment?

4. What type of intake assessment or psychological tests do you (and/or your supervisor) routinely use, and why? How could these approaches be reconsidered and strengthened?

RESOURCES FOR FURTHER LEARNING

Eells TD, ed. *Handbook of Psychotherapy Case Formulation*. New York, NY: Guilford Press; 2011.

Eells TD. *Psychotherapy Case Formulation*. Washington, DC: American Psychological Association; 2015.

Frank RI, Davidson J. *The Transdiagnostic Road Map to Case Formulation and Treatment Planning: Practical Guidance for Clinical Decision Making*. Oakland, CA: New Harbinger Publications; 2014.

Johnstone L, Dallos R. *Formulation in Psychology and Psychotherapy*. New York, NY: Routledge; 2013:21-37.

Liese BS, Esterline KM. Concept mapping: a supervision strategy for introducing case conceptualization skills to novice therapists. *Psychotherapy*. 2015;52(2):190-194.

McGoldrick M. *The Genogram Casebook. A Clinical Companion to Genograms: Assessment and Intervention*. New York, NY: WW Norton & Company; 2016.

Sperry L, Sperry JJ. *Case Conceptualization: Mastering This Competency With Ease and Confidence*. New York, NY: Routledge.2012.

REFERENCES

1. Eells TD. *Psychotherapy Case Formulation*. Washington, DC: American Psychological Association; 2015.
2. Liese BS, Esterline KM. Concept mapping: a supervision strategy for introducing case conceptualization skills to novice therapists. *Psychotherapy(Chic)*. 2015;52(2):190-194.
3. Ridley CR, Jeffrey CE. The conceptual framework of thematic mapping in case conceptualization. *J Clin Psychol*. 2017;73(4):376-392.
4. Eells TD, ed. *Handbook of Psychotherapy Case Formulation*. New York, NY: Guilford Press; 2011.
5. Johnstone L, Dallos R. Introduction to formulation. In: *Formulation in Psychology and Psychotherapy*. New York, NY: Routledge; 2013:21-37.
6. Frank RI, Davidson J. *The Transdiagnostic Road Map to Case Formulation and Treatment Planning: Practical Guidance for Clinical Decision Making*. Oakland, CA: New Harbinger Publications; 2014.
7. American Psychological Association. *Evidence-based Practice Guidelines*. Washington, DC: American Psychological Association; 2005. Available at https://www.apa.org/practice/guidelines/evidence-based-statement. Accessed April 1, 2020.
8. American Board of Psychiatry and Neurology (ABPN). *Core Competencies Outline*. Deerfield, IL: American Board of Psychiatry and Neurology, Inc.; 2011. Available at https://www.abpn.com/wp-content/uploads/2015/02/2011_core_P_MREE.pdf. Accessed April 1, 2020.
9. Berry K, Barrowclough C, Wearden A. A pilot study investigating the use of psychological formulations to modify psychiatric staff perceptions of service users with psychosis. *Behav Cogn Psychother*. 2009;37(1):39-48.
10. Chadwick P, Williams C, Mackenzie J. Impact of case formulation in cognitive behavior therapy for psychosis. *Behav Res Ther*. 2003;41(6):671-680.
11. Aston R. A literature review exploring the efficacy of case formulations in clinical practice: what are the themes and pertinent issues? *Cogn Behav Ther*. 2009;2(2):63-74.
12. Ghaderi A. Does case formulation make a difference to treatment outcome? In: Sturmey P, McMurran M, eds. *Forensic Case Formulation*. West Sussex: John Wiley & Sons; 2011:61-79.
13. Ridley CR, Jeffrey CE, Roberson RB III. Case mis-conceptualization in psychological treatment: an enduring clinical problem. *J Clin Psychol*. 2017;73(4):359-375.
14. Kuyken W, Padesky C, Dudley R. *Collaborative Case Conceptualization: Working Effectively With Clients in Cognitive-behavioral Therapy*. New York, NY: The Guilford Press; 2009.
15. Persons JB. *The Case Formulation Approach to Cognitive-Behavior Therapy*. New York, NY: Guilford; 2008.
16. American Psychiatric Association. *Diagnostic and Statistical Manual of Mental Disorders*. 5th ed. 2013. Available at https://doi.org/10.1176/appi.books.9780890425596.
17. World Health Organization. *International Classification of Diseases for Mortality and Morbidity Statistics (11th Revision)*. Geneva, Switzerland: World Health Organization; 2018. Available at https://www.who.int/classifications/icd/en/. Accessed April 1, 2020.
18. Markowitz JC, Milrod BL. What to do when a psychotherapy fails. *Lancet Psychiatry*. 2015;2(2):186-190.
19. Easden MH, Kazantzis N. Case conceptualization research in cognitive behavior therapy: a state of the science review. *J Clin Psychol*. 2018;74(3):356-384.
20. Flinn L, Braham L, das Nair R. How reliable are case formulations? A systematic literature review. *Br J Clin Psychol*. 2015;54(3):266-290.
21. Gibbons MBC, Rothbard A, Farris KD, et al. Changes in psychotherapy utilization among consumers of services for major depressive disorder in the community mental health system. *Adm Policy Ment Health*. 2011;38(6):495-503.
22. Mosher DK, Hook JN, Farrell JE, Watkins CE Jr, Davis DE. Cultural humility. In: Worthington EL Jr, Davis DE, Hook JN, eds. *Handbook of Humility: Theory, Research, and Applications*. New York, NY: Routledge/Taylor & Francis Group; 2017:91-104.
23. Gierus J, Mosiołek A, Koweszko T, Wnukiewicz P, Kozyra O, Szulc A. The Montreal Cognitive Assessment as a preliminary assessment tool in general psychiatry: validity of MoCA in psychiatric patients. *Gen Hosp Psychiatry*. 2015;37(5):476-480.
24. Nasreddine ZS, Phillips NA, Bédirian V, et al. The Montreal Cognitive Assessment, MoCA: a brief screening tool for mild cognitive impairment. *J Am Geriatr Soc*. 2005;53(4):695-699.
25. Rossetti HC, Lacritz LH, Cullum CM, Weiner MF. Normative data for the Montreal Cognitive Assessment (MoCA) in a population-based sample. *Neurology*. 2011;77(13):1272-1275.
26. Kroenke K, Spitzer RL, Williams JBW. The PHQ-9: validity of a brief depression severity measure. *J Gen Intern Med*. 2001;16(9):606-613.
27. Ben-Porath YS, Tellegen A. *MMPI-2-RF (Minnesota Multiphasic Personality Inventory-2-Restructured Form): Manual for Administration, Scoring, and Interpretation*. Minneapolis, MN: University of Minnesota Press; 2011.

28. First MB, Williams JBW, Karg RS, Spitzer RL. *Structured Clinical Interview for DSM-5 Disorders, Clinician Version (SCID-5-CV)*. Arlington, VA: American Psychiatric Association; 2016.

29. Kaufman J, Birmaher B, Brent D, et al. Schedule for affective disorders and schizophrenia for school-age children—present and lifetime version (K-SADS-PL): initial reliability and validity data. *J Am Acad Child Adolesc Psychiatry*. 1997;36(7):980-988.

30. Kaufman J, Birmaher B, Axelson D, Pereplitchikova F, Brent D, Ryan N. *The KSADS-PL DSM-5*. Advanced Center for Intervention and Services Research (ACISR) for Early Onset Mood and Anxiety Disorders, Western Psychiatric Institute and Clinic; Child and Adolescent Research and Education (CARE) Program, Yale University; 2016. Available at https://www.kennedykrieger.org/sites/default/files/library/documents/faculty/ksads-dsm-5-screener.pdf. Accessed April 1, 2020.

31. Spitzer RL, Kroenke K, Williams JB, Löwe B. A brief measure for assessing generalized anxiety disorder: the GAD-7. *Arch Intern Med*. 2006;166(10):1092-1097.

32. Cervantes RC, Fisher DG, Padilla AM, Napper LE. The hispanic stress inventory version 2: improving the assessment of acculturation stress. *Psychol Assess*. 2016;28(5):509-522.

33. Wegner DM, Zanakos S. Chronic thought suppression. *J Pers*. 1994;62:616-640.

34. McGoldrick M. *The Genogram Casebook: A Clinical Companion to Genograms. Assessment and Intervention*. New York, NY: WW Norton & Company; 2016.

35. Snaith RP, Zigmond AS. The hospital anxiety and depression scale. *Br Med J (Clin Res Ed)*. 1986;292(6516):344.

36. Butcher JN, Dahlstrom WG, Graham JR, Tellegen A, Kaemmer B. *The Minnesota Multiphasic Personality Inventory-2 (MMPI-2): Manual for Administration and Scoring*. Minneapolis, MN: University of Minnesota Press; 1989.

37. Ben-Porath YS. *Interpreting the MMPI-2-RF*. Minneapolis, MN: University of Minnesota Press; 2012.

38. Millon T, Grossman S, Millon C. *MCMI-IV: Millon Clinical Multiaxial Inventory Manual*. 1st ed. Bloomington, MN: NCS Pearson, Inc; 2015.

39. Morey LC. *Personality Assessment Inventory Professional Manual* 2nd ed. Lutz, FL: Psychological Assessment Resources; 2007.

40. Meyer GJ. *Using the Rorschach Performance Assessment System (R-PAS)*. New York, NY: Guilford Publications; 2017.

41. Murray HA. *Thematic Apperception Test*. Cambridge, MA: Harvard University Press; 1943.

42. Derogatis LR. *Brief Symptom Inventory (BSI)-18: Administration, Scoring, and Procedures Mannual*. Minneapolis, MN: NCS Pearson; 2000.

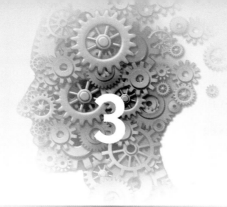

Fitting the Therapy and the Therapist to the Patient

SHIRALI PATEL, MD, MPhil AND ADAM M. BRENNER, MD

HOW DO YOU BEGIN TO SELECT A MODALITY?

There are a number of different therapy modalities to consider when meeting with a patient for the first time. As a new therapist, you might feel overwhelmed when faced with having to decide how best to proceed. Developing a working knowledge of the therapy modalities and their indications can be a helpful starting point. In this chapter, we have two goals:

1. Briefly cover which psychotherapy modalities have been studied and recommended for treatment of common psychiatric disorders.

2. Discuss the practical steps of selecting the most appropriate psychotherapy modality and therapist for a new patient.

We will focus on three particular types of therapy: supportive therapy, psychodynamic psychotherapy, and cognitive behavioral therapy (CBT) and its adaptations. These therapies, as well as systems-based approaches, are covered in greater detail later in this book, and you will find more in those associated chapters about the underlying theories and respective evidence bases. However, we will also mention when other psychotherapies not covered in this book are supported by the evidence base.

EVIDENCE BASE OF PSYCHOTHERAPY FOR COMMON CONDITIONS

Over the years, various psychotherapies have been studied within the research setting, with results that support their efficacy in treatment of mental health disorders. National and international organizations, as well as individual authors, have reviewed and incorporated this growing research into guidelines, with the aim of assisting clinicians in developing evidence-based treatment plans. In this section, we provide an overview of the recommended treatment modalities for different disorders in adult patients.

Limitations

Because this is a brief summary of a vast (and growing) literature, there are a number of limitations to the discussion presented here. While we will mention some important modalities not otherwise covered in this book, we will not name all therapy modalities studied or practiced. We do recommend expanding your knowledge and understanding of the therapy modalities that extend beyond those covered in this chapter and book over time. Additionally, our aim is not to provide an exhaustive review of the psychotherapy evidence base for all disorders within the Diagnostic and Statistical Manual of Mental Disorders (DSM)—that would fill an entire book itself. A further limitation is that supportive therapy is rarely mentioned in guidelines, since it is so rare to find studies aimed at demonstrating its efficacy (see more in Chapter 5). This is one of those places where it is good to remember that absence of evidence is not evidence of absence. Another major limitation of the evidence base is that researchers, in trying to prove efficacy of a treatment, often narrow the pool of subjects to only those with the one diagnosis they are studying. In reality, you will rarely meet patients with a single diagnosis in clinical practice. Most patients report symptoms that meet criteria for multiple different DSM diagnoses or are suffering with complicated behavioral and emotional issues that do not fit well into any of the defined diagnostic categories.

We have primarily drawn upon guidelines published within the United States, Canada, and the United Kingdom and online peer-reviewed references such as UpToDate and Cochrane Systematic Reviews. The particular guidelines that we refer to include those published by the American Psychiatric Association, the Society of Clinical Psychology (Division 12 of the American Psychological Association), Canadian Network for Mood and Anxiety Treatments (CANMAT), and the National Institute for Health and Care Excellence (NICE, United Kingdom). We recommend that you consult these guidelines, as well as the research literature for updates and for more in-depth discussions of the extent and limitations of the studies. It is the nature of evidence-based practice that things are constantly evolving and, unfortunately, textbooks cannot be updated anywhere close to the rate by which guidelines change and new reviews are published. Ultimately, we hope this brief review here will serve as a useful starting point for thinking about which therapies are recommended for specific disorders.

Mood Disorders

Mood disorders encompass a range of diagnoses, including major depressive disorder, bipolar disorder, persistent depressive disorder, cyclothymia, and other related but unspecified areas of concern. Here, we will focus on major depressive disorder and bipolar disorder.

Major Depressive Disorder. The most robust evidence exists for CBT, though psychodynamic psychotherapy and supportive therapy can also be selected to treat patients who are experiencing impairment from depression.[1-5] CBT treats depression by helping the patient learn to correct distorted thinking that has led to hopelessness and low self-worth and by applying behavioral activation to directly combat lethargy and anhedonia. Psychodynamic therapy approaches depression by exploring underlying conflicts or otherwise inaccessible disturbing mental content. Interpersonal therapy (IPT), problem-solving therapy, and acceptance and commitment therapy (ACT) are not focused on in this book but also have a strong evidence base supported by guidelines (see Chapter 12 for a further description of ACT).[3,6-8] Psychotherapies may lead to longer-lasting effects for patients than medication treatment alone, and combined treatment of medication and psychotherapy has advantages over either alone.[2]

Bipolar Disorder. It can be difficult to effectively engage in psychotherapy during an acute manic or mixed phase episode. Nonetheless, patients with bipolar disorder have been shown to benefit from psychotherapy in conjunction with pharmacotherapy for the treatment of their illness. Psychoeducation (an important aspect of supportive therapy) and CBT have both shown useful in helping patients cope with their illness, adhere to treatment, restore stability to their lives, and recover.[9] Other therapies not covered in this text, such as interpersonal psychotherapy, social rhythm therapy, and family-focused therapy, have also been shown to provide therapeutic benefits.[10-15]

Anxiety Disorders

We are including the DSM diagnoses of generalized anxiety disorder, social anxiety disorder, panic disorder, and phobias under this heading of "anxiety disorders." Broadly speaking, variations of CBT have the strongest evidence base for psychotherapeutic treatment of these disorders.[1,16-25] Most forms of panic-focused CBT involve psychoeducation, cognitive restructuring, self-monitoring, exposure, modifications of anxiety-maintaining behaviors, and relapse prevention.[16,22] CBT that includes exposure, social skills training, cognitive restructuring, and relaxation training has been noted to be helpful for social anxiety disorder.[19,20,25] For specific phobias, CBT that focuses on exposure and cognitive restructuring is recommended.[1,23,24]

There are also some studies indicating that short-term psychodynamic psychotherapy (PP) is effective in treatment of anxiety disorders (including panic disorder, social phobia, generalized anxiety disorder).[1,20,21] Likewise, supportive therapy (SP) has also been shown to be helpful for some anxiety disorders.[1,18] It remains unclear, however, how psychodynamic and supportive therapies compare with CBT, given the number of studies with varying results.[18]

Adjustment Disorders

While adjustment disorder is a common diagnosis, especially in outpatient and consult-liaison settings, there is a great dearth of evidence to guide the choice of psychotherapeutic interventions. This may be due to the often self-limiting nature of the disorder. Consensus expert opinion generally suggests brief psychotherapies, which may be supportive, psychodynamic, or cognitive behavioral.[26-28]

Obsessive Compulsive Disorder

CBT with an emphasis on exposure response prevention (ERP) is generally recommended for treating obsessive compulsive disorder (OCD).[1,25,29-33] Psychotherapy helps patients with OCD through learning that resisting the compulsive behavior may be uncomfortable but will not be catastrophic. In addition, psychotherapy teaches patients to see obsessions as ideas that, though disturbing, can be reappraised in terms of their meaning and actual danger. CBT can be administered as the sole treatment for patients who decline medication treatment or are not too depressed, anxious, or severely ill to partake in therapy alone.[30,31] There is also some evidence for ACT as a treatment for OCD.[29,32]

Posttraumatic Stress Disorder

Trauma-focused cognitive behavioral therapeutic approaches have been extensively studied for use with posttraumatic stress disorder (PTSD), resulting in good evidence to support their use. These approaches sometimes focus more on cognitive processing, which others more on exposure/reprocessing.[34-39] The cognitive aspects of these treatments help patients by reexamining problematic ideas about the cause of the trauma or about the ongoing danger and risk. Behavioral exposure can include retelling the traumatic experience, imaginal exposures, virtual reality, and in vivo encounters with triggering situations. In any of these scenarios, the goal is to allow the patient to experience the traumatic memory or reminders in safety and with a decreased fear response. More details on trauma-specific cognitive behavioral therapies, such as cognitive processing therapy and prolonged exposure, are reviewed in Chapter 6.

Supportive therapy has not typically been studied for PTSD, but some elements of supportive therapy including psychoeducation and stress reduction training can be helpful. Psychodynamic therapy is not an evidence-based therapy for PTSD itself, but the long-term distorting effects of trauma on relationships and self-image may be responsive to dynamic therapy. Additional therapy modalities with at least some evidence support, but not covered in this book, include eye movement desensitization and reprocessing (EMDR) and narrative-focused therapy.[25,34-38]

Eating Disorders

CBT, psychodynamic therapy, and supportive therapy approaches all may be helpful for anorexia nervosa, but comparative studies have generally failed to demonstrate differences in outcomes between these three approaches. A variant of CBT for eating disorders (CBT-ED) that focuses on relapse prevention and can include both behavioral (exposure to foods and establishing a more regular eating pattern) and cognitive (motivation for change and experience of body) components has growing support in the literature.[40,41] Psychodynamic approaches focus on the conscious and unconscious meaning of eating and eating symptoms and how these are embedded in important relationships. Supportive approaches emphasize psychoeducation, nutritional education, and praise for any progress toward healthier eating. Family-based therapy can also be useful for adolescents as a treatment aimed at relational difficulties that are contributing to the persistence of eating disorder symptoms.[40,42-44]

For bulimia nervosa, CBT is the recommended treatment, and there is evidence of its superiority compared to other approaches.[41,43,45,46] There is also support for family-based therapy and interpersonal psychotherapy.[42,43,45]

For binge eating disorder, CBT-ED has also been recommended.[41,47] In order to reduce symptoms, CBT treatment includes behavioral strategies aimed at normalizing patterns of eating and monitoring of behaviors, as well as cognitive modifications addressing dysfunctional thoughts about one's body.[41-43,47,48] Interpersonal psychotherapy can also be considered.[43,47]

Schizophrenia

Psychosocial interventions that have demonstrated success for patients with schizophrenia often focus on supportive strategies (though these are not typically referred to as supportive therapy, per se). These include family psychoeducation, social skills training, supported employment, and supported housing. Sometimes, these modalities are bundled together under the rubric of an assertive community treatment team (for more information, see Chapter 9). Cognitive remediation, which is also not covered in this book, has shown value in helping patients with symptoms specific to difficulty with concentration and memory.[49]

CBT has also demonstrated benefit in helping patients decrease both positive and negative symptoms. The cognitive side of the therapy gently helps patients assess the reality or reasonableness of hallucinations and delusions, while behavioral interventions emphasize development of social skills.[50-53] Although individual narratives may provide anecdotal reports of the utility of psychodynamic approaches,[54] research has not demonstrated usefulness of psychodynamic therapy for schizophrenia, and attempting to explore unconscious or conflictual material may actually be destabilizing and harmful.

Personality Disorders

Personality disorders are a diverse group of diagnoses and not all personality disorders have been equally or extensively studied. The literature for Cluster A personality disorders, which include schizotypal, schizoid, and paranoid personality disorders, is particularly limited. In the absence of research evidence, some experts suggest that cognitive therapy can affect change in cognitive and social disabilities for schizoid and schizotypal personality disorders,[55] while others argue that supportive approaches are most likely to be helpful for schizotypal personality.[56]

There is a substantial research literature for borderline personality disorder. Psychotherapy is generally recommended as the core treatment modality for borderline personality disorder (PD), specifically dialectical behavioral therapy

(DBT). DBT, a form of CBT that was originally developed for treating suicidal or self-destructive behaviors, has been very extensively studied, with substantial evidence for its efficacy.[57-61] There is also evidence for the value of psychodynamic approaches to borderline personality disorder, including transference-focused therapy and mentalization-based therapy.[57-61] Supportive interventions, such as validation, psychoeducation, and focusing on achievable life goals, can also help and have been studied with demonstrated benefits in the "Good Psychiatric Management" protocol.[61]

While much has been written about the etiology and conceptual understanding of narcissistic personality disorder, the evidence base is largely limited to case series and reports of supportive therapy and psychodynamic approaches.[62-64] Likewise, the evidence base for histrionic personality disorder is limited, though there is some evidence that short-term dynamic psychotherapy or brief adaptive psychotherapy is helpful for these patients.[65] Little evidence indicates that psychotherapy, particularly psychodynamic or supportive therapy, is of benefit for patients with antisocial personality disorder;[66] CBT may be used or incorporated into treatment programs for patients with mild antisocial personality disorder who possess some insight and reason to improve.[67] Generally speaking, however, it is imperative that therapists remain aware of potential negative feelings they may have toward patients with antisocial personality disorder and mindful of the potential for the patient's manipulation of the therapeutic relationship.[55,67]

The literature for Cluster C disorders, which include avoidant, dependent, and obsessive compulsive personality disorders, is also very limited. That being said, there is some evidence supporting the use of both psychodynamic therapy and CBT for these patients.[1,68] Of note, avoidant personality disorder is frequently thought of as very similar to and often co-occurring with social anxiety disorder; as such, much of the literature studying avoidant personality disorder has been completed in the context of co-occurring social anxiety disorder, with results that support the use of cognitive behavioral techniques.[65,69] Obsessive compulsive personality disorder and obsessive compulsive disorder, however, are thought to be distinct entities with only modest co-occurrence; whereas the OCD patient's world contains obsessive thoughts and compulsive behaviors, the obsessive compulsive personality disorder (OCPD) patient's world does not. Instead, the patient with OCPD uses rigid rules and regulations to maintain control over their internal and external world and often exhibits limited emotional awareness.[70] The recommended treatment for OCD, therefore, cannot be applied to an OCPD patient.

Substance Use Disorders

Substance use disorders encompass a variety of different conditions including use of alcohol, opioids, stimulants, cannabis, and more. Psychosocial interventions that extend beyond individual therapy are often a crucial part of treatment, and therefore recovery programs often build in groups, peer support, and engagement with families. Because ambivalence or denial about their condition can make it hard for patients to engage in traditional individual therapies, a therapy approach called motivational interviewing (MI) may have particular value for those patients. It is a brief approach that utilizes an empathic and nonjudgmental approach to examining the patient's ambivalence about addressing addictive behaviors and has been shown to improve patients' motivation for and commitment to change.[71] In addition, CBT and other CBT-based therapies can be helpful for some patients with substance use disorders. The aim is to help reduce behaviors and modify thinking patterns that increase risk or vulnerability to relapse. For example, CBT for alcohol use disorder might focus on increasing the patient's sense of control or accountability for their drinking.[71-74]

Motivational Interviewing

Ann C. Schwartz, MD

Motivational interviewing (MI) is an evidence-based intervention that uses a directive and patient-centered approach to interacting with patients and enables patients to explore and resolve ambivalence to promote behavioral change (Rollnick and Miller, 1995; Laakso, 2011). You might think of it as the therapy for patients who are not yet sure they want therapy. While originally developed to address substance use disorders (Miller, 1983), the interventions have been used with a variety or presenting concerns (health, fitness, nutrition, treatment adherence, substance use, and gambling), patient populations (eg, age, ethnicity, religion, sexuality, and gender identities), treatment formats (eg, individual, group, telemedicine), and settings (eg, health, corrections, and education) (Center for Substance Abuse Treatment, 1999; Miller and Rollnick, 2013).

MI has been found to be effective in reducing maladaptive behaviors including problem drinking, gambling, and HIV-risk behaviors and generating positive treatment outcomes including reduction in consumption, higher abstinence rates, better social adjustment, and successful referrals to treatment (Center for Substance Abuse Treatment, 1999; Hettema et al, 2005). In addition, MI has been found to be effective in promoting adaptive health behavior change including exercise, diet, and medication adherence (Miller and Rose, 2009).

Stages of Change. The theory behind MI was influenced by Prochaska and DiClemente's *Transtheoretical Model of Change* (Prochaska and DiClemente, 1982). The change process was conceptualized as a sequence of five stages through which people progress when they think about, initiate, and maintain new behaviors (Prochaska and DiClemente, 1984). This model of change highlighted the need for clinicians to be flexible and tailor the methods to the patient's current level of readiness for change (Miller and Rollnick, 2013), as people need and use different kinds of motivational support depending on which stage of change they are in (Center for Substance Abuse Treatment, 1999).

The five stages of the transtheoretical model are precontemplation, contemplation, preparation, action, and maintenance. In the *precontemplation stage*, individuals are not considering change in their problem behaviors and only see costs rather than benefits to the change or new behavior. In the *contemplative stage*, individuals are beginning to consider that they may have a problem and may be able to recognize some benefits of the change or new behavior, but they still see and perceive the costs to be greater than the benefits. In the *preparation stage*, individuals have come to the realization that the benefits of the new behavior outweigh the costs, have a goal to change the behavior in the near future, and make plans to do so. Once individuals decide to put the change into practice and modify the problem behavior, they enter the *action stage*. Individuals enter the *maintenance stage* once they are actively maintaining the new change in behavior for more than 6 months.

Patients will not always make a linear progression through the five stages and instead may regress to previous stages, relapse, or skip stages altogether (Prochaska and DiClemente, 1984). Recurrence of the problematic behavior is the rule, not the exception, and is an event that could occur at any point along the cycle of recovery. The "readiness ruler" is a common approach for assessing where patients are in terms of readiness to quit, as motivation is not static and can change daily. The easiest way to use a readiness ruler is to ask patients, on a scale of 1 (not ready) to 10 (ready), what number best reflects how ready they are now in terms of changing the specific problematic behavior (Sobel and Sobel, 2008).

MI was originally conceptualized as a way to work with patients who were in the early stages of change as a way of initiating treatment (Miller and Rollnick, 2013) as most therapies are designed for patients who are ready for change. The MI approach addresses where the patient currently is in the previously mentioned cycle of change and assists them in moving through the stages toward successful sustained change (ie, the maintenance stage). Framing the treatment within the stages of change can help the therapist better empathize with and understand the patient's treatment progress.

Theoretical Approach. MI can be used when the patient's ambivalence and motivation appear to be obstacles to change. The MI approach acknowledges that ambivalence about problem behaviors and initiating change is normal. However, it also views this ambivalence as an important obstacle in recovery that can be resolved by working with the patient's intrinsic motivations and values (Rollnick and Miller, 1995). The MI techniques help elicit behavior change by helping patients explore and resolve ambivalence. This is accomplished by skillfully increasing a patient's ability to acknowledge discrepancies between current behaviors and desired goals, while simultaneously minimizing resistance to change (Davidson, 1994).

An assumption of the theory is that the responsibility and capability for change lie within the patient and are not imposed by the therapist (Rollnick and Miller, 1995). MI is collaborative, rather than authoritarian, and honors the patient's autonomy, evoking the patient's own motivation rather than trying to install it. The therapist's task is to provide a directive but empathic and supportive environment that will support and enhance the patient's intrinsic motivation for and commitment to change (Miller and Rollnick, 2002). While MI does seek to "confront" patients with reality, it does not involve arguing with the patient or telling them what they should or must do. As with any therapy, MI is most successful when a trusting and collaborative relationship is established between the therapist and patient (Center for Substance Abuse Treatment, 1999).

Skills and Strategies. Skills or strategies of MI that are particularly useful in the early stages of treatment include asking open-ended questions, affirmations that recognize the patient's strengths, listening reflectively to demonstrate understanding of the patient, summarizing what has transpired up to that point in the session, affirming the patient's strengths, motivations, intentions, and progress, and eliciting self-motivational statements. These approaches are used instead of trying to lecture or persuade the patient that the change is necessary (Miller and Rollick, 2002). These MI methods can be remembered using the acronym OARS: Open-ended questions, Affirmations, Reflective listening, and Summaries (Miller and Rollnick, 2002).

Four general principles (Miller and Rollnick, 2002) can guide the therapist in MI and include: (1) express empathy through reflective listening, (2) develop discrepancy, (3) "roll" with the resistance, and (4) support self-efficacy.

Empathy is a key component of MI, as patients are more capable of opening up and sharing and exploring ambivalence when they feel understood and accepted. An important part of expressing empathy is reflective listening, which seeks to understand the patient's frame of reference and communicates acceptance of patients where they are, while also supporting them in the process of change. Normalizing comments are also helpful and may include statements such as "many people have made several attempts to quit" that communicates that the patient is not alone and that others have had similar experiences.

A second principle of MI is *developing discrepancy* between the patient's goals or values and their current behavior. Discrepancy is initially highlighted by raising the patient's awareness of the negative consequences of a problem behavior and helping them confront the behaviors that contributed to the consequences (Center for Substance Abuse Treatment, 1999). Using this approach, the therapist plays the role of a detective who is trying to solve a mystery, but having a challenging time as the clues do not add up (Kanfer and Schefft, 1988; Sobell and Sobell, 2008). Persuasion or argumentation should be avoided, as this tends to evoke defensiveness or opposition and could precipitate more resistance (therefore diminishing the probability of change). Instead, elicit the patient's views on their current behaviors that may be in conflict with their personal goals and let them present the arguments for change.

Resistance may manifest as arguing, interrupting, denying, or ignoring and is predictive of poor treatment outcomes and lack of involvement in the therapeutic process (Center for Substance Abuse Treatment, 1999). Resistance is a signal that the therapist may need to change direction. MI does not meet resistance head on but rather "rolls with" the resistance in an attempt to shift patient perceptions in the process (Miller and Rollnick, 2002). Examples of rolling with resistance include listening reflectively by paraphrasing or summarizing back to the patient in a nonjudgmental way that shows understanding but not necessarily agreement. Developing discrepancy between the patient's views and their wider goals or objectives and encouraging the patient to come up with possible solutions or alternative viewpoints are additional ways of rolling with the resistance. In this way, the patient is the primary source for finding the answers and solutions; the therapist explores concerns and uses the patient's perspectives to explore their views and better understand the struggles of the patient.

The principle of *supporting self-efficacy* is another way to help patients stay motivated to change. Self-efficacy, or the belief that one can change their problem behavior, has been described as a critical determinant/component of behavior change (Bandura, 1982). Many patients find it difficult to believe that they can begin or maintain behavioral change, and the patient's belief or hope in the possibility of change is an important motivator. The therapist serves as a source of encouragement for the patient. The patient must come to believe that change is possible and that they are responsible for carrying out the necessary actions to change. One way to do this is by the technique of asking for permission (eg, "do you mind if we talk about…?"). This communicates respect for patients and may leave the patient more open to talking about change.

Processes and Session Flow. Motivational interviewing has also been conceptualized as four fundamental processes that help simplify the way that MI is delivered. These processes help describe the flow of the conversation and how MI unfolds in actual practice (Miller and Rollnick, 2013). The processes include engaging, focusing, evoking, and planning. *Engaging* is the foundation of MI and is the process by which both parties establish a healthy connection and a working relationship, as therapeutic engagement is a prerequisite for everything that follows. *Focusing* is the process by which you develop, maintain, and clarify direction in the conversation to focus on change. This gives the therapist permission to move into a directional conversation about change. The third process is *evoking*, or the "why" of change, which involves eliciting the patient's own motivations for change and occurs when there is focus on a particular change and the patient's feelings about why and how they might make the change. The final process is *planning*, or the "how" of change, which encompasses the developing commitment to change as well as formulating a specific plan of action (Miller and Rollnick, 2013).

Summary. In summary, MI is a patient-centered psychotherapeutic intervention and evidence-based approach that has been found to be effective in reducing maladaptive behaviors as well as promoting adaptive health behavior change in patients who are ambivalent about therapy and change. MI is a collaborative conversation style that can strengthen a person's own motivation and commitment to change (Miller and Rollnick, 2013). The principles and skills of MI described in this text box can guide the therapist to help elicit patients' own intrinsic motivation to change and ultimately improve treatment outcomes.

References

Bandura A. Self-efficacy mechanism in human agency. *Am Psychol*. 1982;37:122-147.

Center for Substance Abuse Treatment. *Enhancing motivation for change in substance abuse treatment. Treatment Improvement Protocol (TIP) Series, No. 35*. HHS Publication No. (SMA) 12-4214. Rockville, MD: Substance Abuse and Mental Health Services Administration; 1999.

Davidson R. Can psychology make sense of change? In: Edwards G, Lader M, eds. *Addiction: Processes of Change. Society for the Study of Addiction Monograph No. 3*. New York, NY: Oxford University Press; 1994:51-78.

Hettema J, Steele J, Miller WR. Motivational interviewing. *Annu Rev Clin Psychol*. 2005;1:91-111.

Institute of Medicine. *Treating Drug Problems*. Washington, DC: National Academy Press, 1990.

Kanfer FH, Schefft BK. *Guiding the Process of Therapeutic Change*. Champaign, IL: Research Press, 1988.

Laakso LJ. Motivational interviewing: addressing ambivalence to improve medication adherence in patients with bipolar disorder. *Issues Ment health Nurs*. 2011;33(1):8-14.

Landry MJ. *Overview of Addiction Treatment Effectiveness*. HHSPUB. No. (SMA) 96-3081. Rockville, MD: Substance Abuse and Mental Health Services Administration, Office of Applied Studies, 1996.

Miller WR. Motivational interviewing with problem drinkers. *Behav Cognit Psychother*. 1983;11:147-172.

Miller WR, Rollnick S. *Motivational Interviewing: Preparing People for Change*, 2nd Edition. New York, NY: Guilford Press; 2002.

Miller WR, Rollnick S. *Motivational Interviewing: Helping People Change*, 3rd Edition. New York, NY: Guilford Press; 2013.

Miller WR, Rose GS. Toward a theory of motivational interviewing. *Am Psychol*. 2009;64(6):527-537.

Miller WR, Sovereign RG, Krege B. Motivational interviewing with problem drinkers: II. The drinker's check-up as a preventive intervention. *Behav Psychother*. 1998;16:251-268.

Prochaska JO, DiClemente CC. Transtheoretical therapy toward a more integrative model of change. *Psychother Theory Res Pract*. 1982;19:276-288.

Prochaska JO, DiClemente CC. *The Transtheoretical Approach: Crossing Traditional Boundaries of Therapy*. Homewood, IL: Dow Jones-Irwin; 1984.

Rollnick S, Miller WR. What is motivational interviewing? *Behav Cognit Psychother*. 1995;23(4):325-334.

Sobell LC, Sobell MB. *Motivational Interviewing Strategies and Techniques: Rationales and Examples*. 2008. Available at https://www.esrdnetwork.org/sites/default/files/MI_rationale_techniques.pdf. Accessed February 25, 2020.

CLINICAL JUDGMENT IN SELECTION OF THE THERAPY AND THERAPIST

As a clinician, you are charged with the complex task of translating the often limited research findings and guidelines into a workable treatment plan, tailored to address a given patient's unique needs. While it is typical in research trials to limit the number of confounding variables, many patients in clinical practice present with multiple complaints or comorbidities or otherwise present with diagnoses that do not fully align with those studied in the literature. Things are much messier and complicated in real life. For example, a patient may suffer a loss that triggers panic attacks. The panic attacks lead to increased isolation, and the patient then becomes depressed. At the same time, the loss highlights issues of abandonment that have always been a challenging part of the patient's personality. Alternatively, a patient may present in a hypomanic state that is related to substance use. As therapy works on stabilizing these symptoms and behavioral issues, it becomes clear that the patient suffered a terribly traumatic childhood that has deeply scarred their capacity to succeed in work and in intimate relationships. Because of this complexity, it is important to develop an approach to thinking about a patient that allows you to both recognize their complexity, while still making use of the research findings and guidelines. We will start by discussing concerns you should consider in thinking about the patient and then specific questions you should ask the patient about their perspective of therapy.

THE CLINICIAN'S PERSPECTIVE ON CHOOSING A TYPE OF THERAPY

Safety

It is important to consider safety first when choosing a psychotherapy modality. In any initial mental health assessment, we ask about imminent safety concerns, as well as gather information about risk and protective factors for harm. This includes a past history of suicide attempts or nonsuicidal self-harm, violence toward others, family history of suicides and mental illness, and access to weapons, as well as questions about faith and family that provide support and protection from harm (see Chapter 5 for more on safety planning). It is important to maintain a working understanding of the patient's safety risk, since therapy can be both a stressor and a support for a fragile patient. If suicidality, self-harm, or impulsivity is a significant element in a patient's presentation, then it is important to consider forms of therapy that are less confrontational, more supportive, and focused on skill building as the first step in treatment. For example, such a patient may benefit from therapies that focus on the ability to safely cope with perceived stressors or tolerate interpersonal stress, before engaging in other types of therapy that could provoke distressing emotions and thoughts related to past experiences or traumas. Ultimately, no matter what therapy modality you decide to recommend for a given patient, it is always important to reassess safety throughout your time with them. Ongoing life dynamics and stressors can certainly change unexpectedly, leading to new or worsened symptoms.

Capacity for a Therapeutic Relationship

It is also important to consider the degree to which a patient can maintain a relationship with someone, while tolerating confrontation and interpersonal stress. This is because therapy is often a longer term commitment that is interspersed with intense moments. As part of this, we recommend asking about past experiences in therapy and how long they were able to continue with any prior therapist(s). We would also recommend making note of the presence or absence of steady relationships in the patient's narrative, including those with providers, family members, partners, colleagues, or friends. If a patient reports a complete lack of meaningful relationships in their lifetime, this can also be an indication to start with a more supportive stance that helps build a stronger alliance and gives you time to gauge how able the individual is to tolerate interpersonal stress and build a relationship with you as their therapist. Alternatively, you might start with very structured therapy that does not depend quite as much on rapport with the therapist.

Psychological Mindedness

It is also important to assess a patient's level of psychological mindedness, defined as the capacity an individual has for self-examination or self-reflection.[75] As you encounter patients during your training, you will notice that they vary in their level of psychological mindedness.

While supportive therapy can be helpful for individuals of any level of psychological mindedness, certain therapy types, such as psychodynamic psychotherapy and most adaptations of CBT, require greater capacity and willingness to engage in self-reflection, in order to connect the dots between thoughts, emotions, experiences, and a sense of self. Thus, if someone presents with sufficient coping skills to tolerate distressful emotions and some ability to reflect internally on their thoughts and feelings (ie, some degree of psychological mindedness), then the patient may be a suitable candidate for therapies that delve deeper into exploring one's sense of self and the cognitive distortions, painful emotions, and/or life experiences that have affected it. A psychodynamic approach would facilitate this via a less structured, more exploratory method that focuses on affect, while a cognitive-based therapy would use a more structured approach that focuses on thoughts as directly related to feelings and behaviors. Determining which approach to take would rely on a further assessment of the patient's relative strengths and areas for improvement, as well as the patient's preferences. Sometimes, a patient's limited capacity or unwillingness to reflect internally is part of what has led them to their current situation. When this is the case, then adapting either a dynamic or cognitive-based approach to improve the patient's capacity for self-reflection may still be warranted.

PATIENT'S PERSPECTIVE

When deciding on a course of action for a patient, it is imperative to keep the patient's preferences in mind, in addition to your own judgments about their well-being. The patient's goals and expectations of therapy are major considerations and form a significant part of evidence-based practice.

Goals

After learning about the patient's past and present, you will also want to ask about the patient's goals for therapy. It is useful to have a clear understanding of where a patient stands presently and where the patient would like to go in the future in terms of mental health. While providers will have different techniques for opening up this conversation, potential questions to ask include:

- *I am curious to hear what goals you had in mind for therapy?*

- *What do you hope to get out of therapy?*

Sometimes, patients will come in with specific goals or desires, sometimes, they will come in with less clear goals, and sometimes with goals that are impossible.

Occasionally, a patient will respond with, *"I don't know—that's why I came to you."* You can be helpful to the patient by suggesting a possible goal that seems to be implied by their presentation. For example, if a patient described crippling panic attacks, you could offer, *"From what you have told me, one goal might be to help you better control your anxiety. What do you think about that?"*

As you listen to the patient, consider and explore whether the responses align with any of the following types of goals:

- **Coping skills.** Does the patient hope to strengthen coping skills or learn alternate ways of coping with stressful situations?

- **Processing life events.** Does the patient want help in processing a life event that they are struggling to make sense of?

- **Symptom alleviation.** Does the patient wish to alleviate a specific symptom or set of symptoms?

- **Recurrent problematic relationship patterns.** Does the patient wish to explore patterns that keep recurring in life or increase insight into the self?

- **Unclear.** Does the patient recognize a need for therapy but remain unsure of why?

Considering these questions can be helpful in understanding the patient's wishes at the start of therapy. When a patient has a clear goal, it is usually much easier to select a therapy modality. For example, a patient who is looking for help learning to live with a newly diagnosed grave illness may benefit from supportive therapy. As another example, a patient who presents with significant depression and anxiety and whose priority is to directly and immediately lessen these symptoms may be most appropriate for CBT. Alternatively, a patient with the same presentation whose priority is to increase insight into their selves and life experiences would be a good fit with a psychodynamic approach.

Patients will sometimes come to a therapist driven not by a specific goal but with a general need to be helped and will work with the therapist to gain clarity of what feels amiss. Alternatively, the patient may look to the therapist to help create goals based on the therapist's expertise. In these cases, it is usually best to not push the patient too quickly into creating artificial goals. Instead, reflecting with the patient about their experience in a supportive manner and helping them find the right words to describe their struggles will become the starting point and initial goal of the therapy. This can also be useful information in then helping the patient come up with a more informed set of goals for the treatment.

Other patients may express a preference for goals that are not feasible—usually related to changing their external, but not internal, world. In such cases, you can gently point this out by stating a variation of the following: *"While it is not possible for me, as your therapist, to change your current circumstances or control what others say to you in your day-to-day life, I do think we may be able to identify why you keep finding yourself in such situations and how to better cope when things become a struggle."* With patients that have a deeply rooted tendency to externalize their difficulties, it may take time and support before the patient is able to move from externalizing their difficulties to reflecting internally.

Regardless of what goals the patient offers, asking about their hopes for therapy should help foster a stronger therapeutic alliance and set the tone for a collaborative approach to therapy going forward.

Expectations About the Therapy Process

Patients will sometimes come to their first therapy evaluation with preconceived notions about what the therapy process will be like. These fantasies may be drawn from television or movies. Sometimes, they are based on a friend or family's experience of therapy or what they have read about therapy online, as well as cultural norms surrounding mental health care in general. Therapy is likely to be most helpful when the patient and provider are on the same page, so we would encourage you to ask the patient about any expectations or ideas they have about how the process works. One way of opening up this conversation is to ask the patient about past experiences with therapy, either through personal therapy or through stories from friends/family.

Some questions that you might ask the patient are:

- *Have you personally had any prior experiences with therapy? If so, what were they like for you? What was helpful? What was not helpful?*

- *Tell me what you imagine therapy to be like. Is there anything about therapy that you are particularly excited about? Anything you are particularly worried about?*

- *Have any of your friends or family sought out therapy? Did they describe to you what their experience was like? How do you think your family or friends would react if you told them you were interested in therapy?*

These kinds of questions will help you to gain a better idea of how the patient expects therapy to go. They can also help you consider modalities that are more in line with what the patient expects. For example, a patient anticipating a more didactic approach to therapy may feel uncomfortable and lost if the therapist initiates a psychodynamic therapy, without explaining the therapy modality or discussing alternative modalities that might align more readily with their expectations.

It is always important to provide information to a patient about why you are recommending a certain treatment and what to expect. This is an essential aspect of good practice. This is especially important when there is conflict between what a patient wants and imagines and what you think would be the most appropriate therapy modality and process. When you are able to explain and provide a reasonable rationale for your recommendation, the patient is then able to make a truly informed decision about the therapy treatment. You may also decrease the degree of frustration patients feel once they have begun therapy and are discovering the process to be different than what they imagined.

Patient-Therapist Fit

In addition to expectations about the therapy process, patients may also come to therapy with expectations about their new therapist. They may be very anxious about who you are and ask questions about your background, including your educational background or degree status, age, race, gender identity, religion, ability status, sexual orientation, socioeconomic status, and/or national origin. This can sometimes feel uncomfortable, like the patient is questioning your qualifications or challenging boundaries. It can help to remember that these questions are not really about you personally but instead about the patient's concerns about fit between themselves and you as the therapist. They want to know if you will be able to understand what they are going through. They may be afraid that someone who is too "outside" of their life experience will not be able to empathize or help them with their struggles. Or sometimes, patients may ask questions because we just asked them very personal things about themselves, and this just seems like the fair and reciprocal conversational thing to do.

If a patient asks questions about your background that are not related to your clinical training and education, you are certainly not obligated to disclose anything that you would like to keep private. If the content does not fall into that category of professional or educational training background, then the question is whether it will be more or less useful for the therapist to answer a personal question. It is usually a good idea to begin by asking why the patient is curious about this particular aspect of your personal background, if they have not made that clear.

Whether you answer the question will be a judgment call that depends on different factors, including the type of therapy you are recommending. In a psychodynamic therapy where you hope to create the greatest possible freedom of exploration, you might inform the patient why you do not answer questions by stating, "I typically don't answer questions about my personal background, as it can interfere with the therapy process over time. But, it does sound like the answer to this question may be of importance to you. Could you tell me more about that?" The patient's response to your questions can give you additional information about what they find important and/or what their fears and expectations surrounding therapy look like. It can also provide you with important information about the patient's worldview, areas of cultural salience, and how they see themselves fitting in the world, all of which are likely connected to the patient's state of being.

On the other hand, if you are suggesting a more supportive therapy, you might prioritize reducing the patient's anxiety by answering the question. At the beginning of your career (as compared to later), you are in fact less likely to have had many of the experiences that your patient is wondering about, including marriage, raising children, dealing with aging parents, etc. Acknowledging what you do not directly know about life can actually be reassuring and decrease the patient's fear of being misunderstood or judged. For example, you might say, "No, I don't have children, but I want to understand whatever you can share with me about your experience with your children." A word of caution about this approach: self-disclosure by the therapist to one patient does not necessarily go unobserved or undiscussed with other patients the therapist is treating. So if you disclose an aspect of your personal life to one patient, you may find this information shared with other patients with undesired consequences. This occurs more frequently in inpatient or contained settings.

Sometimes, the patient's concerns are not about your experiences but about your identity. Issues of race, gender, sexuality, religion, and immigrant status are among the many aspects of identity that a patient may be wanting to share with their therapist. Sometimes, these aspects of your identity are obvious to the patient (or at least they think so), without asking you anything specific. When these aspects of identity do not align, it can help to reassure the patient that this identity match often is not necessary for a therapist and patient to do good work together. But, it is important to first understand what they are concerned about and let them know that you will be sure to ask about and take into account these differences in identity as they become relevant to the treatment process and goals. For a more in-depth discussion of the importance of cultural identities, see Chapter 8.

Of course, because perceived and actual similarities in culture and background can also affect the therapy process, you can also let the patient know that you will also be taking into account any areas of overlap, in addition to the differences. Sometimes, new therapists can be overconfident about understanding patients who come from similar backgrounds or seem otherwise like them—this is called "over-identifying" with the patient and is also an element to be mindful of, so as not to make inaccurate assumptions about the patient's experience. Ultimately, demonstrating a willingness to acknowledge and discuss both perceived and actual similarities and differences helps build a strong therapeutic alliance.

When the Patient Requests a Different Therapist

For those occasions when the patient remains unsatisfied after discussion of the patient-therapist fit, you might provide them with references to therapists who may better meet their expectations. These are choices that you will consider carefully with your supervisor. On the other hand, if you are working in an area or system in which no alternate options are available, go ahead and acknowledge these limitations and provide reassurance that you will do your best to learn more about their identity including furthering your own education through independent reading or training and also helping them teach you what is important to them about their identity. For example, a straight therapist might say to a gay patient who is struggling with dating again after divorce, "It's true that I don't have direct experience of dating in the gay community. Maybe you can help me learn what the norms and expectations might be?"

When a patient expresses doubt about working with you or chooses not to engage in therapy with you, remember that this does not mean you are a bad therapist. Many new therapists suffer from "impostor syndrome"[76] and are already anxious that they are not qualified for this work. It is understandable that we would then feel a bit shaken when the patient chooses not to work with us. Nonetheless, the experience of being rejected as a potential therapist can feel jarring and shake your already fragile confidence. You may feel like you have made or said something wrong or that being who you are is not enough or "right" in some way. You may even feel resentful toward the patient. It is always helpful to be mindful of your own emotions and reactions during this process and to discuss them with your supervisor, particularly if these feelings are distressing. Recognizing those feelings and reactions can be a fruitful way of learning more about the patient and about your own self.

A different issue is that of the patient who rejects you as a therapist out of their own prejudice and biases. There might be some aspect of your identity (gender, race, age, sexuality, religion, immigrant status, etc.) that the patient has a bias about. In Chapter 8, we discuss ways to think about and respond when faced with overt prejudice coming from your patient.

CLINICIAN EXPERTISE AND LIMITATIONS OF COMPETENCE

On occasion, you may find that it is you who wishes to avoid starting therapy with a particular patient. This could be due to feeling uncomfortable around the patient because of safety concerns, because of the patient's objectionable beliefs, or because the patient reminds you of someone from your own past. Once again, we recommend discussing this with your supervisor as a starting point. In such cases, it is helpful, both for the patient and for yourself as a beginning therapist, to develop a better understanding of why the patient has left you feeling uncomfortable. Whenever possible, and it is often possible, your supervisor will help you learn to tolerate this discomfort while providing good care for the patient. When this is not possible, your supervisor will consider referring the patient to someone else (if that is feasible). When your discomfort stems from an actually dangerous situation, your supervisor will prioritize helping you take the appropriate steps to ensure your own safety.

No therapist is equally skilled in all types of therapy, as literally hundreds have been developed through the years. While it is important to acquire a working knowledge of the main therapy modalities, it is likely that you will develop greater ease and expertise with specific types of therapy. These will become the primary modalities that you generally offer your patients. This ease and expertise might come about because you train in an institution that has particular investment in one approach to therapy or because you are especially inspired by the wisdom and skill of one of your supervisors. If you benefited from being a patient in therapy before or during your training, you might also be influenced by the approach of your own therapist. And finally, you might be drawn to a particular therapy approach because it is a better fit for your temperament, values, or aptitudes.

Let us suppose you meet with a patient whom you think would benefit from a specific type of modality in which you have limited expertise. Be upfront with them about this. If you are certain that the areas in which you are knowledgeable would *not* be a good fit for the patient's current needs, then refer the patient to therapists who would be able to provide the indicated therapy. Alternatively, some patients will request a specific type of therapy that you do not know well. Again, let them know that your particular areas of therapy expertise do not include what they are requesting. When there are multiple modalities that may be helpful for a specific set of symptoms or disorders, then you can let the patient know what therapy modalities you do engage in and how they may prove equally helpful for the patient, based on what you know about the treatment literature, the patient's presentation, and the patient's preferences.

THE IMPORTANCE OF INFORMED CONSENT

When a physician recommends a certain medication to a patient, be it for hypertension, diabetes, or any other ailment, it is considered good practice to walk through the risks, benefits, and alternatives associated with the recommended medication. This is called "informed consent." Similarly, with therapy, it is helpful to walk through what the patient might expect from engaging in therapy. In so doing, remember to state the therapy modality that you are recommending to the patient and why you think this would be helpful. You should include a description of how the specific therapy modality is organized, commenting on how much structure is built into the therapy modality, and the expected length and frequency of therapy. *Benefits* of therapy to discuss include its anticipated impact on symptom relief, behavioral change, and insight into one's self. Indicate these effects can continue to develop and extend, even beyond the end of the therapy.

Risks to discuss as part of informed consent include therapy not working and the patient not showing improvement. We also recommend explaining that it is not uncommon for patients to feel worse before they feel better at times during the course of treatment, given that the process of therapy requires being vulnerable at times and having experiences and ideas that are uncomfortable or painful. And lastly, you should make clear if there are *alternatives* for the patient to choose from, including different modalities of therapy or medication treatment, as applicable to a patient's set of symptoms.

WHAT IS THE CORRECT DOSE OF THERAPY?

Once you have decided on the modality of therapy, another question to consider is the "dose" of therapy. This is an important question because patients understandably like to have an idea of how long treatment will take and what it might cost them!

With some therapies, such as CBT, there is more evidence and clearer guidance available about optimal frequency of treatment, although even CBT is highly flexible in terms of the recommended number of sessions. With other therapies, such as psychodynamic therapy or supportive therapy, there is much less available data or consensus to guide you. In the latter case, we think it makes sense to initially prescribe therapy the way a medical provider would prescribe a medication, eg, the lowest dose necessary to alleviate or control symptoms. For therapy, this means the minimum amount of therapy necessary to achieve the agreed-upon goals. This helps ease the burden, both for the patient and for the healthcare system in which treatment is being provided. Depending on the type of therapy, you might let the patient know that individual therapy is most typically a weekly treatment and encourage them to reflect on what was discussed in-between sessions and to complete any assigned tasks or worksheets. If the system in which you are working is set up for a finite number of treatment sessions, let the patient know upfront how long your work together can last. When you are offering an open-ended treatment (eg, without a session limit), you can let the patient know that you would like to start by working together for a certain number of weeks and then assess what progress has been made and where to go from there at specific intervals.

As the treatment progresses, you might recommend decreasing the frequency of an effective treatment in response to the patient's concerns about side effects. For example, a patient might say, "I know we're working on important stuff but after our last few sessions I had trouble sleeping and I was on edge for days. Maybe we could slow things down?" On the other hand, there are times when you will suggest increasing the frequency of sessions. This could occur when more frequent sessions would allow for more effective support in a crisis or facing an overwhelming new life stressor. Or, it may occur when you feel that an increased "dose" of therapy would foster greater depth in exploration of some current area of concern.

In reality, money and other resources (such as transportation, time off from work, and/or childcare) are factors that will enter into psychotherapy treatment discussions, much like medication cost often becomes part of the decision framework for medical illness. Some patients have ample financial resources, while other patients are limited in what they can afford. However, the availability of ample resources should not change the treatment recommendation. In other words, the dose of therapy should still remain the least amount necessary to achieve mutually agreed-upon goals, even when there are no financial restrictions.

For patients with more limited means, the lack of finances may strongly influence their decisions about frequency and length of therapy. As a provider, we encourage you to acknowledge and keep these concerns in mind, but to first think creatively about alternate solutions that would allow the patient to receive the recommended therapy for the recommended time duration, even within the financial parameters laid out by the patient's situation. You may be working, for example, in a city or academic setting where multiple tiers of therapy costs and providers are available to help offset the cost for the patient. Alternatively, there may be options for teletherapy that can help offset the cost of transportation for the patient. While finances are inevitably an important element in any discussion regarding treatment, be sure to still discuss with the patient the treatment you would recommend, regardless of financial constraints, and to then first consider and explore how to make this recommended treatment type and duration available to the patient. Of course, if you are working in an area where no alternatives are available, then inform the patient of this and work with the individual to come up with a treatment plan that is still beneficial but also within their means. We also hope that situations where no alternatives are available may act as a catalyst for you to advocate for and even develop programs down the road that help shrink the healthcare disparities present between different socioeconomic groups.

HOW DO I KNOW IF I NEED TO CHANGE TREATMENTS?

As therapy progresses, you should periodically ask yourself the questions outlined above in the section "Clinical Judgment in Selection." Sometimes, our initial impression of a patient changes as we learn more about them over time.[77] A patient's goals can also change over time. Because of this, it is imperative to ask the patient how they think therapy is going and to also evaluate progress from your point of view. This is not a topic that needs to be asked at every therapy visit, or even every month, but it is important to check in from time to time. If you and the patient both feel that the current mode of therapy has been helpful and that they are making progress, there is no need to consider a change in modalities. However, patients will sometimes feel that therapy is not working. This raises the possibility that a change in therapies is indicated, but you should be cautious in that conclusion. There can be multiple reasons behind the perceived lack of improvement and it is often complicated.

It is important to respect the patient's experience but to also use your clinical judgment to understand the whole situation. In particular, it is important to consider whether their frustration is not due to a poor fit of therapy modality but is instead a result of the difficulties inherent in becoming a psychotherapy patient. A helpful analogy can be that of learning a new instrument, such as the piano. Learning to play the piano takes time and persistence, as a student must build and maintain a relationship with their teacher, learn a new (musical) language, practice scales and other exercises, and learn to tolerate making mistakes in order to gain a new skillset. Similarly, therapy also takes time and persistent effort, as a patient learns new ways of talking about their problems and new ways of relating. As with any new practice, they will need to tolerate rough patches and plateaus on their road to improved mental well-being.

However, when you find that the patient is struggling to understand the concepts of the therapy or the approach to therapy does not appear to be a good fit with the manner in which the patient learns, you will want to discuss this with your supervisor. Even with the most thoughtful initial assessment, not every therapy works for every patient. Although initial evaluations aim to be comprehensive, it is impossible to fully know a patient and their struggles within a few sessions. Over the course of therapy, you may find that a patient reports new or previously undisclosed symptoms or maladaptive coping habits that change your recommendations. For example, your patient who presents with depression turns out to also have a serious substance use disorder. Alternatively, you may find that a patient's circumstances change in the middle of therapy, leading to new difficulties that are more immediate and would benefit from an alternate mode of treatment. In such situations, it is important to start by discussing your concerns about the patient's presentation with your supervisor. Your supervisor will help you think through the options, so that an informed decision that includes both your input and the patient's input can be made prior to any changes.

Many therapists develop an eclectic style that incorporates elements from multiple different modalities, even while primarily engaging in a single type of therapy. For example, a provider engaging primarily in psychodynamic therapy may incorporate elements from CBT when it seems appropriate for the patient's presentation. In this case, you could, as part of the consent process, inform the patient that you will be engaging primarily in a psychodynamic psychotherapy, but that you may utilize elements from other modalities of therapy if and when it seems appropriate for their ongoing struggles. This provides you, as the therapist, with the flexibility to adjust your therapy modality as you see fit, without leaving the patient in the dark about any treatment shifts that may occur.

Conclusion

When meeting with a patient for the first time, there are a number of factors to consider when deciding on a treatment plan. As a starting point, it is important to be familiar with the literature and guidelines for treatment of mental health disorders. Considering the patient's presentation from both their perspective and your perspective will then allow you to identify the patient's specific symptoms, behaviors, and goals and appropriately prioritize and align them with potential therapy modalities. Moreover, you will also be able to consider the patient's preferences for therapy and therapist, and connect and compare this with your own areas of expertise and potentially available resources. Combining these elements together will ultimately allow you the best chance to find the right fit of therapy modality and therapist for the patient.

Self-Study Questions

1. List at least three acknowledged limitations to the review of psychotherapy literature in this chapter. How would you work to remedy these in your actual psychotherapy practice?

2. Think of the last patient you interacted with or reviewed in seminar. Based on their primary diagnosis, what type(s) of psychotherapy would be supported by the literature?

3. List and describe at least two clinician perspectives and two patient perspectives that influence the choice of psychotherapy type.

4. When might you consider changing psychotherapy treatment type?

5. How might you proceed if your patient requests a different therapist? How might you react to that internally, and how might you get support?

RESOURCES FOR FURTHER LEARNING

American Psychiatric Association (guidelines). Available at https://www.psychiatry.org/psychiatrists/practice/clinical-practice-guidelines

Society of Clinical Psychology, Division 12, American Psychological Association (guidelines). Available at https://www.div12.org/diagnoses/

Up To Date. Available at www.uptodate.com

Cabaniss DL, Holoshitz Y. *Different Patients, Different Therapies.* New York, NY: W.W. Norton & Company, Inc; 2019.

Cochrane Database of Systematic Reviews. Available at www.cochranelibrary.com

REFERENCES

1. Gabbard GO. *Textbook of Psychotherapeutic Treatments*. Arlington, VA: American Psychiatric Publishing, Inc; 2009.
2. Gelenberg A, Freeman MP, Markowitz JC, et al. *Practice Guideline for the Treatment of Patients With Major Depressive Disorder*. American Psychiatric Association Website. Available at https://psychiatryonline.org/pb/assets/raw/sitewide/practice_guidelines/guidelines/mdd.pdf. Published October 2010. Accessed February 17, 2020.
3. *Treatment Target: Depression*. Society of Clinical Psychology, Division 12, American Psychological Association Website. Available at https://www.div12.org/diagnosis/depression/. Updated 2015. Accessed February 17, 2020.
4. Gabbard GO. *Long-Term Psychodynamic Psychotherapy, A Basic Text*. Washington, DC: American Psychiatric Publishing, Inc; 2010.
5. Simon G. *Unipolar Major Depression in Adults: Choosing Initial Treatment*. UpToDate Website. Available at https://www.UpToDate.com/contents/unipolar-major-depression-in-adults-choosing-initial-treatment?search=depression&source=search_result&selectedTitle=2~150&usage_type=default&display_rank=2#H21696480. Updated November 13, 2019. Accessed February 13, 2020.
6. Powers MB, Zum Vorde Sive Vording MB, Emmelkamp PM. Acceptance and commitment therapy: a meta-analytic review. *Psychother Psychosom*. 2009;78(2):73-80.
7. Parikh SV, Quilty LC, Ravitz P, et al. Canadian Network for Mood and Anxiety Treatments (CANMAT) 2016 clinical guidelines for the management of adults with major depressive disorder: section 2. Psychological treatments. *Can J Psychiatry*. 2016;61(9):524-539.
8. *Depression in Adults: Recognition and Management*. The National Institute for Health and Care Excellence (NICE) Website. Available at https://www.nice.org.uk/guidance/cg90. Published October 2009. Accessed February 17, 2020.
9. Hirschfeld RMA. *Practice Guideline for the Treatment of Patients With Bipolar Disorder*. 2nd ed. American Psychiatric Association Website. Available at https://psychiatryonline.org/pb/assets/raw/sitewide/practice_guidelines/guidelines/bipolar.pdf. Published April 2002. Accessed February 17, 2020.
10. Hirschfeld RMA. *Guideline Watch: Practice Guideline for the Treatment of Patients With Bipolar Disorder*. 2nd ed. American Psychiatric Association Website. Available at https://psychiatryonline.org/pb/assets/raw/sitewide/practice_guidelines/guidelines/bipolar-watch.pdf. Published November 2005. Accessed February 17, 2020.
11. *Treatment Target: Bipolar Disorder*. Society of Clinical Psychology, Division 12, American Psychological Association Website. Available at https://www.div12.org/diagnosis/bipolar-disorder/. Accessed February 17, 2020.
12. *The NICE Guideline on the Assessment and Management of Bipolar Disorder in Adults, Children, and Young People in Primary and Secondary Care*. The National Institute for Health and Care Excellence (NICE) Website. Available at https://www.nice.org.uk/guidance/cg185/evidence/full-guideline-pdf-4840895629. Published 2014. Accessed February 17, 2020.
13. Yatham LN, Kennedy SH, Parikh SV, et al. Canadian Network for Mood and Anxiety Treatments (CANMAT) and international society for bipolar disorders (ISBD) 2018 guidelines for the management of patients with bipolar disorder. *Bipolar Disord*. 2018;20(2):97-170.
14. Salcedo S, Gold AK, Sheikh S, et al. Empirically supported psychosocial interventions for bipolar disorder: current state of the research. *J Affect Disord*. 2016;201:203-214.
15. Bobo WV, Shelton RC. *Bipolar Major Depression in Adults: General Principles of Treatment*. UpToDate Website. Available at https://www.UpToDate.com/contents/bipolar-major-depression-in-adults-general-principles-of-treatment?search=bipolar%20disorder&topicRef=15267&source=see_link#H4080527171. Updated March 28, 2019. Accessed Retrieved January 19, 2020.
16. Stein MB. *Practice Guideline for the Treatment of Patients With Panic Disorder*. American Psychiatric Association Website. Available at http://psychiatryonline.org/pb/assets/raw/sitewide/practice_guidelines/guidelines/panicdisorder.pdf. Published January 2009. Accessed February 17, 2020.
17. Mitte K. Meta-analysis of cognitive-behavioral treatments for generalized anxiety disorder: a comparison with pharmacotherapy. *Psychol Bull*. 2005;131(5):785-795.
18. Hunot V, Churchill R, Silva de Lima M, Teixeira V. Psychological therapies for generalized anxiety disorder. *Cochrane Database Syst Rev*. 2007;2007(1):CD001848.
19. Heimberg RG. Cognitive-behavioral therapy for social anxiety disorder: current status and future directions. *Biol Psychiatry*. 2002;51(1):101-108.
20. *Social Anxiety Disorder: Recognition, Assessment and Treatment Clinical Guideline*. The National Institute for Health and Care Excellence (NICE) Website. Available at www.nice.org.uk/guidance/cg159. Published May 22, 2013. Accessed January 10, 2020.

3

21. *Cognitive and Behavioral Therapies for Generalized Anxiety Disorder*. Society of Clinical Psychology, Division 12, American Psychological Association Website. Available at https://www.div12.org/treatment/cognitive-and-behavioral-therapies-for-generalized-anxiety-disorder/. Accessed January 10, 2020.

22. Treatment Target: Panic Disorder. Society of Clinical Psychology, Division 12, American Psychological Association Website. Available at https://www.div12.org/diagnosis/panic-disorder/. Accessed January 11, 2020.

23. Exposure Therapies for Specific Phobias. Society of Clinical Psychology, Division 12, American Psychological Association Website. Available at https://www.div12.org/treatment/exposure-therapies-for-specific-phobias/. Accessed January 12, 2020.

24. Treatment Target: Social Anxiety Disorder and Public Speaking Anxiety. Society of Clinical Psychology, Division 12, American Psychological Association Website. Available at https://www.div12.org/treatment/cognitive-behavioral-therapy-for-social-anxiety-disorder/. Accessed January 12, 2020.

25. Katzman MA, Bleau P, Blier P, et al. Canadian clinical practice guidelines for the management of anxiety, posttraumatic stress and obsessive-compulsive disorders. *BMC Psychiatry*. 2014;14(suppl 1):S1.

26. Casey P, Bailey S. Adjustment disorders: the state of the art. *World Psychiatry*. 2011;10(1):11-18.

27. Casey P. Adjustment disorder: new developments. *Curr Psychiatry Rep*. 2014;16(6):451.

28. Carta MG, Ballestrieri M, Murru A, Hardoy MC. Adjustment Disorder: epidemiology, diagnosis and treatment. *Clin Pract Epidemiol Ment Health*. 2009;5:15.

29. Treatment Target: Obsessive Compulsive Disorder. Society of Clinical Psychology, Division 12, American Psychological Association Website. Available at https://www.div12.org/diagnosis/obsessive-compulsive-disorder/. Accessed February 19, 2020.

30. Koran LM, et al. Practice Guideline for the Treatment of Patients with Obsessive-Compulsive Disorder. American Psychiatric Association Website. Available at https://psychiatryonline.org/pb/assets/raw/sitewide/practice_guidelines/guidelines/ocd.pdf. Published July 2007. Accessed February 16, 2020.

31. Koran LM, Simpson HB. Guideline Watch (March 2013): Practice Guideline for the Treatment of Patients With Obsessive-Compulsive Disorder. American Psychiatric Association Website. Available at https://psychiatryonline.org/pb/assets/raw/sitewide/practice_guidelines/guidelines/ocd-watch.pdf. Published March 2013. Accessed. February 16, 2020.

32. Obsessive-Compulsive Disorder and Body Dysmorphic Disorder: Treatment. The National Institute for Health and Care Excellence (NICE) Website. Available at www.nice.org.uk/guidance/cg31. Published November 29, 2005. Accessed February 19, 2020.

33. Simpson HB. Pharmacotherapy for Obsessive-Compulsive Disorder in Adults. UpToDate Website. Available at https://www.UpToDate.com/contents/pharmacotherapy-for-obsessive-compulsive-disorder-in-adults?search=OCD&source=search_result&selectedTitle=2~149&usage_type=default&display_rank=2. Updated Jan 07, 2020. Accessed February 19, 2020.

34. Treatment Target: Posttraumatic Stress Disorder. Society of Clinical Psychology, Division 12, American Psychological Association Website. Available at https://www.div12.org/diagnosis/posttraumatic-stress-disorder/. Accessed September 25, 2019.

35. Ursano RJ, et al. Practice Guideline for the Treatment of Patients With Acute Stress Disorder and Posttraumatic Stress Disorder. American Psychiatric Association Website. Available at https://psychiatryonline.org/pb/assets/raw/sitewide/practice_guidelines/guidelines/acutestressdisorderptsd.pdf. Published November 2004. Accessed September 23, 2019.

36. Benedek DM, et al. Guideline Watch (March 2009): Practice Guideline for the Treatment of Patients With Acute Stress Disorder and Posttraumatic Stress Disorder. American Psychiatric Association Website. Available at https://psychiatryonline.org/pb/assets/raw/sitewide/practice_guidelines/guidelines/acutestressdisorderptsd-watch.pdf. Published March 2009. Accessed February 17, 2020.

37. PTSD Treatments. American Psychological Association Website. Available at https://www.apa.org/ptsd-guideline/treatments/index. Published July 31, 2017. Accessed February 19, 2020.

38. Post-Traumatic Stress Disorder. The National Institute for Health and Care Excellence (NICE) Website. Available at www.nice.org.uk/guidance/ng116. Published December 5, 2018. Accessed February 17, 2020.

39. Bisson JI, Roberts NP, Andrew M, Cooper R, Lewis C. Psychological therapies for chronic posttraumatic stress disorder (PTSD) in adults. *Cochrane Database Syst Rev*. 2013;2013(12):CD003388.

40. Treatment Target: Anorexia Nervosa. Society of Clinical Psychology, Division 12, American Psychological Association Website. Available at https://www.div12.org/diagnosis/anorexia-nervosa/. Accessed August 10, 2019.

41. Eating Disorders: Recognition and Treatment. The National Institute for Health and Care Excellence (NICE) Website. Available at www.nice.org.uk/guidance/ng69. Published May 23, 2017. Accessed August 11, 2019.

42. Yager J, et al. Practice Guideline for the Treatment of Patient With Eating Disorders, 2nd ed. American Psychiatric Association Website. Available at https://psychiatryonline.org/pb/assets/raw/sitewide/practice_guidelines/guidelines/eatingdisorders.pdf. Published May 2006. Accessed August 10, 2019.

43. Yager J, et al. Guideline Watch (August 2012): Practice Guideline for the Treatment of Patients With Eating Disorders. 3rd ed. American Psychiatric Association Website. Available at https://psychiatryonline.org/pb/assets/raw/sitewide/practice_guidelines/guidelines/eatingdisorders-watch.pdf. Published August 2012. Accessed August 10, 2019.

44. Hay PJ, Claudino AM, Touyz S, Abd Elbaky G. Individual psychological therapy in the outpatient treatment of adults with anorexia nervosa. *Cochrane Database Syst Rev.* 2015;2015(7):CD003909.

45. Treatment Target: Bulimia Nervosa. Society of Clinical Psychology, Division 2, American Psychological Association Website. Available at https://www.div12.org/diagnosis/bulimia-nervosa/. Accessed August 10, 2019.

46. Wonderlich SA, Peterson CB, Crosby RD, et al. A randomized controlled comparison of integrative cognitive-affective therapy (ICAT) and enhanced cognitive-behavioral therapy (CBT-E) for bulimia nervosa. *Psychol Med.* 2014;44(3):543-553.

47. Treatment Target: Binge Eating Disorder. Society of Clinical Psychology, Division 12, American Psychological Association Website. Available at https://www.div12.org/diagnosis/binge-eating-disorder/. Accessed August 10, 2019.

48. Hay PJ, Bacaltchuk J, Stefano S, Kashyap P. Psychological treatments for bulimia nervosa and binging. *Cochrane Database Syst Rev.* 2009;2009(4):CD000562.

49. Dixon L, et al. Guideline Watch (September 2009): Practice Guideline for the Treatment of Patients With Schizophrenia. American Psychiatric Association Website. Available at https://psychiatryonline.org/pb/assets/raw/sitewide/practice_guidelines/guidelines/schizophrenia-watch.pdf. Published September 2009. Accessed February 16, 2020.

50. Lehman AF, et al. Practice Guideline for the Treatment of Patients With Schizophrenia 2nd ed. American Psychiatric Association Website. Available at https://psychiatryonline.org/pb/assets/raw/sitewide/practice_guidelines/guidelines/schizophrenia.pdf. Published April 2004. Accessed February 16, 2020.

51. Treatment Target: Schizophrenia and Other Severe Mental Illnesses. Society of Clinical Psychology, Division 12, American Psychological Association Website. Available at https://www.div12.org/diagnosis/schizophrenia-and-other-severe-mental-illnesses/. Accessed February 15, 2020.

52. Psychosis and Schizophrenia in Adults: Prevention and Management. The National Institute for Health and Care Excellence (NICE) Website. Available at www.nice.org.uk/guidance/cg178. Published February 14, 2014. Accessed February 17, 2020.

53. Bighelli I, Salanti G, Huhn M, et al. Psychological interventions to reduce positive symptoms in schizophrenia: systematic review and network meta-analysis. *World Psychiatry.* 2018;17(3): 316-329.

54. Saks ER. *The Center Cannot Hold: My Journey Through Madness.* New York, NY: Hachette Books; 2008.

55. Bateman AW, Gunderson J, Mulder R. Treatment of personality disorder. *Lancet.* 2015;385(9969): 735-743.

56. Rosell DR. Psychotherapy for Schizotypal Personality Disorder. UpToDate Website. Available at https://www.UpToDate.com/contents/psychotherapy-for-schizotypal-personality-disorder?sectionName=Supportive%20psychotherapy&search=schizotypal%20personality&topicRef=116590&anchor=H196283614&source=see_link#H196283614. Updated May 24, 2018. Accessed February 10, 2020.

57. Treatment Target: Borderline Personality Disorder. Society of Clinical Psychology, Division 12, American Psychological Association Website. Available at https://www.div12.org/diagnosis/borderline-personality-disorder/. Accessed February 10, 2020.

58. Oldham JM, et al. Practice Guideline for Treatment of Patients With Borderline Personality Disorder. American Psychiatric Association Website. Available at https://psychiatryonline.org/pb/assets/raw/sitewide/practice_guidelines/guidelines/bpd.pdf. Published October 2001. Accessed February 17, 2020.

59. Oldham JM. Guideline Watch: Practice Guideline for the Treatment of Patients With Borderline Personality Disorder. American Psychiatric Association Website. Available at https://psychiatryonline.org/pb/assets/raw/sitewide/practice_guidelines/guidelines/bpd-watch.pdf. Published March 2005. Accessed February 17, 2020.

60. Borderline Personality Disorder: Recognition and Management. The National Institute for Health and Care Excellence (NICE) Website. Available at www.nice.org.uk/guidance/cg78. Published January 28, 2009. Accessed January 15, 2020.

3

61. Skodol A. Psychotherapy for Borderline Personality Disorder. UpToDate Website. Available at https://www.UpToDate.com/contents/psychotherapy-for-borderline-personality-disorder?search=borderline%20personality%20disorder%20treatment&source=search_result&selectedTitle=3~70&usage_type=default&display_rank=3. Updated September 06, 2018. Accessed February 05, 2020.

62. Ronningstam E. Narcissistic personality disorder: a current review. *Curr Psychiatry Rep.* 2010;12(1):68-75.

63. Dhawan N, Kunik ME, Oldham J, Coverdale J. Prevalence and treatment of narcissistic personality disorder in the community: a systematic review. *Compr Psychiatr.* 2010;51(4):333-339.

64. Caligor E, Petrini MJ. Treatment of Narcissistic Personality Disorder. UpToDate Website. Available at https://www.UpToDate.com/contents/treatment-of-narcissistic-personality-disorder?search=narcissistic%20personality%20disorder%20treatment&source=search_result&selectedTitle=1~25&usage_type=default&display_rank=1. Updated May 17, 2018. Accessed January 10, 2020.

65. Gabbard GO. Psychotherapy of personality disorders. *J Psychother Pract Res.* 2000;9(1):1-6.

66. Meloy JR, Yakeley J. Antisocial personality disorder. In Gabbard GO, ed. *Treatments of Psychiatric Disorders.* Arlington, VA: American Psychiatric Publishing, Inc; 2014:1015-1034.

67. Black DW. Treatment of Antisocial Personality Disorder. UpToDate Website. Available at https://www.UpToDate.com/contents/treatment-of-antisocial-personality-disorder?search=treatment%20of%20antisocial&source=search_result&selectedTitle=1~41&usage_type=default&display_rank=1. Updated May 23, 2019. Accessed February 20, 2020.

68. Simon W. Follow-up psychotherapy outcome of patients with dependent, avoidant, and obsessive compulsive personality disorders: a meta-analytic review. *Int J Psychiatry Clin Pract.* 2009;13(2):153-165.

69. Lampe L, Malhi GS. Avoidant personality disorder: current insights. *Psychol Res Behav Manag.* 2018;11:55-66.

70. Skodol A, Bender D. Approaches to the Therapeutic Relationship in Patients With Personality Disorders. UpToDate Website. Available at https://www.UpToDate.com/contents/approaches-to-the-therapeutic-relationship-in-patients-with-personality-disorders?search=OCPD%20and%20OCD&source=search_result&selectedTitle=5~149&usage_type=default&display_rank=5. Updated March 14, 2019. Accessed February 18, 2020.

71. Treatment Target: Mixed Substance Abuse/Dependence. Society of Clinical Psychology, Division 12, American Psychological Association Website. Available at https://www.div12.org/diagnosis/mixed-substance-abuse-dependence/. Accessed November 11, 2019.

72. Kleber HD. Practice Guideline for the Treatment of Patients With Substance Use Disorders. 2nd ed. American Psychiatric Association Website. Available at https://psychiatryonline.org/pb/assets/raw/sitewide/practice_guidelines/guidelines/substanceuse.pdf. Published May 2006. Accessed November 11, 2019.

73. Connery HS, Kleber HD. Guideline Watch (April 2007): Practice Guideline for the Treatment of Patients With Substance Use Disorders, 2nd ed. American Psychiatric Association Website. Available at https://psychiatryonline.org/pb/assets/raw/sitewide/practice_guidelines/guidelines/substanceuse-watch.pdf. Published April 2007. Accessed November 11, 2019.

74. McKay J. Psychotherapies for Substance Use Disorders. UpToDate Website. Available at https://www.UpToDate.com/contents/psychotherapies-for-substance-use-disorders?search=substance%20use%20disorder%20treatment&source=search_result&selectedTitle=5~150&usage_type=default&display_rank=5. Updated March 01, 2019. Accessed February 20, 2020.

75. Grant A. Rethinking psychological mindedness: metacognition, self-reflection, and insight. *Behav Change.* 2001;18(1):8-17.

76. Seritan AL, Mehta MM. Thorny Laurels: the impostor phenomenon in academic psychiatry. *Acad Psychiatry.* 2016;40(3):418-421.

77. Cabaniss DL, Holoshitz Y. *Different Patients, Different Therapies.* New York, NY: W.W. Norton & company, Inc; 2019.

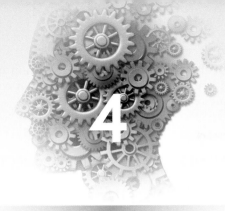

How to Begin: Empathy, Alliance, and Boundaries

ADAM M. BRENNER, MD

INTRODUCTION

In this chapter, you are going to learn how to begin individual psychotherapy. Many beginning therapists are very nervous about this process. You might wonder how you can conduct a treatment when you are just beginning your training and still have so much to learn about the theory and technique of psychotherapy. How can you launch an actually helpful and ultimately successful treatment if you are going to be learning as you go? Although it is normal to feel anxious and even a bit overwhelmed, getting your treatments off to a good start is very attainable. Instead of expecting yourself to understand everything and have mastered all the relevant interventions before getting started (which would be impossible, as you have to learn by doing!), we are going to suggest that there are three essential tasks in the opening phase of therapy.

These three essential tasks are relevant to all psychotherapies and include (1) making an empathic connection; (2) establishing a therapeutic alliance; and (3) setting up boundaries and a frame for therapy. Although these three elements require attention and adjustment throughout the whole course of the treatment, they are especially crucial in the earliest meetings, when you and your patient are just starting your work together. In this chapter, we will break these tasks down to their smallest, most manageable units and give you the practical tools to help patients successfully begin therapy.

In learning and teaching therapy, we have also found that many hypothetical concerns tend to come up when getting started. We will refer to these as "What If" questions and have used real-world feedback from our own trainees to create numerous text boxes throughout the chapter that discuss common questions that relate to therapy. These can be a reference for you to read now, or come back to later, when these questions become relevant to you.

MAKING AN EMPATHIC CONNECTION

What Is Empathy?

Empathy is a complicated topic to learn about, because the term encompasses several different mental and interpersonal activities. Any survey of the literature would quickly reveal that there is no absolute consensus about its definition.[1-7] This may be because different authors tend toward greater or lesser emphasis on the different components of empathy, sometimes in the context of what is most important for the kind of clinical situation they are writing about.

There are actually at least four distinct things happening that make a patient feel their therapist has successfully empathized with them. First, there is a cognitive element. The therapist has to imagine her way into the patient's state of mind. In order to do this, the therapist will draw on their own experiences, their knowledge of human nature, their understanding of the patient's cultural context, and what the patient can tell us explicitly about what they are thinking and feeling.

Second, the therapist will allow herself to resonate emotionally with what the patient is feeling. This is the affective component. The therapist tries to feel some small part or echo of what the patient is feeling. We do this largely by adopting a receptive emotional state. Much as we would do when watching a film or a play, we let our guard down and allow ourselves to be moved by the material we are experiencing.

Third, there is an interpersonal element of empathy. The therapist communicates back to the patient what she is understanding and feeling. In other words, the success of the empathic activity lies in whether the patient feels you have empathized with them. Empathy that is completely internal to the therapist, with no communication back to the patient, is of little use to a beginning therapy (although there may be extended periods of time later on when good therapeutic technique in different approaches calls for the therapist's silence).

And finally, there is an attitudinal element—true empathy requires an attitude of concern and caring. The patient should feel that they are with someone who not only understands their thoughts and their feelings, but also intends to address the patient's vulnerability with compassion and kindness.

The Importance of Identifying and Naming Feelings

How will you actually know what your patient is feeling so that you might then empathize with that feeling? This is a harder question than it might seem at first glance. Of course, some patients will tell you directly what they are feeling. But even then, they may not be able to tell you the whole truth immediately. They may tell you one feeling of several they are experiencing, because they think that one makes more sense or is more socially acceptable. Or, they may tell you a watered-down version of their feelings so that you do not think they are overreacting, or because they think intense feelings are inappropriate. Early in a therapy, you might need to emphasize to a patient that you welcome their feelings and that connecting with what they are feeling is an important part of therapy.

An important first empathic step is just to be aware when the patient is starting to feel something. It is a good idea to pay attention to physical changes and to gently ask about them. These responses are sometimes referred to as "process comments" in therapy and emphasize an attention to the here-and-now experience of the patient within the therapy session. For example, the patient's eyes may become a bit red or slightly watery and you might say, "*Your eyes looked a little sad just now—were you aware of feeling something? Can you tell me more about the feeling?*" Or, a patient may physically stiffen or cross their arms across the chest or begin fidgeting, and you might say, "*You look like you might have gotten a bit more uncomfortable as we talked just now. Were you aware of feeling (uncomfortable, anxious, troubled, etc.)? Can you tell me about that?*"

In general, the first step is usually to tell the patient what you are tentatively noticing. We do not want the patient to think we have some magical mind reading talent— this will either make them more anxious or raise their expectations of us beyond what we can fulfill! At the same time, we are already helping the patient learn that they can observe and notice their own emotions and eventually reflect on them.

Sometimes it is not easy to orient yourself to what the patient is feeling. Some patients avoid their own feelings and tend to speak very abstractly and intellectually. Other patients lose themselves in a wealth of details or tangents as they tell their stories. Even though the question, "How did that make you feel?" has become a cliché of psychotherapy, it can be helpful to ask the patient directly about their feelings. Here are some ways to draw out the emotional experience from a patient's story: "*What did you feel when that happened? How did you respond inside?*"

When the material the patient is presenting is complicated or confusing, it may be helpful to remember something Elvin Semrad, MD, an eminent psychotherapy teacher, used to say: "Most of the time the patient is either mad, sad, or scared."[8] This may seem like a huge oversimplification, but when you feel caught up in something that you do not understand, or cannot find your bearings, it does help to have a few fixed points to help you navigate.

When the patient cannot seem to find words for what they are feeling, you can draw on your own experience of the world and make an educated guess. If the experience sounds like one that would generally provoke anger, you might say, "*I imagine you might have felt angry at that moment.*" Some patients, however, will find that too direct. They may need you to give them some more wiggle room, and some implicit permission for feeling angry. For such a patient, the following may be more useful: "*That sounds like the kind of moment that would make most people angry.*" Another way to help your patient find the feeling in their story is to direct their attention to what they are feeling in the moment as they talk with you. You might ask, "*Are you feeling something right now while you're telling me this story?*"

There are times where our patients are clearly talking about something meaningful and significant, and you will try to imagine your way into the experience, but still feel at a loss. Perhaps the experience is too confusing for the patient to narrate clearly. Or perhaps the patient is talking about some kind of emotional state that is (to this point in your life) beyond your experience or education. There is nothing wrong with saying to a patient something like the following: "*You're telling me about something important, something that had a real impact on you. Tell me more about what it felt like for you.*"

You will find that patients do not expect you to be omniscient or to understand everything or to pick up on every underlying emotion. This is worth emphasizing because beginning therapists often seem to expect this of themselves. Your patients, however, will deeply appreciate that you are giving them your full emotional attention, that you are trying to connect with what they are feeling, and that you see emotional understanding as a process that you can grow toward together.

Developing your emotional vocabulary will also help you connect with patients. As noted above, Semrad's "mad, sad, and scared" is a very useful rubric, but the more specific you can be in naming your patients' feelings, the more truly understood they will feel. For example, although all of the following words are in the anger family, each tells us something distinct about the patient's experience: irritated, frustrated, resentful, bitter, sullen, seething, indignant, enraged, furious. Like in art or design, it would be a much less interesting world if we were limited to primary colors and could not make use of all the shades of the spectrum and the complex fusions of colors. Sadness also comes in many varieties. Think of the difference between someone whose feelings are bittersweet versus someone who is desolate. The patient who is disappointed and demoralized is in a different place than the patient who is heartbroken and dejected, although both would fall under the umbrella of sadness.

We do have to include one very important addition to the triad of "mad, sad, or scared"—shame. Sometimes shame is the central, presenting complaint. More often, patients have something that they think of as their primary problem (behavior, romance, academics, work, a psychological symptom, etc.) and then they are secondarily ashamed of having the problem and ashamed of what the problem might mean about them. When a person feels shame, they may feel defective, disgusting, repulsive, or pathetic, to name a few specific shades of the emotion. They feel all kinds of things that bring them to anticipate that you will not want to be with them, to listen to them, to be close to them. They expect, on some level, for you to recoil. One of the most important things you will do as a new therapist for a patient is really what you do not do. You do not recoil. When they tell you something painful or disturbing, you find some way to make clear that you want to hear more. How you do it does not matter as much as the intention. People will pick up on your intentions, and they will forgive (or not notice) all kinds of awkwardness or confusion or verbal stumbling.

One of the striking things is that patients often feel grateful for your willingness to listen to the things that are so disturbing to them. And yet, on the therapists' side, we often feel grateful ourselves. It is an incredible privilege to have a person let you into their life and especially to the corners of their world and their self where they feel most vulnerable.

Why Are Some Patients Reluctant to Know or Speak Feelings?

So far, we have been discussing this as if the patient wants you to know what they are feeling and just needs help finding the words to share their experience. However, this is often not the whole picture. Most people are ambivalent about sharing feelings when they begin therapy. They want to express their feelings and have you understand them, but they may also feel very reluctant to have this happen. This can lead to some awkward or tense moments. Sometimes you may feel certain you clearly understood the patient and simply reflected this back, only to find your patient rejecting the empathy. Perhaps the patient even becomes irritable or withdrawn. Why may that have happened?

There are a number of common reasons why a patient may be less than eager to express their feelings or to have you perceive them. First, some patients may find their feelings frightening. They might be afraid that if they let themselves feel, then the floodgates will open, and they will be overwhelmed by emotion. Or, they might be worried because their feelings have sometimes led to impulsive actions with bad outcomes.

Second, some patients might want to avoid feelings out of shame. They may have been taught that the expression of emotion is inappropriate and embarrassing. Specifically, some male patients may have the idea that showing or expressing feelings is "unmanly" or violates some code of masculinity. Patients with these concerns will be watching you to see if your response shows any disgust or disapproval.

Third, your patient may not be afraid of their feelings directly, but may be afraid that they will be showing "weakness" if they show emotion. Somewhere in the past, they may have learned the painful lesson that letting down their guard emotionally leads to others thinking they are vulnerable, and therefore targets for attack or exploitation.

Finally, different cultures have different rules about whether, when, and how much emotion should be displayed. In addition, there can be enormous variation within any cultural group, whether it is due to race, ethnicity, generation, gender identity, religion, sexual orientation, education, politics, or economic factors. As a result, an attitude of "cultural humility"[9,10] is generally more useful than aspiring to "cultural competence." Whenever you are uncertain about cultural influences and expectations (which will likely be often), you can ask your patient, *"How were feelings expressed and shared in the world you grew up in?"* Your openness to learning about your patient's world and worldview is just as important as how much you already know about the patient's culture at the outset of the therapy. You will learn more about this topic in Chapter 8.

How to Respond Empathically

Earlier, when we were defining empathy, we saw that there was an element of communication involved. So, no matter how sensitive, tuned in, or discerning you might be in the moment, it is still essential to reflect this back to the patient in a way that they can feel comfortable with.[11,12] Ultimately, what matters is whether the patient feels that their therapist empathized with them. How do effective therapists do this?

Facial expression and body language. At its most basic, the empathic response begins with what you show through your own facial expression and body language. Sometimes all that is required to convey your empathy for their sadness is the sadness that will naturally appear on your own face. Of course, this is not generally something the therapist does intentionally. In fact, the task for many beginning therapists is to relax and not try to control this process too much. After all, one of the first ways babies learn to engage with people and to play is through matching facial expressions.[13] Given how much culture shapes communication, it is remarkable that facial expression corresponding to the basic emotions is actually so consistent around the world. People separated by different languages or cultures can still convey basic and crucial information about emotions with several universally common facial expressions.[14]

Body language can also convey important empathic information. An open, nondefensive posture can help allay concerns that empathy will be twisted and used for exploitation. A patient who is afraid that their therapist will withdraw in disgust may find the therapist's shift to an open or leaning forward position as reassuring as any words.

Informal verbal expression. The verbal expression of empathy begins with sounds that are not yet even words (also known as paralanguage). A simple "*Hm*" or "*Mmm*" or "*Uh-huh*" can say a lot to a patient. It can underline the moment and convey that the patient said something significant. Just knowing that the therapist is following along and gets that something mattered can be very validating for a patient. How much or how little of this you do as a therapist is really a matter of your own style and temperament. This is again one of those places where it is best to just be yourself.

Similar advice applies to the kind of spontaneous response you make when someone says something profoundly sad or shocking, such as "*Oh my!*", "*No!*", etc. These informal expressions of empathy can feel more real to the patient than the most beautifully crafted and sophisticated formulation of their situation, because they can sense that it came from your heart. Again, allowing yourself to respond as one real person to another will generally be much more supportive than an artificial reserve meant to mimic someone's idea of a therapeutic demeanor. Of course, there are limits, which we will touch on more when we discuss therapeutic boundaries. For example, if your own style and spontaneous expressions include profanity, you will want to weed that out; while it will certainly feel real to the patient, it might also raise a lot of anxieties for some patients that are not going to be helpful.

Verbal reflection. When a patient directly expresses a feeling or a state of mind, simply echoing the content can also be powerful. Without adding any interpretation or inference, you try to reflect back just what you are hearing. There is no one right way to do this.

For example, a patient might say: "I can't tell anyone about my fears; I'm all alone with them." The therapist could respond with any of the following, depending on what they wanted to emphasize:

- "*You can't tell anyone about your fears.*"
- "*Your fears can't be spoken.*"
- "*You feel so alone.*"
- "*Frightened, and also alone.*"

Labeling feelings directly when you hear them is another helpful way to let patients know they are understood. There are lots of different ways to do this. At its most simple, saying "*Sad,*" when you hear a sad story is a fine response. "*How sad!*" would be a bit stronger. "*That's one of the saddest things I've heard*" would of course be even stronger. You are trying to find the degree of emphasis that matches where the patient is emotionally. Remember the goal here is to help the patient feel you understand, not to ratchet up the emotion past where they feel comfortable.

When you sense that the patient can only handle very little of the emotion you are reflecting back, you can create a little more distance for them with phrases like "*That sounds sad*" or "*I imagine that might have been sad.*" Alternatively, you might help them tolerate the feeling by normalizing it: "*No wonder you felt sad*" or "*Of course you felt sad.*" When a patient feels particularly ashamed of the feeling, you might alleviate their embarrassment by saying "*I imagine if I were in your shoes I'd have felt sad.*"

What if My Patient Is Really Angry With Me?

Because therapy entails the process of eliciting and giving space for emotions, it will invariably entail anger (and the related spectrum of emotions, including irritation, resentment, and rage). Many times, the anger is not directed toward the therapist directly, but is instead one of a myriad of emotions that finds its voice within the context of therapy.

You should be aware that most patients will become frustrated, irritated, and even angry with you, if the relationship lasts long enough. This may be in response to something you do that disappoints them. Other times the anger may not be about you, but might be about another important relationship or an experience from the past. All these kinds of anger are relatively common and provide useful grist for the therapy mill, if you are willing to pay attention to this possibility and address it within the session. This may be the first time a patient has been able to express anger toward another person that does not result in destruction or rejection, which provides them a new way to view and deal with this emotion. However, in our experience, trainees often recoil from expressions of anger during therapy and either avoid provoking any anger in their patient, or become overly soothing. It is vital to increase your tolerance for angry emotional expression, similar to the same way therapists must become accustomed to tearfulness.

Of course, patients can cross the line into becoming abusive and/or dangerous during periods of intense anger. Being a "good therapist" *does not* mandate that the therapist continue to place themselves in treatment relationships that are abusive or imminently physically dangerous. Concern that your patient may act on their anger toward you is always to be discussed with your supervisor, and can be a reason to end a session early. This is another reason that attending to the therapy space is important. Always be aware of proximity to your patient, seating arrangements, and ways to have easy access to an exit. These are more common issues when working in specific treatment environments, but are not limited solely to inpatient or forensic settings.

Challenges to Empathy

With some patients, you might feel that they are giving you very little to empathize with. They may not show much affect and when asked they cannot report any feelings. What can you do with that? One option is to consider that they may feel uncomfortable expressing what they are feeling; perhaps what they are feeling is not what they are "supposed to feel." For example, a patient talking about their new baby believes that they should be feeling loving and grateful, but is actually feeling frightened and resentful. If you think this might be the case it can help to say, "*I wonder if you say that you feel nothing because you think your actual feelings are inappropriate.*" By noting the patient's concern about appropriateness, you convey that you are likely to be more accepting of their feelings than they are. Much effective empathy involves inviting the patient to share their feelings even when they are anxious about how they will be received.

Just as some feelings are harder for patients to feel comfortable with than others, some feelings are harder for therapists to empathize with. We might think of these as lying along a spectrum of acceptability. Many people are more comfortable, for example, connecting with sadness than with anger. Anger can lead to aggressive wishes and impulses, and the therapist might be nervous about stirring these up. Will the patient have the impulse control to feel such urges and not act on them? In addition, most of us are more comfortable with anger that seems justified; it can feel good to help a patient feel their righteous indignation in response to the world's hurts!

Moving a little further down the spectrum, we come to anger that seems inappropriate or unjustified.[15] The patient is holding an old grudge, or nursing a bitter, intense resentment over small or unintended slights. These festering old wounds can incubate vengeful feelings. Revenge usually means making the other person feel what we have been through—and is the source of a great deal of the destructiveness in the world.

Further down the spectrum, and especially hard for new therapists, is the patient who presents at ease with his/her sadism. Cruelty has become part of who they are and operates independently of any possible causes. Often the best you can do is to listen patiently and carefully to their history, in an attempt to find an empathic position. An adult patient may seem completely unsympathetic initially as you learn about their sadism, but this can change as you hear about childhood experiences that left them feeling vulnerable, helpless, and abused.

What if I Just Do Not Like My Patient?

This is another one of those problems that is inevitable if you treat enough patients over time. It is certainly much less comfortable than meeting with someone you like. It is very natural to worry that you will not be able to do your job—to offer empathy and establish an alliance—if you do not like the patient, but this is often not true.

The first thing to do is allow yourself to feel what you feel. Your reactions to the patient (called "countertransference") may teach you a lot about the patient and about yourself. This is one of the times when supervision is invaluable! Not liking someone can follow from a variety of negative feelings that you feel when with the patient—irritation, scorn, disgust, disapproval, impatience, guilt, embarrassment, envy, to name just a few. Try to identify exactly what the patient does, or fails to do, that elicits the particular reaction. You might find some valuable clues to understanding the presenting problem that brought the patient to therapy in the first place.

Sometimes unlikeable traits become easier to tolerate when they are part of the larger issue you are working on, as opposed to feeling that they are just an obstacle. A severely unlikeable patient is often similarly unlikeable in the rest of their lives, and thinking we will find another therapist who will enjoy being with them is probably unrealistic.

On a related note, learning the patient's developmental history can help. Your reactions may lessen when you have some context for understanding what pressures shaped these unlikeable qualities, and your capacity for empathy may increase. Alternatively, you might learn something important about your own psychology. Perhaps you tend to dislike patients of a certain type because they tap into your own personal experiences with someone important in the past.

So, it certainly is possible to do therapy with someone you do not like. On the other hand, it is okay to realize that every therapist cannot treat every patient. Some patients push buttons that are too deeply personal, and we cannot work around it to find a position of empathy. This is not an absolute; it can certainly change over the course of your career. When you are in training, these are decisions that you will reach in consultation with your supervisors.

FORMING A THERAPEUTIC ALLIANCE

What Is a Therapeutic Alliance?

You will often hear it said that the relationship between the therapist and the patient is one of the most important predictors of therapeutic success.[1] But what do we mean exactly when we refer to the "relationship"? Through decades of work, psychotherapy researchers have been refining the concept of the "therapeutic alliance" and how to measure it in order to answer this question. Therapeutic alliance has been "defined broadly as the collaborative bond between therapist and patient."[16] This is a helpful definition, as the phrase "collaborative bond" neatly sums up two of the most important and most well-studied aspects of the alliance. First, there is the idea that therapist and patient are working together—they are collaborating. Second, there is the appreciation that this work occurs in the context of an emotional and interpersonal connection—they have a bond.

Many studies with very different kinds of therapy have demonstrated that this "collaborative bond" is important no matter what modality is being used. Measuring the therapeutic alliance early in the therapy or over time correlates with treatment success. A brief glance at the literature will show that there are many measures of alliance and no established standard, although they generally share a consensus about the key ideas and the value of measuring the alliance from the perspective of the patient. The Working Alliance Inventory, Vanderbilt Therapeutic Alliance Scale, and California Psychotherapy Alliance Scale (WAI, VTAS, CALPAS) are among the best studied and validated of the many scales.[17]

These scales all aim to capture something of the interpersonal and affective bond between the patient and therapist. In order to get at the strength of the bond, the patient is typically asked questions relating to feeling appreciated, liked, and trusted by the therapist, as well as reciprocal questions about appreciating, liking, and trusting the therapist. In order to assess the quality of the collaboration, the patient is asked whether the pair share the same goals, understand the problem the same way, and are working together toward the goals.

In this section, we are going to explain what you can do to give you and the patient the best chance of establishing a healthy and productive therapeutic alliance. First, we will look at the question of treatment goals, and then we will turn to the challenge of building a trusting bond with different kinds of patients.

Agreeing on Goals

One of the essential aspects of a therapeutic alliance is that the patient and the therapist agree on what they are doing together. This is easier said than done and is one of the most common reasons why psychotherapies do not succeed. One problem is that both therapist and patient are prone to making assumptions. The patient thinks it is obvious what kind of help they are looking for. The therapist thinks it is equally obvious what kind of help they are offering. And, unfortunately, neither is at all obvious to the other.

Given that most people who train to be psychotherapists are already psychologically minded, students and residents generally appreciate that psychotherapy is a process that helps by changing something in the patient's own mind. It is within the "internal world" that therapy is able to have an impact.

But, if we ask patients what they are hoping for from therapy, we will get an array of very different kinds of answers. Some of these will indeed focus on a change internal to the patient. Here are some examples:

- *Remove or diminish symptoms* ("I need to stop having these awful anxiety attacks"; "I want to feel like I can enjoy my life again and not see everything as so bleak.")

- *Change their character* ("I can't seem to let anyone get close to me. Can therapy help me let people in?"; "I'm filled with envy and self-doubt all the time. I don't want to be this kind of person.")

- *Mourn* ("It's been a year since she broke my heart and I still can't stop thinking about her"; "I need to accept that since the surgery I'm never going to be the same again, but I can't.")

When the patient comes to therapy with these kind of goals, your job as a collaborator is much more straightforward. You listen carefully to what the person is hoping for, reflect it back to them to make sure you understood correctly, and talk with them about how a psychotherapy can help them achieve this goal.

However, there will be many patients whose hope is that therapy will result in a change in their external world. From their perspective, the problems they suffer from come from outside themselves, not from within. Their experience of their world is colored by the lament, "if only." If only other people could appreciate their talents. If only their spouse would give them what they need. If only they had not been traumatized long ago. If only they did not have to live with bipolar disorder. There is an endless variety of such laments, but they all contain the hope that somehow the therapist will help them in putting the world to right.

These kinds of wishes are certainly understandable. As a therapist you can sympathize with the hope that one could find a guide who will tell you how to turn your world around. Unfortunately, this is beyond what any therapist can actually do. Therapists are not experts in the workings of the world. No one could be—the world, and all its different families, workplaces, and cultures, is vastly too complex for any one's expertise. In fact, the patient is often going to be far more informed, and sometimes even wiser, about the working of their particular external world than you are. Instead, we should think of therapists as expert helpers who are concerned with the inner world of the patient.

This is a good thing because, after all, anything you think you know about the patient's external circumstances is ultimately filtered through the patient's inner world. For example, if you are hearing about your patient's difficult spouse, you are really only hearing about the image and construction of that spouse that resides in the patient's mind. And in turn, any influence you might have on the external relationship will first go through the internal relationship that the patient has in their mind.

If the therapist's business then is with the patient's inner world (including the choices and behaviors generated there), then the kinds of goals we can truly help patients with are ones that involve changing something within the patient. These kind of goals might include, for example:

1. Building up some aspects of the mind, such as self-esteem or self-control

2. Learning new ways of coping or responding to people

3. Increasing understanding of some internal conflict or of some way that the patient holds themselves back from what they say they want

4. Mourning a loss that the patient cannot move beyond

There is then some education we might need to do to help a patient understand what we actually can offer. That can often be accomplished by reframing the patient's lament about the world into a task that involves changing the patient's internal world. For example, "If only people would appreciate me at work" might lead to the therapist suggesting, "*We could work together on understanding why you don't let people see your strengths,*" or "*We could work together on understanding why it is so hurtful when you don't get the praise you feel you deserve.*"

Similarly, the lament "My spouse won't give me what I need" might become "*We could work together on learning to be more clear and assertive about what you hope for,*" or "*We could work together to understand the choices that led to a relationship that is so disappointing to you.*" In all of these examples, the therapist is conveying to the patient "*I know you feel very hurt by the world, but what I can do is help you to understand or change how you react to that world. And that can make a very real difference.*" Sometimes it helps to be explicit about that to the patient. For example, "*There is very little the two of us can do to change the people outside of this room. However, we can work together to help you handle those situations in a healthier way.*"

One last thing worth noting is that sometimes the patient's stated goal—whether it is an internal or externally directed one—does not turn out to be the most deeply held and important hope they have for psychotherapy. This hope may be too precious and may leave them too vulnerable to share in the initial meetings with you. That is alright. As you and the patient work together and mutual trust grows, you will learn about these more fragile and guarded therapeutic wishes. This then brings us to the second aspect of the therapeutic alliance, or collaborative bond. How does that bond begin and then grow in therapy?

What if My Patient Is Older or Has Had Experiences That I Have Never Had?

There is no need to pretend that life experience is not valuable to a psychotherapist. As you grow older, you learn about different aspects of adult development through your own experiences—sometimes joyous, sometimes painful. You will certainly draw on that experience to deepen your understanding of your patients. But even when you are a therapist at the end of his/her career you will not have had every kind of experience that your patients have lived with. Your particular racial, economic, and ethnic background will provide exposure to some aspects of the world, while limiting your contact with other spheres. In addition, your own choices will lead you to accumulate some kinds of experience but will also cut off other possibilities.

It is important to remember that a therapist is not a guru. You are not offering yourself as a source of ultimate wisdom or as an expert in all the ways that humans can live. In fact, experience as a therapist may lead you to a healthy skepticism that anyone could live up to such expectations! Instead, a therapist offers their services in helping a person better understand their own mind and better shape and regulate their own behavior.

The therapist does not need to know more about the patient's world than the patient does; the therapist instead needs to be a student who is eager and open to learning what the patient knows. I remember one patient early in my career, a middle-aged woman with a grown but very troubled son, trying to help me understand the persistence of her depression in the face of all our therapeutic efforts. She finally said, "You know, you're generally only as happy as your least happy child." It would be many years before I would confirm this from my own experience but being open to learning this from my patient sufficed for me to continue being a useful therapist to her.

Building Trust to Build Alliance

Some part of the bond between patient and therapist rests on the experience of empathy. As we saw in Chapter 1, we are built for attachment, and empathy fosters attachment. If the patient feels that you are sincerely interested in understanding and helping, they will naturally begin to feel connected to you. If they then feel that you are working on a shared set of goals, this bond will take a further leap forward. But, at many points along the process, the patient will be asking themselves (sometimes explicitly and sometimes less consciously), whether they really can trust this new therapist. How do patients begin to know if they can trust you?

First, they will draw on their previous experience. Patients who grew up with trustworthy families and have had treatment in the past with trustworthy caregivers will tend to generalize from those experiences, and you will be given the benefit of the doubt. For such patients, new therapists (or helpers of any kind) are trustworthy until proven otherwise.

Second, patients will make some inferences based on your position and your credentials. If you are in training at a reputable school, program, or healthcare center, they may appreciate that you had to prove yourself to be there. There were criteria for acceptance which included being of good character and demonstrating professional responsibility, and you cleared those bars. This is part of the reason why sharing your credentials with new patients is a specific form of "self-disclosure" that is appropriate and helpful to establishing a therapeutic process (see below for further discussion under "Boundaries").

And third, while you are focused on learning about the patient, the patient will also be learning a great deal about you in the early meetings. Some of the most important things that patients hope to learn early in the process are that you are reliable and dependable. Reliability and dependability—therefore consistency—are building blocks of trust. Things you may take for granted might mean a great deal, especially for patients who have not experienced much consistency in their past relationships. You set aside a time for them, you held that time, and you didn't schedule something else for your convenience. You are there when you say you are going to be there. Punctuality is valuable because it removes the possibility of the patient waiting for you. Early in a relationship, if someone is waiting for you, they are usually also worrying about whether you are going to be there. Finally, you offered your attention to their problems, and they found that you are indeed attentive and focused on their concerns.

Being open and responsive to a patient's feedback also builds trust. If your new patient is not bringing it up themselves, then it is a good idea to ask them how well this new process is going. Is it what they expected? Do they feel you are understanding them? Are they finding what they had hoped for? Are they feeling comfortable? This is not to say that you expect your new patient to feel totally comfortable or to be happy with everything you are doing. Therapy is a difficult process. Nor does it mean that you can change or remove everything that makes them uncomfortable. However, your interest and efforts to be flexible within appropriate limits may mean a great deal to the patient in building their trust.

Suppose, for example, that the patient says they are uncomfortable because they do not know what you are thinking as they talk. This is a fairly common piece of feedback. Some of us have less expressive and reactive faces than others. Some of us also are very anxious when we are starting as new therapists, and this can make us stiffen and become less expressive than usual. Your patient does not need or expect you to become a different sort of person. It is the fact that you are interested in their experience and make efforts to adjust that will ultimately matter the most.

Some Obstacles to Building Trust

Some patients will have a harder time trusting a new therapist. One of the reasons for this might be a history of trauma. Abuse that came at the hands of those who are supposed to care for us (such as parents, teachers, spouses, etc.) can be especially poisonous. The patient cannot bring to you the expectation that authorities in helping roles are generally trustworthy, because they have learned the exact opposite lesson in the past. The first step in building trust, then, is appreciating and acknowledging this. You might say something like, "*It makes sense that you're feeling anxious as we get started. Being nervous with someone new is understandable given what you've been through in the past.*"

Patients who have been traumatized have often been helpless and experienced feelings that were out of control.[18] So, it is important that you make clear that in therapy, they will be the ones in control. There are going to be many choice points in every session, with decisions about how deep to go, how much painful feeling for the patient to bear, how much risk to take in talking about unexplored topics, etc. Therapists build trust with traumatized patients by making it very clear that all such decisions will be in the patient's hands. We can say things like, "*As we talk, painful things may come up. I want to make sure you know that what to talk about will always be up to you and I don't have any expectations about how fast we're supposed to go.*"

This kind of intervention can prevent the patient from imagining that therapy is supposed to be an immediate dive into the deepest, darkest, and most turbulent waters of their mind. If the patient thinks that is what the therapist requires, they may comply and find themselves in a flood of overwhelming feelings or anxiety. Unfortunately, this just tends to retraumatize the patient.

Another challenging experience is establishing an alliance with a paranoid patient. Even a mild degree of nonpsychotic paranoia, the kind that can be part of personality and not necessarily something like schizophrenia, is enough to pose a significant obstacle to trust. There are some things that you can do to increase the chance of therapy taking hold. First, transparency is key. You should make sure your patient understands exactly what you are doing and why. When a person is paranoid, every ambiguity in an interaction can seem like an opportunity for someone to take advantage of them. If you find this pattern occurring in therapy, you can try being even more explicit than usual in "narrating" what you are trying to do. For example, in the absence of explanation, the patient might think "Dr. M just wants to know about my past so he has something to hold over me." To preempt this concern, you might say, "*I was wondering if I can ask you more about your childhood and family, because if I understand better where you're coming from I might be more helpful about your coping with the current situation.*"

A certain degree of interpersonal distance and affective coolness can also help with paranoid patients.[11] This means possibly turning down the intensity of your empathy, at least at the beginning of your work together. People who are paranoid may misinterpret your attempts to connect emotionally as something more intrusive or invasive. A little bit more formality may be reassuring.

There is an additional challenge when the patient's paranoia also includes specific concerns about plots or recent events in their life. You wonder how you can build trust when someone is telling you something that you do not believe. The patient may even ask whether you believe them. Again, transparency and humility are helpful touchstones. For example, you can tell a patient that what they have said is very hard for you to believe, but you want to hear more about why they are convinced it is the best explanation for what they have experienced. It is worth remembering that when the "delusion" is not bizarre, it may be highly unlikely yet still turn out to be true. Just as being a hypochondriac does not protect a patient from getting an actual illness, so being paranoid does not protect against the possibility of being actually threatened in the world.

What if I am Sleepy and Doze Off in a Session?

Patients deserve a therapist's alert and undivided attention, but therapists are fallible human beings. Over the course of a career it is unfortunately quite possible that you will be sleepy or doze off during a session. Usually this means the therapist is simply exhausted—perhaps you were on call, or were up with a baby, or are fighting off some illness. When the therapist is too tired, the quiet and soothing environment of the therapy office can have the unwelcome effect of bringing on drowsiness. You might notice this yourself as you catch your head nodding or your eyes closing, or more likely it will be the patient who brings it to your attention. What to do then?

First, simply acknowledge the drowsiness and apologize. Avoiding the reality just makes things worse, and as with so many things in life the "cover up" becomes as big a problem as the original lapse. After all, therapy is based on a relationship of honesty and trust. A therapist might say, "I'm very sorry, I hadn't realized how tired I was today." Most patients do not need any more of an explanation than that, and in fact many would find it unhelpful to hear more details about your recent hardship. Remember, this hour was supposed to be about them. This brief exchange may be all you need to be jolted back to wakefulness. If that does not suffice, you can consider excusing yourself for a few minutes while you splash some water on your face, or do whatever you find helpful to return to an alert and attentive state.

Patients' reactions to their therapist's sleepiness vary. Once you have acknowledged the lapse and apologized, it is a good idea to listen for the patient's reaction. Some are understandably angry. Other patients are sympathetic and want to take care of you. And others blame themselves—they must not be interesting enough to hold their therapist's attention. This may be an important opportunity to deepen your understanding of the patient's inner life, or to reinforce the value of the patient's authentic feelings, whatever they are.

ESTABLISHING BOUNDARIES IN PSYCHOTHERAPY

Why Boundaries?

There is a famous line from a Robert Frost poem called *Mending Wall:* "Good fences make good neighbors."[19] Frost seems to suggest that boundaries not only set people apart or create limits, but also contribute positively to good relationships. This line is often quoted whenever someone wants to make a point that we need boundaries.

But there is another crucial line in that poem, which is not so often repeated: "Before I built a wall I'd ask to know/What I was walling in or walling out." In other words, what is the purpose of the wall? Is it meant to prevent something? Is it meant to contain something? These are the very questions to ask as we learn about boundaries in psychotherapy.

Boundaries, also sometimes called the "frame" of the therapy, are essential to the success of the treatment.[20,21] They include the ethical rules for therapy, but they are more than that. The boundaries of the therapy also include the roles assigned to therapist and patient, the physical setting, the way time is scheduled, how payment is arranged, the questions of physical contact and self-disclosure, and how to respond to gifts. There are three major reasons for boundaries, and understanding these reasons will help you maintain the frame of the therapy, explain this frame to the patient when necessary, and decide with your supervisor when exceptions should be made.

First, boundaries help prevent exploitation of the patient. Therapy is always conducted to serve the interests of the patient. The therapist's interests are met primarily by being paid (although also by the professional growth of learning to do therapy). Other than being paid or being trained, the therapist is expected to set their own desires to the side. It is important to acknowledge that therapists have the same desires as anyone else. We want to find sexual excitement and romantic fulfillment, to be praised and appreciated, to be entertained, and to acquire material rewards. But, we understand that meeting any of those needs through the patient would be exploitation (even if the patient appears to feel or act otherwise). By engaging in psychotherapy, the patient has agreed to put themselves in a very vulnerable and emotionally intimate position, in order to allow you to provide some kind of help for their emotional, psychological, and/or behavioral problems. They have placed their trust in the idea that you, their new therapist, will not allow yourself to benefit from or take advantage of this vulnerability.

Second, boundaries help the patient let down their guard and engage in therapy. As therapy begins, we are asking the patient to talk about difficult topics and try new ways of relating and behaving. Cordoning off the therapy session as something separate from the rest of life's relationships can be reassuring and freeing. The patient does not have to be so careful to not offend the therapist or hurt their feelings, because we have established that this relationship is not here to make the therapist feel better. The patient knows that this relationship will always only be therapy—the therapist is not going to become a mentor, or a religious advisor, or a friend, or a lover. Because of those boundaries, the patient can (at least partly) let go of their efforts to make the right impression or put their best foot forward. In fact, in order for the therapy to be as helpful as possible, therapists want to understand what their patient is like when they are not their "best" self.

Third, the boundaries also help make it possible for the therapist to do a very unusual and demanding kind of work. Knowing that this relationship is limited to the therapy session makes it much easier to bear the challenging, irritating, or even offensive aspects of the patient's behavior. Unlike the patient, we are supposed to bring our best self to this work, or at least a particular professional version of ourselves. It is not unusual for patients to express their appreciation of how patient and kind they find their therapist. It would not be possible to bring this "best self" if we had to keep it up indefinitely, hour after hour, or if we felt too vulnerable ourselves.

Boundary Crossings, Violations, and the Slippery Slopes in Between

Some experts in psychotherapy boundaries have made the useful distinction between boundary crossings and boundary violations.[22] A violation is a major rupture of a boundary that leads to exploitation of the patient or serious harm to the efficacy of the treatment. By comparison, a boundary crossing is a minor break in the frame of the treatment that is done with the intention to be therapeutic.

Boundary crossings might sound like they would pose little problem then, if it were not for the accompanying concept of the "slippery slope." When major boundary violations such as sexual relationships with patients occur in therapy, and the case is carefully reviewed, it often becomes clear that the damage did not occur all at once. The trouble was usually slowly brewing for some time and often began with very minor boundary crossings that seemed benign or even kind at first. For example, the patient expresses how lonely he is and how hard it is to leave at the end of the session. The therapist begins by occasionally extending the therapy session by a few minutes. This starts to become a regular occurrence and the therapist and patient decide it would be best if they met at the end of the day so that other patients' schedules were not impacted. What began as an attempt by the therapist to be flexible in support of a patient's aloneness has become a special arrangement that now blurs the distinction between the professional work day and the therapist's personal time in the evening.

It would be simplest if we could simply teach you that a therapist should never, ever cross any boundaries and treat them all as absolutely untouchable. Unfortunately, human beings are much too complicated and psychotherapy is too ambiguous a process for these "absolutes" to be effective for all patients all the time. There are times where flexibility is called for and the therapist needs to adjust something about the limits of their role, the extent of their anonymity, or the constraints of time and schedule (to name just some possibilities). This is done in order to meet some pressing need of the patient or because the particular patient is having a negative experience of the boundaries and their progress in therapy is threatened.

The decision to allow a boundary crossing is not to be taken lightly and should never be taken without discussion with your supervisor (including *after* it occurs). This is important to emphasize because sometimes you will be caught by surprise and will not have had the opportunity to consider the decision-making process in supervision in advance. For example, your generally withdrawn, isolated, and defensive patient has had an emotional breakthrough in the session, and turning to you at the door with tears in his eyes, he throws his arms around you in gratitude. Is the hug an isolated boundary crossing in the service of maintaining the alliance with a fragile patient, or a boundary crossing that will lead to the erosion of the frame and result in eventual harm to the patient? (For more guidance, see section Managing Physical Contact.)

It is not easy to know in the moment, and it is very common for therapists to be embarrassed by boundary crossings, as well as being embarrassed by any moment where they feel they lost control of the therapeutic frame. It is a natural and understandable reaction to embarrassment to avoid talking about these kinds of moments, but this is exactly what is needed in your next supervisory interaction. It may help to know that your supervisor is not going to be shocked that you experienced this and other uncomfortable moments. All therapists, no matter how experienced, face challenging boundary dilemmas and cannot know for certain whether they did the right thing in the moment. This is one of the reasons that psychotherapy should not be practiced in professional isolation, even by the most seasoned professional. Even well after finishing our training, we all need to have a consultant or peer to call on for supervision from time to time. Boundary crossings are too complicated and too impactful, and psychotherapy too difficult to practice, for any of us to manage these scenarios by ourselves. In fact, I have often called on some of the coauthors of this book for just such help.

Creating Privacy and the Sense of Safety

As we discussed earlier, the therapeutic alliance depends on the patient feeling safe enough to be quite vulnerable with their therapist. This is not something that is established in one or even several sessions; it will grow and build over time, as trust in any relationship would grow. However, what we do at the beginning can have a great impact on setting the tone for therapy and getting off on the best foot. There are things therapists can do from the beginning that show the patient how seriously we take their privacy.

Privacy begins with confidentiality.[23] Most patients assume that their therapist will not be talking about their problems or stories outside of the session; those who need some specific reassurance about this have usually been betrayed in the past when they confided in someone. Additionally, many patients in today's context of electronic medical records will be worried about what you put in their file and who has access to it. Those who are not concerned about this may simply be unaware of how easily electronic medical records are shared among providers within healthcare settings. Therefore, it is important to tell a new patient what they can expect in terms of confidentiality and limitations to confidentiality. The issue of access to the patient's record will vary depending on how the clinic or healthcare system has set up their medical record, so this is something your supervisors will need to explain to you. Patients also may wonder how much detail goes into the medical record. You should discuss the specific policies at your clinical setting with your supervisor. In the author's clinic, a new therapist might then say, "*Your other medical providers can see the medications I provide for you and diagnosis I enter into the record, but only your other mental health providers (if there are any) can read my notes. I want you to know that I don't put the details of our conversations in the note. Generally, I'll just note how any symptoms are progressing and that we used psychotherapy to continue working on problems we identified at the start. The only exception is if I am worried about safety, and if the details are relevant to your or others' safety.*"

Privacy does not consist only of the issue of what information might leak out of therapy. Another part of privacy is the patient's ability to be in control of what they share in the first place. This is one of the reasons that it is generally unwise to treat people in individual therapy who are friends, family members, or coworkers of your existing individual therapy patients. We do not want the patient to have to worry about what other people are saying to you about them. Even if the patient does not think this is a cause for concern, that can shift over time as more sensitive material is discussed or as those other relationships change. Similarly, we want the patient to feel as free as possible in telling you everything relevant about their own relationships. This can be hard enough without worrying that they will damage your impression of their friend (or spouse, partner, parent, etc.) who is also your patient.

These same considerations should also keep therapists from having social media connections with their patients, using Google or other search engines, or using other social media platforms to check on or investigate their patients' lives. It is best if the patient and therapist limit their relationship to what happens in the office during the scheduled therapy times. This helps avoid the slippery slope of the relationship becoming more casual, social, or romantic. This also supports the patient's sense of safety, as they directly decide in each encounter what they want to share with you about their life. There are rare times when an urgent concern about the patient's or someone else's safety might mean crossing this boundary. However, this is something you would only do in consultation with your supervisor.

4

What if My Patient Tells Me They Are Suicidal?

This is one of the biggest worries of many beginning therapists and it is an important one. Over time if you treat enough patients you will have a session with someone who is acutely thinking of suicide. Sometimes the patient will bring this up, and sometimes you will broach the subject in response to something about their affect, behavior, or the content of the session that has gotten you worried. Once you are aware of the patient's suicidality, this of course becomes your top priority. All other treatment tasks and goals can be set to the side as you address the patient's safety. Trying to work on other therapeutic issues when you are unsure if the patient will survive the week will not be helpful.

One way to think of it is that your more general training and identity as a mental health provider now comes to the fore. You set aside your "therapist hat" and put on you "suicide assessment hat." This just means doing what you have already been taught to do as a trainee in social work, psychology, psychiatry, etc. Sometimes new therapists feel under some pressure to seamlessly integrate the suicide assessment into the flow of the therapy session, but this is not necessary and often just impossible. If it is helpful, you can say directly to the patient that you are changing the mode you are in: *"I'm worried about you, so I'm going to pause our usual kind of work today and ask you some questions to make sure you're in a safe situation."*

How this assessment of safety will be supervised depends on your level of training and the supervisory system set up in your program. This is something that should be explained to you as you are oriented to any new training setting. Regardless of how the supervision is arranged, a trainee therapist should always reach out for supervision whenever worried about a patient's safety. I learned from a very wise psychotherapy teacher and forensic psychiatrist, Tom Gutheil MD, the valuable rule "Never worry alone."

Just as in any outpatient suicide assessment, an important question is whether it is safe for the patient and the clinician to manage the suicide risk outside of a hospital. If your assessment leads you to the conclusion that it is safe, then the session will end with some contingency plan in place should the situation become more dangerous before the next time you meet. Although notes of therapy sessions in the formal medical record can generally be quite brief, it is important for therapists to use the same kind of documentation of suicide assessment that they would use in any other mental health encounter.

Sometimes the result of the assessment is that the patient should go to a hospital. And sometimes this is not just a recommendation, but a mandate. How the clinician and the supervisor or clinic setting can enforce this mandate differs in different states and different healthcare systems. When this is the case, new therapists are often afraid that the patient will be so angry with them that the therapeutic relationship will end. This can happen and is a painful outcome, but still far better than the patient's death. Fortunately, this outcome is less common than you might think. Even therapy patients who are furious at the time and feel that you have betrayed their trust might see things very differently even a few days later. When symptoms have subsided or the acute suicidality has passed, the patient may instead be grateful for your action and the result is an even stronger therapeutic alliance.

THERAPIST SELF-DISCLOSURE

How do you decide what to share about yourself and your own experiences with your therapy patients? This is a very difficult question. Most previous experience you have had with relationships this intense and intimate have included at least some degree of reciprocal openness. Even your experiences of being professionally mentored have probably included learning from your mentor's stories about their own lives. In therapy, however, you are going to need to be much more cautious about what you say about yourself. There are two reasons for this. One is the slippery slope that we have already discussed. Sharing about yourself can confuse the limits of what kind of relationship this is (therapeutic vs. social). But, it can also lead to confusion about which direction the therapy is aimed. The patient is there to get help, and the therapist's role is to provide it. In some instances, telling the patient about your own past struggles may be intended to help the patient see that there is hope or that you are able to understand what they are going through. Unfortunately, this can easily backfire, leaving the patient feeling that they should offer you some support or at least be careful that they do not add too much to your own burdens.

The second reason for caution is it turns out that the therapist's privacy, like the patient's, is also an important condition of successful therapies because it helps to maintain the nonreciprocal therapy framework. Over time you will find that patients appreciate that you bring a degree of attention, compassion, and understanding that is very rare to find in this world. You are able to offer that, and to sustain it over long periods of treatment, because your professional self is not as vulnerable as your personal self. Your privacy is part of what keeps you feeling secure enough to consistently offer your best self to the patient.

Psychotherapy and Social Media

Lia Thomas, MD.

Social media is now an ever-present part of our society. The questions we answer in this text box deal with professionalism and patient care, and the interactions of social media. As social media is a rapidly evolving platform, the guidance here is to be applied broadly.

Many trainees come with a vast knowledge of social media and can use that knowledge for betterment of their program and institution. Social media can be used to provide education on mental health to the broader community—decreasing stigma, demystifying psychotherapy, encouraging self-care. Social media can also connect you with experts both within and outside your local training area, providing for additional supervisors and future collaborators. However, as trainees transition from perhaps undergraduate or medical school into beginning their training as a treating provider, further consideration is required regarding how social media can be used or misused.

As a trainee, you should first begin by knowing the rules of your program institution. Does your department or university have a social media policy? Does your GME office or graduate program have one? Many programs are drafting such rules and you need to be aware of them, lest you run afoul of them. If you choose to identify yourself as a resident, student, or intern of a certain program, be advised that you now serve as a representative of that program on these global platforms, including email. Think before you hit send or create a post! As a general rule, do not post negative comments about your program. If you have a grievance or a concern, use the appropriate channels.

Although much of the world is on some form of social media, data suggest that there are different types of users on different social media platforms. For example, while you may use Instagram regularly, your supervisor's knowledge of social media may be limited to Facebook and YouTube. Have open conversations with your supervisor about social media platforms and their role in psychotherapy. Think of them as opportunities for mutual growth and discovery.

If your intention is to continue with your social media profiles, take some time to answer the following questions:

How visible are you on platforms currently? Have you recently "Googled" yourself to see what shows up publicly? What information are you sharing with the world? What information are those in your social media network sharing about you in the world? Are you comfortable with that information being shared? How would you feel if a patient brought up this information in the therapy session?

When was the last time you checked your security settings on your social media platforms? This might be the time to reassess those. Do you want to consider a personal versus a professional profile? Perhaps you use social media to connect with family and friends. Do you want to consider having a more restricted account for those persons? Again, no system is 100% private; there is always the possibility that some of your information may be more visible than you intended it to be.

As you take this time to reflect on your personal relationship with social media, let us now address the issues of how to address your use of social media in your therapeutic relationships. Three questions often come up regarding social media and psychotherapy: (1) Should I look up a patient? (2) What do I do if a patient "friends" me or otherwise reaches out to connect with me via social media? (3) What do I do when a patient looks up my social media information and brings it into the therapy session? We shall explore these questions independently.

First, should I look a patient up or "Google" them? First, ask yourself—what is the purpose of getting this information? Is it out of curiosity? For example, did the patient make a comment about something they said on Facebook, but chose not to disclose further? Or, is there perhaps a medical emergency? For example, did the patient leave a concerning message, is not answering their phone, and you need to access additional contact information. This is a good time to bring your supervisor into these conversations. For example, is your interest in searching out the patient a part of the transference and countertransference of the ongoing therapy work?

The American Psychiatry Association produced a 2017 Resource document entitled "Ethical Considerations Regarding Internet Searches for Patient Information" that was later published in the peer-reviewed literature (Dike et al., 2019). To summarize, it recommended that—unless there is an emergency—it is not recommended that you conduct an online search of your patients without prior discussion/obtaining of consent.

The second common question is, "what to do when a patient 'friends' you or otherwise reaches out to connect with you via social media?" This response may depend on the platform and your settings. Some platforms—like Twitter—have a default setting where persons can connect to you without the need for you to reciprocate. Other platforms (eg, Facebook) will have your content shared immediately once a friend request is accepted. Again, this returns to the early conversation—what information about yourself do you want to share?

You need to return to discussions of professional ethics in these circumstances, particularly those surrounding professionalism and the doctor-patient relationship. Your patients are not your friends and as such, you must maintain professional boundaries. Although this process of maintaining boundaries should be a shared process, situations like these may require you to be more firm in your approach.

Should a patient send a friend request or other request to connect via social media, we advise you do not accept it. Instead, bring this up in supervision and discuss this request with the patient at the next therapy session. Gently query the patient's motivations—What did they want to know about you? What were the reasons for choosing to search for you online? This is an opportunity to deepen the therapeutic work with your patient within the appropriate boundaries for the therapeutic session. And remember—every interaction is part of the therapeutic process.

Now let us address the third common question, which is what to do if a patient brings information about you into the therapy session that they discovered online. This is likely to bring up a myriad of feelings in you—embarrassment, surprise, anger, to name a few. The content of their query may also drive your feelings. For example, did they look up where you went to college or read a recent publication? Did they bring up something you posted about your personal life and recent weekend outing with friends? Regardless of the content, you may feel overexposed and uncertain how to proceed.

In the moment of the experience, try to separate your immediate feelings with the need to maintain therapeutic rapport. Assume no malice on the patient's part, and engage them in a discussion as to why they brought this information to you. Many patients are curious about their therapist and struggle with the one-sided process of disclosure. You may not need to answer questions or expound further on the information your patient brought to your session. Exploring the patient's motivations for searching for additional information about you may be sufficient and can lead to greater work in the therapy session. Again, you will need to bring these events—and your feelings about them—into supervision. Your supervisor can help you navigate the feelings that will arise from these situations.

We do not wish to leave you alarmed at the prospect of using social media while you engage in your work as a therapist. Instead, we want you to be intentional in your choices, discuss your thoughts with supervisors, and develop your own processes.

Reference

Dike CC, Candilis P, Kocsis B, Sidhu N, Recupero P. Ethical considerations regarding internet searches for patient information. *Psychiatr Serv.* 2019;70(4):324-328.

However, there is some information about you that the patient is entitled to know as they decide whether to consent to this treatment. This includes your status as a trainee, where you have or are receiving your training, whether you have prior experience in providing the treatment, and that the content of their sessions will be shared with a supervisor (including possible video and/or audio recordings). Some patients will take the initiative in asking about all of this, but I would argue that all patients should be offered this information as part of the process of informed consent.

A more difficult question is raised when the patient wants to know something about your identity as a precondition for deciding whether to proceed with therapy. Some common examples include LGBTQ patients asking about the therapist's sexual or gender identity, religious patients asking about the therapist's faith, patients in recovery asking about the therapist's history of addiction, and patients who are parents wanting to know if the therapist also has children. Often these questions really mean, "Are you someone who can understand what I need to talk about?" It is a good idea to respond by asking the patient to tell you more about the reason for the question. Sometimes, just finding that they can talk to you about the concern is reassuring. You can also tell the patient that in some kinds of therapy (eg, psychodynamic psychotherapy) there is value in not knowing the answer to such questions; it can leave the patient freer to wonder, fantasize, and explore their own experience. Sometimes, however, the patient will make clear that the answer to the question is a "deal breaker." They may have too much anxiety about the risk of judgment or misunderstanding to move forward unless they know the therapist has the specific personal qualification they are looking for. What do you do then?

Some therapists who specialize in treating a specific population may be upfront about the relevant aspect of their own identity. Their website, for example, might make clear that they are a Christian therapist or that they are in recovery from addiction. For others, the question might simply feel too personal and have too much of a cost to the therapist's need for privacy. If that is the case, the therapist should straightforwardly say to the patient, "*I understand why you want to know but unfortunately that is not something about myself that I share with my patients.*" For all of us, there are no doubt some questions that will feel too invasive, while there might be some questions where our comfort in disclosing depends on what kind of feeling we already have with this specific patient. In our experience, there are very few personal questions that have not been asked by a patient, with a variety of motivations. It is an important part of your training to begin thinking about what questions might be too invasive or set off warning bells, in advance of any patient needing to ask. In addition, what your colleagues might self-disclose may not be what you feel comfortable self-disclosing. It is never a good idea to override your own gut feelings of warning.

However, your supervisors may have different views on this topic. Some will feel that a question about your religious identity or about your sexuality should never be answered with a disclosure. Others may feel that if the question does not feel too personal to you and it allows the patient to start a therapy (when otherwise they would not), answering is an acceptable boundary crossing. Once again, this is something to discuss with your supervisor and to begin thinking about as a therapist in training. And in that regard, it is always reasonable to say to a patient, "*I'm really not sure whether that is a question I feel comfortable answering (or whether answering that question would be good for your therapy) and I'm going to need to give this some thought. Let's come back to it at our next session.*"

What if My Patient Starts to Cry? or What if I Start to Cry?

If your patient begins to cry, you may not need to do anything. Your patient may expect that therapy will include crying and that therapists are okay with this. Some patients, however, will be embarrassed or anxious that you expect them to remain "professional." At the beginning, it can help to simply reassure such a patient, "*It is okay to cry in therapy.*" If your patient is sobbing so hard that they are unable to continue talking, then you might need to wait until they gather themselves. Letting a patient know that you are not pressuring them, that they can take their time and cry, is itself a valuable intervention. It is also a good idea to have tissues available and already in easy reach of the patient throughout your therapy space; it is a courtesy and means one less thing for the patient to worry about.

What if the session provokes your own tears? This can be a troubling experience for a new therapist, especially if you believe that this work requires absolute control of your emotional reactions. In fact, that is not possible. Therapists do respond emotionally to our patients' pain; this is part of being empathic. Your capacity to contain these responses grows with practice. But, it is not always possible to calibrate that response so exactly that you will not ever become tearful when listening to stories of tragedy or sitting with a patient who is tormented and suffering.

Sometimes, the patient will experience your tearfulness as a moment of validation and affirmation. At other times, the patient may become anxious that you will be overwhelmed. It will be helpful to acknowledge your reaction while keeping the focus on the patient. For example, the therapist could say, "*Yes, what you have been describing has touched me. I think this might mean that we are talking about something that is really important to you (or painful to you, or confusing to you, etc.). Can you tell me more about your own thoughts and feelings about this?"*

New therapists are sometimes afraid that reddened eyes or a single tear will open the floodgates, and they will lose control of their feelings while with the patient. This is very rare. Of course, the patient does need their therapist to retain their own balance during the session; if the patient's material is stirring your own emotions past the point of containment, this should be discussed in supervision. In addition, many of us have found that our own therapy is an invaluable part of our development as a therapist. It can help you understand and regulate your emotional reactions to patients, increase your empathy for the vulnerability of being a patient, and give you the opportunity to watch an experienced clinician do their work.

The Importance of Physical Setting

The physical setting of the therapy should first of all convey a sense of privacy. People walking by outside the room should not be able to see inside. Some windows are located where this would be an impossibility, such as a 10th floor room with a window to the outside. But, other windows can present a problem, and if so, the therapist should arrange to have shades or curtains that cover them. The room should also be quiet. The patient should not be able to hear conversations outside the room. This is vital for two reasons. First, it is distracting and we need to provide a space where the patient and the therapist's attention can be undivided. Second, if the patient can hear conversations from outside, they will assume that this works both ways, and that people outside can hear what the patient is saying. This is also why we do not meet patients for therapy in public places such as restaurants and cafes. (In addition to the reason that meeting in such places can confuse patients about the possibility that therapy might evolve into a social or intimate relationship.) Of course, physical setting is sometimes limited by health or other conditions (see Chapters 9-12). However, even in those settings, great care should be taken to maximize and convey a sense of privacy, including drawing curtains, keeping voices low, and minimizing distractions or other persons present.

Seating should be comfortable. Again, we do not want the patient to be distracted by physical discomfort. It is hard enough to tolerate the emotional discomfort of starting therapy. Some therapists have recliners or ottomans so the patient can put their feet up. This is just a matter of the therapist's preference. It is also nice if chairs can be arranged so that they are facing each other, but not directly head on. This can help lessen a feeling of being interrogated or examined. The distance between the chairs is also a matter of your preference and what works for your patient population. At a minimum, however, the chairs should be far enough apart that you can both stretch out your legs without kicking each other and extend your arms fully without physical contact. In addition, your office should be accessible and comfortable for individuals with a variety of physical needs and disabilities.

It is also a good idea to have a clock visible where you will be able to see it without having to turn your head. Some patients are concerned that they will bore their therapist and too much of a show of checking the clock feeds into that worry. Some therapists have multiple clocks in their office. Another helpful provision is tissue boxes within reach of the patient's seating. This will help minimize disruptions when your patients become tearful and will also convey the message that tears are acceptable and expected.

Decoration is also a matter of personal preference, but there a few good rules of thumb. You might be spending a lot of time in your therapy office, and you should have things that you like to look at, including wall art. The art should not be particularly provocative or disturbing. Working again on the understanding that starting therapy is going to generate plenty of disturbing material from within the patient, you want to have a relatively clear field for this to come into view. One way that therapist offices are often different from other professional offices is the absence of therapist family photos. This practice probably has its origin in psychodynamic therapies, which want the patient to be free to have whatever fantasies might come to mind about the therapist's personal life. These fantasies can be very valuable in learning about the patient's inner world. But, supportive therapists and cognitive behavior therapists also sometimes refrain from displaying family photos, in order to emphasize that the therapy is about the patient's life and not about the therapist's. It can help to discourage the idea that therapy is reciprocal or involves self-disclosure by the therapist.

Time as an Important Boundary

One of the most important elements of the frame is time. A therapy session generally is scheduled in advance and is planned for a set length of time. The length can vary depending on the type of therapy, scheduling constraints, and the preference of the therapist. Whatever the details, the more the therapy time is predictable and dependable, the more the patient will feel supported by the therapeutic process and frame. The more the patient can rely on the therapy session having an expectable beginning and ending, the more they will be able to relax into the process.

Punctuality matters. Some patients will tell you how they feel when you are late. Other patients will squelch their feelings of anger or resentment. This may be a characteristic way they have of relating to people, and it may be magnified if the patient is paying a reduced fee to be seen by a trainee. They may feel they have no right to any expectations, but whether they share their reaction or not, it is having an impact on the treatment.

It is important to end the session on time. Although a few patients will be watching the clock themselves and will announce when it's time to stop, mostly the therapists will need to say something such as, *"It's time for us to stop for today."* Knowing that the time has limits serves both as motivation to the patient to make the most of it and also allows them to tolerate the discomfort of emotional pain and vulnerability. Nonetheless, it is not unusual for beginning therapists to let the time run over. There are a lot of reasons you might be tempted to do this. Perhaps you feel nothing useful has happened in the session and you are hoping for something else to occur. Or the patient might be in the middle of a story and you worry that it will be rude to interrupt. Maybe the patient has become emotional and you feel it would be unkind to expect them to leave while stirred up or tearful. Most patients have their own sense of the rhythm of the session and they will begin to wind things down on their own. For those who do not, however, what do you do?

The first time it happens that the patient is in the middle of a story or is still emotional, it is probably best to run a bit over, while saying "*Usually we would stop now, but let's take a few more minutes for you to gather yourself*" or "*for you to finish sharing this story with me.*" After that, it is a very good idea to give the patient a "heads up" 5 minutes or so before the end of the session. You can say, "*We're coming to the end of our time so we might want to bring things to a good stopping point,*" or "*I can see that this session has been hard on you. Let's take a few minutes to wind down before we have to stop for the day.*"

The question of contact between sessions is related to the boundary of time and should be covered early in therapy. Should the therapist be available by phone or email between appointments, and if so, to what end? What expectations should the patient have if and when they reach out to the therapist via phone or other means? There is no one answer to this question. Some therapists have a great deal of capacity for this kind of contact, while others find that they would quickly burn out and be of no use to any of their patients if they made themselves too available. In addition, how this is handled will depend on the type of therapy and the agreed upon goals. A therapy aimed at creating a safe space for very intensive interpersonal work might need much stricter boundaries about contact. A brief phone call will not provide adequate structure to process intense feelings and an email lacks the nuances of tone and facial expression that convey warmth and acceptance when talking about hard things. On the other hand, a therapist intending to support the patient in restraining dangerous impulses might very effectively use brief check in or "as needed" phone calls to bolster the patient's developing capacity for self-restraint. Your psychotherapy supervisor (and the type of therapy provided) will help guide you toward how much and what kind of availability to offer each patient. Over the years I have seen therapists with many different approaches, but all successful therapists are clear and consistent about their availability. Unpredictable or unreliable availability is much harder on patients, and sometimes more dangerous, than very clear limits.

Managing Physical Contact

When we discussed how therapy works in the first chapter, we saw that all humans are born with attachment systems. When we are distressed as babies and children, we need to be held and we cry out to draw our caregiver to us. Reciprocally, as adults we have a natural inclination to reach out to a crying child with an embrace. The experience of having a "holding environment" is crucial in development, and it is crucial in psychotherapy as well. However, in psychotherapy, this holding needs to be accomplished with language, and not physically. Our patients will feel "held" by us when there is a therapeutic alliance in place and when we respond to their distress with empathy.

Therapists are generally a lot more cautious about physical touch than other doctors or mental health clinicians. This is because it is so easy for patients in therapy to misinterpret the meaning of the touch. It might also be that the therapy encounter is so emotionally intense that interactions that would be otherwise benign become supercharged. For example, a hand on the patient's arm or shoulder, or a hug at the end of the session, might seem helpful. It is meant to convey our concern and support. But, in the intensity and ambiguity of psychotherapy, it might inadvertently suggest something potentially romantic or sexual to the patient. This may frighten some patients and may excite others, but in either case, it is not going to be good for the treatment.

The best rule of thumb as a beginning therapist is to avoid physical contact with patients.[24] How strictly to adhere to this guideline will differ among schools of therapy, the context in which you practice (eg, hospital-based vs. outpatient mental health care), and probably among your supervisors. On a very practical level, this means that I do not initiate shaking hands with patients myself, although when patients extend their hand I do respond with a firm, brief handshake. My sense has been that the risk of misinterpreting that handshake is less than the disruption caused by rejecting it. In addition, it is important to recognize not all patients come from cultures where handshaking is used to begin or end meetings, so it is best for the therapist not to initiate.

On the other hand, when a patient asks for a hug or simply moves to hug me at the end of a session, I do try to stop them. It is important to offer an explanation, or your patient may feel hurt by what they read as a personal rejection. You might say, *"It's very natural for you to want a hug when you're feeling so poorly. (Or: It's very natural for you want to express feeling close to me with a hug). This may be hard to understand right now, but we find it's better for the therapy in the long run if we don't hug our patients."* That sort of statement is generally all that is needed. Most patients will feel at worst a bit awkward and at best reassured that you are once again thinking about their long-term interests. If the patient wants more of an explanation, you might tell them that given the intensity of the kind of work we are going to do together it is going to be important to put everything into words and not into physical expression. On the rare occasion when a patient has caught me by surprise and hugged me, I have just said something similar for future reference after the hug. Again, different schools of therapy may draw their lines differently, so discuss with your supervisor about what they advise.

What if My Patient Is Sexually Provocative?

Laura Howe-Martin, PhD

It is very likely that over the course of your career at least one patient will make a sexual or flirtatious comment, or even attempt to engage in inappropriate sexual behavior. This is more common in some environments than others (eg, within facilities that treat a high percentage of delirium or dementia, inpatient psychiatric facilities, and prison settings). However, even in outpatient clinics with high-functioning patients, these incidents can and do occur. So, what can you do to manage these situations and how can you become more prepared to cope effectively?

Sexual behavior in therapy can be understood as falling into three categories. The first is unintentional inappropriate sexual behavior (eg, general disinhibition or accidental nudity). This may occur when a patient is overtly delirious, manic, or experiencing other significant psychiatric symptoms. In these cases, the uncharacteristic sexual behavior is understood to be a manifestation of the underlying illness.

The second is flirtation that is characteristic of a more persisting personality or developmental disorder. For example, patients with histrionic tendencies can become flirtatious with their therapist (and potentially office staff or other patients). Other personality pathology such as antisocial personality disorder can entail superficially charming and manipulative behaviors that can emerge as sexual innuendo (eg, "Thank goodness you're smarter and hotter than my last therapist."). Some patients with developmental disorders such as autism spectrum may engage in attempts at flirtation due to difficulties assessing and using appropriate social communication rules.

The third category consists of sexual flirtation that is an overt attempt to cross a boundary with the therapist. This can occur when a patient appears to overtly desire a different, more intimate relationship with the therapist. This can emerge out of feelings of loneliness, lack of appreciation of the boundaries in psychotherapy, or can represent types of transference enactment (more on that in Chapter 7). In addition, flirtation may help the patient avoid the vulnerability that goes with being a patient. This type of flirtation can sometimes start with seemingly benign comments that are meant to be flattering or coy and increase to involve sexual innuendo. It can progress to fairly overt requests for information about relationship status, personal phone numbers, and/or a date (eg, "How about going for a drink when this whole therapy thing is over?").

Categorizing these three types can help us think through the potential motivations surrounding patient behavior and can also help with our case formulation. However, understanding *why* these behaviors occur does not always help with resulting feelings of discomfort, vulnerability, and/or guilt and shame. It is our experience that female therapists are at particular risk of experiencing feelings of vulnerability, self-blame, and fear. Sometimes therapists question what they did to prompt this response from a patient, and even change both their typical demeanor and manner of dress in an attempt to "ward off" these situations. This results in hypervigilance and a lack of being oneself that makes therapy far more arduous than it need be.

However, there is wisdom in recognizing that the therapist (and their demeanor) acts as a stimulus for patients, for all sorts of responses. As such, it is important to recognize that your professional self will also be a stimulus, and you should be aware of what you are bringing into the room that could prompt various patient responses. This is precisely why the boundaries of the professional frame (discussed in this chapter) are so necessary to managing boundary crossings that involve sexual innuendo. Your supervisors and trusted mentors can discuss with you what kind of clothing and overall professional presentation are appropriate for your specific clinical setting.

Our recommendation is to constantly seek good supervision and mentorship around these situations. You are hardly the first therapist who has encountered these situations, and you can learn from others how to explore and manage your own reactions to these situations. Another recommendation is to be firm regarding inappropriate boundary crossings that involve flirting. Even if a flirtatious comment or inappropriate sexual behavior is due to underlying pathology and readily "understandable," these situations can provide very teachable moments within therapy. One response may be as simple as stating, "*Those comments aren't appropriate here.*" Another response to a patient who continues to make jokes that are flirtatious might be, "*It's not okay for you to keep asking me out on a date, even in a joking way. I wonder why you keep doing it?*" Both responses set a clear boundary for what therapy entails, and what it clearly does not.

As a final note, of course, you *should resist the sometimes natural inclination to flirt back*. Some behaviors such as smiling or laughing have been reinforced throughout our lives as synonymous with being "polite" and may occur spontaneously in response to a patient's flirtatious behavior. If you find yourself pulled to respond this way, you are not alone. However, we suggest that you seek useful supervision from a trusted supervisor, with whom you can discuss such difficult topics.

Regardless of your intentions, level of skill, and masterful boundary setting, there are patients who are unable to successfully work within the therapy framework. Sometimes when sexually provocative behavior persists, it has moved into the realm of sexual harassment or aggression. You should never handle these situations alone or persist in treating patients who make you feel unsafe. Again, this is where supervision and potentially consultation with your training director are invaluable.

Managing Payment and Gifts

Part of the frame of the treatment is that the therapist is paid for the service. It may seem strange at first to think of this as something that actually supports the treatment. During many training experiences, billing and payment go on either behind the scenes, or before or after we see the patient. In some settings, such as state hospitals, correctional institutions, or homeless shelters, fees are not paid and no billing is generated. It is not something that we often think much about, except perhaps that we have learned that there are certain elements of documentation that will need to be in the chart in order for billing to follow. In some settings, trainees see patients and insurance is billed; in other clinic settings, the patient may pay directly, usually a reduced fee or a fee on a sliding scale. If we do think about this as trainees, we might experience some doubt about whether we are worth whatever fee is being charged.

Nonetheless, the payment is important because it allows both the patient and the therapist to be clear about what each is getting out of this relationship. The therapist is doing a job, and the patient is getting treatment. The patient is entitled to the therapist's full attention and all the best efforts to provide psychotherapy. The therapist is getting a fee or a salary. Knowing this makes it possible to accept that the therapist will not be getting any care from the patient or other compensation. The patient does not have to feel like they are a burden or imposing on you or in your debt. In addition, the therapist does not have to suppress the inevitable feelings of resentment that will accumulate in anyone who works hard without being paid.

This straightforward frame is challenged when the patient offers the therapist a gift. Receiving a gift can constitute a crossing of the boundary of the payment arrangement. Are there times when this is a benign, or even therapeutic, boundary crossing, or is it always a boundary violation? Most therapists are comfortable accepting small gifts that are not of significant financial value. Such gifts are better understood as gestures of appreciation, not as attempts to provide some kind of additional compensation to the therapist. This is especially true around holiday seasons, when many patients will think it obvious that they would include you on the list of people who receive some small holiday token or treat. Depending on cultural background, the patient might actually think it a breach of the expected frame to not give such a gift to a teacher or doctor that they value (a reasonable enough analogy for this new and unusual relationship with a therapist). In addition, it may be offensive for you to outright refuse such a gift. However, in some therapeutic approaches, it would nonetheless be better if the patient expressed their appreciation in words. This can be conveyed by asking the patient to reflect with you on the meaning of the gift: "*What did you mean to say to me with this gift? Did you have any hopes or any worries about what I might think or feel in receiving the gift?*" It is also helpful to reiterate the nonreciprocal expectations of therapy, in that the patient has no obligation to "take care" of the therapist through gift-giving.

In contrast, some offers are clearly boundary violations, such as a patient wanting to let you in on the opportunity to invest in a financial opportunity or give you an insider stock tip. Other times, it can be less clear, such as the patient who offers extra tickets to a charity event or concert. Aside from the potential difficulties of being at a social event that your patient is attending, it is wise to refuse the offer of any gift whose content—as opposed to meaning—you would actually feel excited about receiving (such as those tickets). Paying attention to your own feelings about the gift is a reasonable way to differentiate something small that expresses appreciation, from something that changes the balance of your own compensation. In general, it is good to err on the conservative side.

Conclusion

In this chapter, we covered some of the basics about starting a psychotherapy. Hopefully, you were able to see that you do not have to be an expert in psychotherapy to successfully launch a new treatment. Your patient will feel less alone and less ashamed simply because you offer your full attention to the patient and make a real effort to elicit and understand their feelings. The experience of empathy is very powerful and something with which you already have valuable experience. Similarly, establishing a therapeutic alliance with the patient also decreases their aloneness and generates hope. This alliance is built around a developing sense of trust and collaboration on goals and therapeutic tasks. You also learned that the capacity for the patient to take the risks needed to deepen their treatment, and for the therapist to safely offer this, depends on the establishment of appropriate boundaries. These boundaries call for a solid frame around the therapy, judicious flexibility, and ongoing supervision.

Self-Study Questions

1. Write three different statements or questions that might help a patient identify and name their feelings, using your own words.

2. Think about conversations you often have with those around you. What are examples of informal verbal expressions that you typically use?

3. What is the therapeutic alliance and why is it so vital to psychotherapy?

4. Think of your last patient or a patient you learned about in psychotherapy class or didactic. Articulate at least two goals central to their treatment.

5. Why are boundaries important in psychotherapy? What is the difference between a boundary crossing and a boundary violation?

6. Review the various ways boundaries are discussed in this chapter (eg, time, gift-giving, self-disclosure). Which ones might you struggle with maintaining and why?

RESOURCES FOR FURTHER LEARNING

Elvins R, Green J. The conceptualization and measurement of therapeutic alliance: An empirical review. *Clin Psychol Rev.* 2008;28:1167-1187.

Gutheil TG, Appelbaum PS. *Clinical Handbook of Psychiatry and the Law.* Philadelphia, PA: Lippincott Williams & Wilkins; 2019.

Herman JL. *Trauma and Recovery: The Aftermath of Violence–From Domestic Abuse to Political Terror.* London: Hachette UK; 2015.

Kandel E. *The Disordered Mind: What Unusual Brains Tell Us About Ourselves.* New York, NY: Farrar, Straus, and Giroux; 2018.

Wachtel PL. *Therapeutic Communication: Knowing What to Say When.* 2nd ed. New York, NY: The Guilford Press; 2013.

Wampold B. How important are the common factors in psychotherapy? An update. *World Psychiatry.* 2015;14:270-277.

REFERENCES

1. Wampold BE. How important are the common factors in psychotherapy? An update. *World Psychiatry.* 2015;14:270-277.
2. Elliott R, Bohart AC, Watson JC, Murphy D. Therapist empathy and client outcome: an updated meta-analysis. *Psychotherapy.* 2018;55:399-410.
3. Watson JC. The role of empathy in psychotherapy: theory, research, and practice. In: Cain DJ, Keenan K, Rubin S, eds. *Humanistic Psychotherapies: Handbook of Research and Practice.* Washington, DC: US: American Psychological Association; 2016:115-145. http://dx.doi.org/10.1037/14775-005.
4. Watson JC, Steckley PL, McMullen EJ. The role of empathy in promoting change. *Psychother Res.* 2014;24:286-298.
5. Gerdes KE, Segal EA, Lietz CA. Conceptualising and measuring empathy. *Br J Soc Work.* 2010;40(7):2326-2343.
6. Gibbons SB. Understanding empathy as a complex construct: a review of the literature. *Clin Soc Work J.* 2011;39:243-252.
7. Macfarlane P, Anderson T, McClintock AS. Empathy from the client's perspective: a grounded theory analysis. *Psychother Res.* 2017;27(2):227-238. doi:10.1080/10503307.2015.1090038.
8. Rako S, Harvey M, Rako S. *Semrad: The Heart of a Therapist.* Lincoln, NE: iUniverse; 2003.
9. Tervalon M, Murray-Garcia J. Cultural humility versus cultural competence: a critical distinction in defining physician training outcomes in multicultural education. *J Health Care Poor Underserved.* 1998;9(2):117-125.
10. Hook JN, Davis DE, Owen J, Worthington EL Jr, Utsey SO. Cultural humility: measuring openness to culturally diverse clients. *J Couns Psychol.* 2013;60(3):353.
11. Havens L. *Making Contact.* Cambridge, MA: Harvard University Press; 1988.
12. Wachtel PL. *Therapeutic Communication: Knowing What to Say When.* 2nd ed. New York, NY: The Guilford Press; 2013.
13. Leclère C, Viaux S, Avril M, et al. Why synchrony matters during mother-child interactions: a systematic review. *PLoS One.* 2014;9(12):e113571. doi:10.1371/journal.pone.0113571.
14. Kandel E. *The Disordered Mind: What Unusual Brains Tell Us About Ourselves.* New York, NY: Farrar, Straus, and Giroux; 2018.
15. Vaillant GE. The beginning of wisdom is never calling a patient a borderline; or, the clinical management of immature defenses in the treatment of individuals with personality disorders. *J Psychother Pract Res.* 1992;1(2):117-134.
16. Krupnick JL, Sotsky SM, Elkin I, et al. The role of the therapeutic alliance in psychotherapy and pharmacotherapy outcome: findings in the National Institute of Mental Health treatment of depression collaborative research program. *Focus.* 2006;4(2):269-277.
17. Elvins R, Green J. The conceptualization and measurement of therapeutic alliance: an empirical review. *Clin Psychol Rev.* 2008;28:1167-1187.
18. Herman JL. *Trauma and Recovery: The Aftermath of Violence—From Domestic Abuse to Political Terror.* London: Hachette UK; 2015.
19. Frost R. Mending wall. In: *North of Boston.* Vol 12. New York, NY: Holt and company; 1914.
20. Gabbard GO, Crisp-Han H. Teaching professional boundaries to psychiatric residents. *Acad Psychiatry.* 2010;34:369-372.
21. Glass LL. The gray areas of boundary crossings and violation. *Am J Psychother.* 2003;57:429-444.
22. Waldinger RJ. Boundary crossings and boundary violations: thoughts on navigating a slippery slope. *Harv Rev Psychiatry.* 1994;2(4):225-227.
23. Gutheil TG, Appelbaum PS. *Clinical Handbook of Psychiatry and the Law.* Philadelphia, PA: Lippincott Williams & Wilkins; 2019.
24. Gutheil TG, Gabbard GO. The concept of boundaries in clinical practice: theoretical and risk-management dimensions. *Am J Psychiatry.* 1993;150(2):188-196.

4

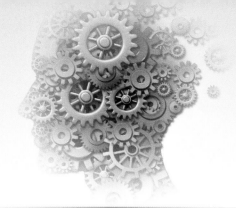

Section 2

LEARNING SPECIFIC PSYCHOTHERAPIES

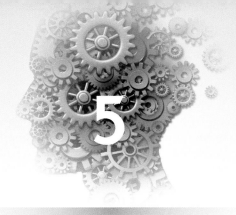

5

Supportive Psychotherapy

RANDON S. WELTON, MD AND ERIN M. CROCKER, MD

Case Study—Overview

Ms. A is a 22-year-old admitted to a medical unit following an overdose of acet-aminophen. Earlier that day, she arrived home from work as her boyfriend was leaving to go out with friends. She had accused him of ignoring her. He had called her "insecure and crazy." She said, "Well if you are not happy with me why don't you move out?" After he said that he might, she stormed upstairs and came back down with a bottle of pills that she proceeded to take in front of him. He called 911. Evaluated in the intensive care unit (ICU) by the psychiatry C&L team, Ms. A reported intense sadness, hopelessness, and a continuing desire to "get it over with and die." She complained of frequently altered sleep and energy. Her appe-tite was usually stable, although she had periodically gone on extreme diets or engaged in purging behavior when she felt that she was "fat and disgusting." She reported chronically low self-esteem. She has had some previous problems with alcohol and experimentation with numerous illicit drugs, as well as a history of three previous psychiatric hospitalizations over the past 3½ years, each of which had been preceded by turmoil in a relationship.

On day 3 of her current medical admission, she was voluntarily transferred to an inpatient psychiatric unit. While on the unit, she was initially withdrawn; she did not engage in group activities and was often angry at staff. She expressed doubt that anyone cared about her or wanted to help. She felt that the providers ignored her pain and just wanted her to take a pill and go away. Her course and response during this admission was similar to past hospitalizations. Over time, she started to open up to her inpatient providers and her suicidality diminished. She was connected with an outpatient therapist and psychiatrist. However, her pattern after previous admissions has been to stop taking prescribed medication and stop attending to appointments shortly after discharge.

INTRODUCTION

Supportive psychotherapy (SP) is a practical and flexible psychosocial intervention, based on an understanding that all patients possess strengths that can at times be tested and even overwhelmed by circumstances. SP helps patients make the best use of their strengths, support systems, and available resources to navigate these difficult times. The problems addressed in SP may arise from temporary situations, such as severe acute stressors, or from ongoing difficulties, such as chronic mental illness.

The theory behind SP emphasizes that all patients have characteristic ways of functioning that help them to manage stress, maintain their sense of self-worth, engage effectively with others, and solve daily problems. These can be thought of as the patient's available "reserves" to maintain effective functioning and modulate emotions. However, in times of crisis, these reserves can be overwhelmed leading to emotional distress, diminished self-esteem, withdrawal from social supports, or difficulties in dealing with challenges. As a supportive psychotherapist, you must first assess the patient's reserves and then help them strengthen existing positive coping strategies or develop new ones. Through the work, patients can gradually become more adept at strengthening their reserves or recognizing their own value and self-worth despite ongoing stressors.

The available evidence-base supports SP's efficacy for a wide variety of psychiatric diagnoses and has also shown its benefit in helping patients with medical illnesses. Because SP is a highly flexible and adaptable form of treatment, it can be provided in a wide variety of treatment settings. SP can become the therapy of choice for a broad array of patients with highly diverse needs and goals. Your tasks as a supportive psychotherapist follow naturally from the goals of therapy outlined above and have been organized by a chapter author (E. Crocker) according to the acronym HOPE[1] which is represented in *Figure 5.1.*

In this chapter, you will be provided with a brief history of SP, a summary of the evidence for the use of SP in a variety of treatment settings, and an overview of the interventions used in SP. These interventions range from the common elements of psychotherapy (CEP) to relatively specific SP interventions to interventions shared with other therapy approaches.

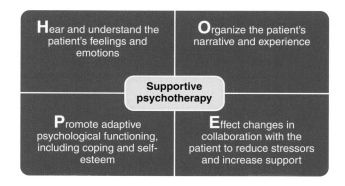

FIGURE 5.1 HOPE acronym of supportive psychotherapy.

A BRIEF HISTORY OF SUPPORTIVE PSYCHOTHERAPY AND ITS USE IN PATIENT CARE

SP is very likely both the most commonly used form of psychotherapy, as well as the most underappreciated. Sullivan once commented, "Supportive therapy is the Cinderella of psychotherapies. Considered a simple-minded endeavor, it seldom evokes theoretical conceptualizations, and neophyte psychiatrists are usually left to develop their own techniques intuitively."[2] For decades the "Cinderella of psychotherapies" was provided to most patients, yet garnered little credit or recognition for being a useful, effective, or important form of treatment. Because SP techniques developed alongside psychodynamic psychotherapy, SP was often considered to be the default approach for patients who were not deemed suitable candidates for a more expressive therapy.[3] This has led to the stigma of SP being considered a lesser therapy for lesser patients.[4,5] While it is true that patients who have cognitive difficulties, intense or unmanageable emotions, or those who have problems with abstract thinking and introspection would certainly be appropriate for SP, there are many other suitable candidates as well. In fact, SP may be the best approach for many patients, including high-functioning individuals.[6,7]

Even in academic settings, SP receives relatively little emphasis in teaching or research, despite its widespread use. For example, a 2012 survey of US psychiatry residencies showed that compared to cognitive behavioral therapy (CBT) and psychodynamic psychotherapy, SP is the most widely practiced but receives the least amount of didactic time and supervision.[8] It has been noted that there is a need for increased attention to SP within psychiatry training programs, both in the form of didactic teaching and clinical supervision.[5,9,10] The extremely limited data available on SP training within psychology and social work training programs indicate a need for increased emphasis in these professions as well.

THE EFFICACY OF SUPPORTIVE PSYCHOTHERAPY

SP is rarely studied as the primary treatment for a mental illness.[11] More commonly, it is used as the comparator or control group within psychotherapy efficacy studies. These studies typically seek to demonstrate the superiority of other psychotherapies but often find SP to be surprisingly effective.[4] These findings are even more notable when one takes into account that researcher bias plays a strong role in the outcome of therapy efficacy studies.[12-14]

SP has been shown to provide benefit to patients suffering from a wide variety of psychiatric disorders, including patients with anxiety disorders,[15-18] depressive disorders,[19-21] depression after traumatic brain injury,[22] psychotic disorders,[23,24] personality disorders,[25-29] eating disorders,[30] and dysthymia with comorbid alcohol use disorder.[31] SP is also effective in combination with medical treatment for alcohol dependence.[32] Patients being treated for substance use disorders are more likely to remain in treatment and attain sobriety when their providers utilize SP-friendly approaches such as developing a strong and affirming therapeutic alliance with the patient early in treatment[33] and demonstrating "empathy and supportiveness."[34]

The use of SP, however, should not be limited to patients who have a psychiatric diagnosis. Patients struggling with medical illness can also benefit significantly from SP. SP is the type of psychotherapy that is most often used in medical treatment settings,[35,36] and primary care providers can realistically integrate brief SP interventions into a busy clinical practice.[10,37-39] Indeed, "the value of supportive interventions in decreasing morbidity and length of stay for medical and surgical patients is impressive…"[10] Studies have shown its benefits in patients with coronary artery disease,[40,41] peptic ulcer disease,[42] irritable bowel syndrome,[43] chronic pain,[44,45] breast cancer,[46-49] ovarian cancer,[50] and those patients who are coping with organ loss.[50] Using SP as part of a comprehensive biopsychosocial approach can maximize patients' medical outcomes as well as their psychological functioning.

One of the major goals of SP is helping patients increase their social support, and "the positive effect of social support on health has been well documented for several decades."[51] Social support has been shown to reduce the body's physiologic response to stress[51-53] and decrease individuals' perceived severity of pain.[54,55] Individuals with greater social support have also been shown to have lower blood pressure, a stronger immune response,[56] improved wound healing,[57] and decreased morbidity and mortality rates.[56,58,59] In fact, "the evidence linking social relationships to mortality was comparable to the evidence linking standard risk factors such as smoking and physical activity to mortality."[56] When you provide SP to your patient, you can improve their physical health by helping them to increase their social support.

PRACTICE OPPORTUNITIES FOR SUPPORTIVE PSYCHOTHERAPY

Because of the breadth of suitable patients and its inherent flexibility, SP can be practiced anywhere that patients are seen. Its utility in consultation and liaison psychiatry is obvious from its benefits in patients who are medically ill. Providers in emergency departments and crisis centers can use it to set short-term, achievable goals for patients. Maximizing problem-solving skills and effective engagement with available social support can make a tremendous difference for patients in crisis. Patients on both medical and psychiatric inpatient units can have their overwhelming distress partially ameliorated through the deliberate application of SP. Patients can be taught to identify and tolerate emotions more productively and to cope with stressors more adaptively. Busy medication management clinics can return to a biopsychosocial model through the use of SP-based psychosocial interventions such as behavioral activation and social skills training. In outpatient therapy practices, the structured provision of SP can benefit individuals presenting with a myriad of problems as they emphasize existing strengths and newly gained skills to address overwhelming situations and stresses.

ADDRESSING THE COMMON ELEMENTS OF PSYCHOTHERAPY WITHIN SUPPORTIVE PSYCHOTHERAPY

CEP have been addressed in Chapter 4, but we will highlight the application of a few of these specifically to SP. The Y Model of psychotherapy, mentioned in Chapter 1 and proposed by Plakun et al, depicts CBT and psychodynamic psychotherapy as being the arms of a "Y," which rest on the solid base of SP.[60] It would be consistent with the model to see the CEP sitting beneath SP on the stem. Attention to these common elements may lead to 30% of the change seen during psychotherapy.[61,62] Focusing on the common elements also aids the practitioner in using other forms of intervention. However, in SP, the common elements become the primary target of therapy.[4] The patient leaves the therapy feeling less isolated, more secure, more hopeful, and better equipped to deal with the stresses that are confronting them. To demonstrate the use of the CEP and SP techniques, we will follow a single patient through a hospitalization.

Empathy

Within SP, empathy is one of the therapist's primary tools for initiating the "H" in HOPE—helping the patient hear and understand their feelings and emotion. Empathy has been defined as "the act of correctly acknowledging the emotional state of another without experiencing that state oneself."[63] As outlined in Chapter 4, empathy involves imagining the patient's state of mind, resonating with the patient's emotional state, and communicating back to the patient what the therapist understands and feels. Empathy helps patients feel understood and over time helps the therapist and patient to understand the patient's less obvious feelings and responses.[64]

Case Study—Using Empathy

Ms. A is discussing the perceived ineffectiveness of her previous mental health treatment with a psychiatry resident on the consultation and liaison team.

Ms. A—I don't think any of it really helped. The therapists were nice, but they were so busy they could hardly keep their patients straight. I never really had the sense that they knew who I was. I was just "self-harming borderline number three" for that day. And the psychiatrists…They were even worse. They would not even try to remember who I was. I would see one of them for 15 minutes every few months, but it always seemed to be a different doctor.

Therapist—I can sense your frustration with a system that did not seem to care about you.

Ms. A—Exactly. How are you supposed to work with a doctor who doesn't seem to want to know you?

Respect

Recipients of SP have often been treated in mental health systems that they perceived as impersonal and uncaring. This can be gradually internalized as feelings of worthlessness. Respect is another important way of helping the patient hear and understand their feelings and emotion. Having a provider who seems happy to work with the patient and respects the patient's time and ideas can be a valuable and therapeutic new experience. Asking about patient's strengths and past successes acknowledges what they have already accomplished. Displays of respect can be as simple as referring to them as "Mr." or "Ms." (or other preferred formal title) rather than by their first names. Asking about current, but noncontroversial, events shows an interest in their opinions and thoughts.

Therapeutic Alliance

The therapeutic alliance is commonly considered to have three basic components: (1) a warm, emotional bond; (2) collaborative goals for treatment; and (3) agreed upon tasks and roles.[65] Therapeutic alliance was discussed in detail in Chapter 4 and is a critical component of SP. Failing to foster or maintain a good therapeutic alliance is associated with a poor clinical outcome,[66] while a positive therapeutic alliance is one of the best supported sources of improvement in psychotherapy.[61,62,67] Developing a strong therapeutic alliance creates the secure environment necessary for patients to develop new coping strategies or to strengthen existing ones.

GOALS AND INTERVENTIONS OF SUPPORTIVE PSYCHOTHERAPY: USING THE HOPE MODEL

Hear and Understand Your Patient's Feelings and Emotions

As a provider of SP, you can help patients improve function and minimize distress by helping them identify and express their emotions. Emotions that spring from mental illness or extreme life circumstances may seem overwhelming. The sufferer may be unable to even name or identify these emotions, much less hope to control or moderate them on their own. SP helps the patient identify and name their feelings, which eventually creates a shared emotional vocabulary between you and the patient, and also helps identify targets for subsequent interventions.

Once the emotions have been named, you then collaboratively create a strategy to help the patient manage or tolerate them. Individuals dealing with chronic emotional pain often go to great lengths to avoid feeling their distress. Avoidance can be demonstrated through denial, unhealthy distractions, or the misuse of substances. These attempts to avoid emotions stem from a belief that the pain is literally unbearable. Patients may worry that once they start feeling and expressing these emotions, they will be unable to shut them down. In SP, patients will be encouraged to experience, accept, and express their emotional response to conscious memories or events, ie, catharsis. Patients will gradually learn that feeling and expressing emotions will not overwhelm them.[4,7,68]

Case Study—Identifying and Expressing Emotions

While in the ICU, Ms. A is interviewed by the resident on the psychiatry consultation and liaison team. She is asked about how she was feeling when she took the pills.

Ms. A—I wanted to die.

Resident—So that is what you were hoping for, but what were you feeling? Were you sad, angry, or scared?

Ms. A—Yes, all of those. I felt everything all at once.

Resident—I realize it was an overwhelming time, but which emotions were the most prominent when you grabbed the pill bottle?

Ms. A—Well I couldn't believe he would do this to me. So, I guess I felt angry at him and then felt like I would always be alone.

Resident—So it sounds like you felt angry and then rejected.

Ms. A—Yes, I suppose so.

5

Many of the techniques to hear and understand the patient's feelings and emotions have already been mentioned in the introductory chapters of this book. Frequent use of empathy (see Chapter 4) helps both you and the patient understand their emotional experience. Exploring the therapist's attempts at empathy will help the patient-therapist dyad come to a more accurate understanding of the patient. Sometimes this new understanding challenges the patient's previous viewpoint. With patients who are defensive or lacking in insight, the provider might contradict what patients have previously said. However, you must do so in a tactful and understanding way (eg, *You discuss it as if it is no big deal, but having your mother move out of the house when you were a teenager must have been very upsetting for you*).

Another part of hearing and understanding a patient's experiences involves *validation* and *normalizing*. Any particular event may elicit a number of differing emotional reactions in your patient. Once the patient identifies and expresses their emotional experience, you can then help validate their experiences and reactions, through acknowledging the reasonableness of the emotional response (eg, *That sounds like a scary experience.*). You can also work to normalize experiences (eg, *I think anyone going through something like that would be terrified*). Normalizing experiences leading to a recognition that others might feel the same thing helps individuals "own their feelings" and decreases a sense of isolation.

One technique that will help the patient feel heard is working with the patient to *develop a vocabulary and mutual understanding* of what they are feeling. Recognizing that others have had similar experiences and that there are specific words for their experiences may decrease isolation and instill hope. Having a shared language aids in monitoring treatment as both parties are using terms the other recognizes. An example of this is the therapist asks a patient if they are falling into "the black hole," which the patient had previously used to describe their depression.

Organize Their Narrative and Experience

SP can help patients develop a narrative that makes their situation understandable. This narrative should consider the patient's preexisting vulnerabilities, the psychosocial circumstances that contributed to the situation, the choices they faced, and the decisions they made. Seeing their current situation as the almost inevitable outcome of numerous factors can make their distress less random and mysterious. Once their decisions and experiences are understandable, the patient and therapist can start to plan the next steps in order to address the underlying, modifiable factors that contributed to the crisis. A more accurate understanding of the factors at play also allows the patient-therapist dyad to determine which factors can be addressed and modified and which need to be accepted and tolerated.

Patients often focus on the aspects of their lives that they see as the most problematic. Still others may assume the therapist already knows the pertinent details of their history. Therefore, it is important to obtain a full psychosocial and developmental history. You can explain, "I want to get to know you, not just hear about your illness." This systematic approach to information gathering will help patients put their illness into perspective. Their illness and/or crisis may be a large part of their life, but it is not the entirety of their life. Below are a variety of techniques that can help the patient organize their experiences.

- *Encourage elaboration*—This can be as simple as asking the patient, "Tell me more about that," echoing what the patient has just said, saying "uh-huh," or even providing nonverbal encouragement such as nodding and waiting. You should attend carefully to nonverbal cues and comment when you have noted a significant change in the patient's affect.[64] This elaboration helps the therapist-patient dyad understand the context and contributors to the patient's emotional state.

- *Offer summary statements*—By occasionally paraphrasing the patient's story, you help create a narrative that explains the current symptomatology. These summaries should be followed by permission for the patient to correct misunderstandings or to fill in gaps. This will not only clarify events but might help the patient look at situations in a different light. For example—*Your parent's separation and divorce made your household very tense. Things got so bad that you ended up moving in with your uncle and aunt. While you were there, they seemed to treat you poorly, a lot differently than they treated their own kids, so you decided to run away from home. Did I get that, right?*

- *Provide psychoeducation*—Patients may not automatically or correctly link their life and emotional experiences to the mental illness and could benefit from psychoeducation (see Box 5.1). The fact that a lack of motivation is a part of depression and amenable to treatment may not be as obvious to patients as providers think. These characteristics may be attributed by the patient or others in their life to a lack of effort, rather than a product of a disease. Elderly patients might be relieved to know that their problems with memory and

Box 5.1   Common Topics in Psychoeducation

- Review the standard signs and symptoms of their illness

- Demonstrate how the general diagnostic criteria have been demonstrated in their life

- Educate them on the biopsychosocial nature of their mental illness including genetic and stress vulnerabilities

- Describe the typical course and prognosis of illness

- Discuss treatment options

- Review the relative risks and benefits of a variety of treatments including psychopharmacological, psychosocial, and complementary/alternative medicine options

- Warn of common comorbid conditions

- Discuss the value of limiting/eliminating the use of alcohol or other illicit substances

- Discuss the connection between stress, their behaviors, and relapse. They should be able to identify behaviors that make relapse more or less likely

- Identify warning signs of relapse[69]

concentration may be related to depression and are not necessarily a sign of dementia. Even those who have been treated for many years may be uninformed about some aspects of their illness. The existing literature supports the importance of psychoeducation in patients with severe mental illness. Psychoeducation, when given repetitively over time, has been associated with decreased symptom relapse in bipolar disorder, reduced relapse, readmission rates, and increased medication adherence in schizophrenia and improved clinical course and medication adherence in depression.[70]

- *Help find a new perspective*—Our personal narrative directs the meaning and significance we place on the events of our life. Patients influence their distress through the stories they tell about themselves. Stories that emphasize guilt, powerlessness, or helplessness exacerbate depression, while themes of the unpredictable nature of life and their illness generate anxiety. Distress can be heightened by internally repeating negative stories. The process of reframing or reauthoring personal narratives changes problems and lives.[71] This can be perfomed in a way to make the narrative more accurate or to generate a more hopeful interpretation of events. As their life is seen as a connected sequence of circumstances, choices, and consequences, the possibility arises that current and future decisions could positively impact the ongoing course of their life. They now play an active role in determining their future. Of note, other treatment approaches such as narrative therapy[71] build upon this approach.

Case Study—Helping Find a New Perspective

Ms. A and her therapist are reviewing her academic history.

Ms. A—I mean, I couldn't even finish college after I stopped taking the meds. I just couldn't get out of bed at that point or go to class. I know it's not Mom's fault she lost her job and our insurance, but still, I never seem to finish anything.

Therapist—You said you were a failure and flunked out of college. What I heard was that your parents lost their insurance that made it impossible for you to stay on your medication. Without your medications, your depression returned and you were unable to focus on your studies so you had to withdraw from school.

Ms. A—Yeah, that's right.

Therapist—You were pulled out of school, but it was not because you weren't trying or you weren't smart enough. You had an illness that made it impossible for you to succeed. That's very different than just saying you were a failure.

Promote Adaptive Psychological Functioning, Including Coping and Self-Esteem

Coping strategies that had once been adaptive can become problematic as circumstances change. The emotional lability and cognitive impact of many mental illnesses further decrease patients' ability to respond adaptively to even normal life stresses. Additionally, a track record of being unable to cope with problems can diminish your patients' confidence in their ability to cope in the present. Through SP, you can help the patient identify and assess their past and current coping strategies. Whereas insight-oriented approaches seek the origins of the current coping mechanisms and ask the patient to wonder about their impact on their life, as a supportive therapist, you take a more active stance in directing the patient toward making effective use of their current coping strategies. Through discussion, praise, encouragement, or suggestion, you can help the patient explore the possibility of using more adaptive approaches. When in crisis, people often focus exclusively on their failures and weaknesses. In their life, however, they will most often have survived and dealt with numerous problems prior to seeking treatment. Once these past successes have been acknowledged, you can offer realistic praise for these talents and abilities. You can then help the patient consider how they might apply these same strengths to their current problems and stressors.[68] These strengths are also included in your case conceptualization (see Chapter 2) and comprehensive treatment plan. The goal for the therapist is to intervene in ways that are familiar to the patient and/or compatible with their personality and past experiences.[7] Although you are assisting the patient, they are the ones doing the majority of the work, so they can take pride and self-satisfaction in their improvement.[1]

Adaptive psychological functioning can also be promoted in the following ways:

- *Instill hope*—Individuals who struggle with mental illness are often saddled with hopelessness about their condition and the future, which constricts their ability to see possibilities and options for themselves. While being careful not to present unrealistic outcomes, you can at least reassure the patient that you will be with them through the struggle. As opportunities for change and improvement arise, reasonable hopefulness can also be shared. This could focus on the possibility of improved future relationships, employment, or living arrangements. Just realizing that there are options available and that you are there to work with them can increase hope.[66]

- *Promote lifestyle regulation*—Promoting proper sleep hygiene, helping patients engage in regular exercise, limiting intoxicating drugs, increasing medication adherence, and improving diet can all result in benefits to mood and function. These have the added advantage of being within the patient's control.

- *Enhance coping strategies*—Coping strategies can be thought of as volitional or habitual responses to external stresses. Often the coping strategy is one that has been successful at some times or in some situations. Problems arise when this approach becomes too broadly generalized or is used inappropriately. After defining the coping strategy through developing the patient's narrative, you can challenge the continuing effectiveness of the strategy. If the patient does not spontaneously come up with a new strategy, you as the therapist can ask about specific options or even tentatively make suggestions to help the patient consider alternate approaches. Whether the proposed coping strategies are familiar or new, they can be practiced in the session using role-play.

5

Case Study—Develop Healthier Coping Strategies

The inpatient resident is discussing Ms. A's response to feeling rejected.

Therapist—How do you normally respond when you feel your boyfriend is ignoring you?

Ms. A—I usually end up yelling at him, storming out, and going to a bar, or I just do something to hurt myself.

Therapist—And how do you feel after that?

Ms. A—Usually worse. I realize that maybe I overreacted and that makes me feel stupid. Plus, if I went to a bar I probably drank too much so I feel lousy, and I spent money that I could not afford.

Therapist—So I wonder if there is some other way to handle feeling rejected that won't make you feel as bad?

Ms. A—Well, there was one time when I just sat there and cried.

Therapist—And how did your boyfriend respond?

Ms. A—He eventually sat by me and held me and we watched a movie.

Therapist—And how did that feel?

Ms. A—It felt nice. And I didn't have a hangover.

Therapist—So it sounds like you've already found a helpful way to deal with feelings of loneliness.

- *Highlight strengths, achievements, and assets*—Past achievements and successes should be highlighted. Ask the patient how those strengths have been used to overcome troubles in the past. To keep your honest praise of their successes from being seen as flattery or as being patronizing, praise should be based on observable achievements or effort.[67] In more psychodynamically oriented therapies, praising the patient might be seen as distracting or potentially problematic, but as long as it is honest and based on achievements, praise can increase the likelihood of further positive changes in behavior.[69] You can collaborate with the patient to create strategies for using these identified skills and talents to address current problems, eg, *Last time you had problems at work, you ended up asking your coworker for advice and that really helped. I wonder if you could try something like that this time.* The most direct way to increase a patient's self-esteem is for them to develop a sense of competency. Therapy can promote this by improving social and interpersonal skills, problem-solving, and coping strategies. As patients learn to accept their emotional responses and generate narratives that better explain their symptoms and behaviors, they will feel more prepared to engage in healthy activities.[66] All of these increase the likelihood of enhanced, realistic self-esteem.

Case Study—Identifying and Using Existing Skills and Strengths

On the psychiatric inpatient unit, Ms. A is discussing her emotions. She initially describes them as wild horses that cannot be tamed. When asked what has helped Ms. A feel more in control in the past, she mentions yoga and meditation as being helpful. Those interventions are possible on the unit and become part of her treatment plan.

- *Use therapeutic confrontations*—Despite the name, therapeutic confrontations (see *Figure 5.2*) are not adversarial or argumentative. A therapeutic confrontation can be thought of as a comparison. You are pointing out the difference between the patient's stated goals and their current attitude or behavior. Therapists can then tactfully discuss the likely outcomes of the patient's ongoing actions. Exploring the discrepancy between the path they are on and where they want to go can help you lead the patient to the development of a plan to change.[64]

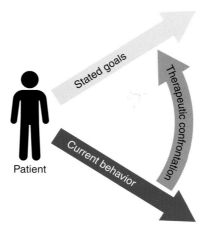

FIGURE 5.2 Therapeutic confrontation.

- *Develop a crisis response plan*—Minimizing the risk of relapse can be part of psychoeducation or a separate intervention. The Safety Planning Intervention by Stanley and Brown has been described as a "best practice" and consists of a prioritized list of coping strategies and people who can be contacted in the case of an impending suicidal crisis.[72] Through the creation of a safety plan, patients should be able to describe the likely symptoms they would experience if their illness worsens. Observable "red flags" should be specifically identified. You then collaborate with the patient to develop a list of responses to these "red flags." Role-playing can be used during the session to practice when they should act and what they should say. Usually, these will culminate in the patient's reporting to an emergency department for acute safety issues, but there are generally preliminary steps that occur first and may prevent emergency department visits. Common steps include:

  - *Distractions* (listening to music, watching a favorite show)

  - *Positive activities* (going for a walk, praying, meditation, journaling)

  - *Contacting a support team* (talking to the spouse, calling a friend)

  - *Contacting medical personnel* (calling a hotline, calling the therapist)

5

Case Study—Creating a Basic Crisis Response Plan

The therapist has worked with Ms. A to develop a list of activities she can try if she begins to feel neglected, abandoned, or suicidal. These are written down and saved as a note in the patient's cell phone.

1. Watch an episode of my favorite show

2. Go to the park and walk for 2 miles

3. Call a close friend and invite them over

4. Call my therapist

5. Go to the emergency department

- *Enhance mentalization*—Mentalization consists of the ability to reflect on and develop an understanding of the beliefs, feelings, attitudes, desires, hopes, and knowledge of others.[73] Mentalization allows the patient to consider the world from the point of view of others. By understanding other people's perspectives more accurately, the patient can respond more appropriately. In addition, repetitive, maladaptive responses can be identified and reconsidered. You can offer tentative alternate explanations for the motivations of others. While this may include references to previous relationships, the focus in supportive therapy remains on making changes in the present not just understanding the past.

Case Study—Using Mentalization to Consider the Behavior of Others

Ms. A discusses an interaction with a coworker that had led her to quit a job she otherwise enjoyed.

Therapist—I understand that you think Nancy dislikes you because she was always interrupting you at work. She never wanted to hear what you had to say. I remember that your father also never wanted to hear your side of the story.

Ms. A—If I tried to explain myself, he said I was talking back and arguing. That made the punishment much worse.

Therapist—So I can see why you might think that Nancy was trying to shut you up. From what you have been saying, though, it sounds like Nancy interrupts everyone. I wonder if maybe she was just inconsiderate, and that it is not about you at all? Maybe she is just more interested in hearing her opinion than in hearing anyone else's opinion.

Ms. A—You mean Nancy is just kind of a jerk, and she is a jerk to me because she is a jerk to everyone.

Therapist—What do you think about that idea? Does that sound like a possible explanation?

- *Increase self-observation*—Initially helping the patient understand the causes and impact of their decisions and responses might lie solely with you as the therapist. Patients may not understand why they behave in the way they do or grasp how their conduct impacts those around them. You will need to help the patient reach conclusions they could not reach on their own.[7] Gradually, however, patients can start stepping back and observing their own emotional responses, decisions, and behaviors in light of what they have learned in therapy. Developing this observing ego allows the patient to gain some emotional distance and monitor themselves in a more objective fashion. As the therapist, you then ally yourself with the patient's observing ego and support its functioning. Gradually, the patient will develop more confidence in their ability to act in a manner consistent with their goals.[66] Through repetition, the patient will gradually be able to do for themselves what they had previously relied on you to do. So, rather than turning to the therapist for validation, patients can explicitly validate their own responses.

Case Study—Enhancing Self-Observation

Ms. A is discussing an upsetting encounter at a grocery store.

Therapist—So let's see if I understand. You were in line at the store, but one of your items did not have a price on it, and it took a long time for the manager to find the price. While you were standing there, the people in line behind you looked annoyed with you. You initially felt sad and stupid, but then something changed.

Ms. A—I asked myself what you would have said if you were there.

Therapist—And what do you think I would have said?

Ms. A—You would probably have said that it was not my fault they did not have the price on the item, and it was not my fault that it took so long to find the price. The people behind me might have been annoyed, but that was not my fault either.

Therapist—And how did you feel after thinking that?

Ms. A—Less upset.

5

Effect Changes to Help Reduce Stressors and Increase Support

Some forms of psychotherapy seek to improve current symptoms by evaluating long-standing patterns in an indirect fashion. CBT helps alleviate depression by looking for maladaptive thinking patterns. Psychodynamic psychotherapy may address anxiety by looking at unconscious patterns of relationships and expectations. In SP, the focus is on the current problem.[7] The immediate goal of alleviating current distress and improving current functioning remains the constant focus of SP. As a supportive psychotherapist, your primary focus on making an impact in the patient's life in the near future will require the selection of treatment goals that are specific, measurable, and time-limited (see Box 5.2). Selecting circumstances or symptoms that are immediately bothersome to the patient ensures that the goals will be specific and relevant.

Box 5.2   Good Collaborative Goals are SMART Goals

Specific

Measurable

Achievable

Relevant

Time-limited

Case Study—Setting Collaborative Goals

While in the ICU, Ms. A and the psychiatry resident discussed the events leading up to her admission. They generated a narrative that focused on Ms. A's series of unstable relationships. These fluctuating relationships led to labile moods that she feels unable to control. Optimizing her social support (relationships) and learning to control her moods became general goals for treatment. They agreed that she could make some changes in how she views and chooses her relationships, and that she could start this work while on the inpatient psychiatric unit. She also indicated she tends to make poorer decisions when she has not had enough sleep or when she has had more to drink than she planned to. She and the resident identified sleep stabilization and improved sleep hygiene as two additional, specific goals. This led her to agree to the psychiatric admission.

It is also important in supportive therapy to focus on ways to *increase social support.* Individuals with severe mental illness or those who are overwhelmed by circumstances may feel separated from social connections. They may isolate themselves or turn to unhealthy relationships because they are easier, more familiar, or result in more immediate benefits. While providing SP, you can help patients evaluate the nature and quality of their current relationships. Nurturing and supportive relationships can be optimized while exposure to toxic relationships is minimized. If there is an absence of positive relationships, strategies can be developed to create them. You can discuss a variety of social options based on which would be most beneficial to the patient. This could include formal group therapy, self-help groups, religious meetings, community classes, and/or interactions with family and friends. These interactions can provide socially acceptable means of asking for, receiving, and providing support. Patients in a group setting can use these skills to develop healthier means of relating to others.[68] Patients can be encouraged to join these groups while in individual therapy, so that the benefits and drawbacks can be discussed.

Your treatment relationship with the patient is also an important and meaningful source of support. All forms of therapy include supportive elements. In SP, these are paramount. The aim is to create a structured and trusting relationship. By creating an environment of safety and security, you enable patients to be honest and forthcoming regarding their most painful emotions and distressing conflicts. With the support of their therapist, patients can then choose to take the risk of making meaningful changes in their relationships.[64] As an SP provider, you also model effective interpersonal and communication skills for the patient. Through active engagement, demonstrating respect and acceptance, and asking and answering questions directly but tactfully, you serve as an example for the patient to follow.[7,74] Modeling these behaviors improves the treatment relationship and can also be generalized by the patient to improve their other relationships.

Supportive psychotherapists should keep their focus on the "here and now" aspects of the patient's life. Ideally, each session involves discussions and interventions that could potentially diminish distress, improve functioning, or enhance social support by:

- *Optimizing treatment adherence*—Discussions of treatment adherence can start with the benefits and proper way of taking medications. The patient should have a clear understanding of the difference between regular medications and "PRN medications." Adherence is improved when providers discuss likely side effects and inquire about them regularly. Adherence also includes the importance of regular attendance at therapy sessions and completing homework assignments.

- *Improving reality testing*—Enhanced reality testing is needed when a patient's decisions or mood are determined by delusions, hallucinations, or other mental distortions. Random events in the environment can be ascribed undue significance, or the motivations and intentions of others can be grossly misinterpreted. A more subtle form of altered reality testing can show up in the pessimism of depression or the risk avoidance of anxiety.[64] With patients whose lives are being directed by delusions or hallucinations, the initial goal is to create a "double awareness" in which the patient's belief is unchallenged, while the therapist simultaneously introduces some doubts about the patient's perceived reality. You must compassionately acknowledge the patient's beliefs and emotional response while expressing a differing experience or understanding, to offer an alternate explanation for the patient's experience. The individual in this stage may accept or reject your explanation or may try to suppress or conceal their experiences. As the patient starts to question the reality of their experience, the provider can strengthen the likelihood and benefits of a more reality-based decision,[75] eg, *Mr. Jones, I know that you hear your mother's voice telling you that you should kill yourself and join her in Heaven, but I can't hear her. No one else hears that voice. It is coming from within your own head. I believe it is part of your illness. The reason you are hearing it more now is because you stopped your medication. If you were to restart your medication, I believe the voice would not bother you as much.*

- *Collaborative problem-solving*—Patients with severe mental illness or catastrophic circumstances often feel powerless. They may never have learned efficient problem-solving techniques or may be hindered in using them. You can work collaboratively with your patients to help improve their problem-solving skills. Problem-solving starts with a realistic assessment of the resources that are at hand and a recognition of what is, and is not, within the patient's ability to control. Initially, your intervention could be as straightforward as listing all of their options and weighing the pros and cons of each. Alternately, you and the patient can generate a list of possible actions and weigh the chances of success for each option. These techniques can be taught and practiced. You can help the patient develop a strategy to research choices and to address the barriers that limit available options. Developing these skills will help the patient address current problems and teach a rational and reproducible approach to managing future difficulties.[76]

- *Directly enhancing social skills*—Many chronically ill patients lack the basic social skills to seek services or engage with others. They can be instructed in techniques, and these techniques can be practiced in the sessions and through homework. Targeted skills can be as simple as maintaining appropriate eye contact, starting and maintaining social interactions, recognizing social cues, using appropriate self-assertion, using the telephone, or asking questions of health workers.[64] After practicing with you, the patient can be guided to try these new skills on others. The results can be discussed in subsequent sessions.

- *Role-playing situations in therapy*—Role-playing is an essential component of SP. It can be used to enhance social skills, prepare for difficult situations, or challenge dysfunctional thoughts. When patients are unsure of what to do, different approaches can be developed and practiced through role-playing.[77] Often the role-play will start with a discussion of how the patient would like to respond. You can then play the role of the patient and try various responses until working together you reach an acceptable "script." You can then shift roles and have the patient play themselves and practice the script that was developed. Resistance to role-playing can sometimes be overcome by emphasizing the importance of practice in developing any skill. Analogies can be developed that are meaningful to the patient and that highlight the importance of practicing a skill to perfect it, eg, batting practice in baseball, rehearsals for musicians.

- *Offering anticipatory guidance*—Anticipatory guidance helps patients prepare for potentially problematic future events. Based on your understanding of the patient's story, you can anticipate interactions and situations that will likely cause the patient difficulty. These problems could involve issues with scheduling, finances, relationships, or anniversaries. After discussing the problem, you will work with the patient to develop possible strategies for dealing with the situation. Once a strategy has been determined, the response can be practiced in the session, allowing the patient to gain a sense of mastery.[74] For example, *in a month it will be the anniversary of your son's death. I think we should start thinking about how you are going to handle that day. Is it best to distract yourself, or should you spend the day deliberately thinking about and remembering your son?* Over time, the patient can learn to perform all of these functions on their own and begin to anticipate and assertively respond to potential future problems.

- *Assigning and reviewing homework*—The benefits of all of these techniques can be heightened by the addition of homework, which vastly increases the amount of time the patient spends on therapeutic activities. Following through with homework in CBT is associated with increased progress,[76] and the same is likely true for SP. There should be an intimate connection between what happens in the therapy session and the homework that is assigned. The therapy session should allow the patient to master the skill required for the homework, while the homework should be a continuation of what has happened in the session. Part of assigning homework is ensuring that the patient understands what is being asked of them and why it is important for them to complete the assignment. The patient should be asked to collaborate on the amount and type of homework assigned. Ask them to identify potential barriers to completing the homework. Potential barriers should be addressed proactively.

If the homework is not completed, this becomes a focus for discussion in the following session. Often there might have been miscommunication about the homework. Did the patient understand what was being asked? Were they able to complete the homework? Did they understand why it was important? Patients can be asked if there were unexpected barriers to completing the homework that could be modified in the future. Finally, if possible, incomplete homework should be completed during the sessions to give them further experience with the skills required.[78]

INTERVENTIONS SHARED BY SP, CBT, AND PSYCHODYNAMIC THERAPY

In the "Y Model of psychotherapy," both CBT and psychodynamic psychotherapy exist on a continuum, where "pure" CBT or psychodynamic psychotherapy exist at one end and "pure" SP sits at the other[60] (see Chapter 1 of this book as well). In reality, many therapists combine SP with CBT or psychodynamic psychotherapy. A review of three studies assessing techniques used by therapists found the widespread use of supportive techniques in both CBT and psychodynamic psychotherapy.[79] Many CBT patients will not be able to acquire or use new cognitive or behavioral skills unless CBT takes place in a supportive, empathic relationship with their therapist.[80] Practitioners of psychodynamic, or expressive, psychotherapy had once been guided by the motto "Be as expressive as you can be, and as supportive as you have to be."[81] More recently, however, there is growing recognition of the intimate connection between psychodynamic and supportive approaches. An intensive study of patients followed for expressive or supportive psychotherapy through the Menninger Clinic found that efforts to "categorically distinguish the purely expressive from the truly mixed from the purely supportive treatments…would have been neither possible nor truly helpful."[26] Rather than referring to psychotherapy as either expressive or supportive psychotherapy, it might be more accurate to describe it as an expressive-supportive (or supportive-expressive) psychotherapy.[68,81] Supportive psychotherapists can use a broad array of therapeutic interventions including those also useful in CBT or psychodynamic psychotherapy.

Interventions/Approaches Shared by Supportive Psychotherapy and Cognitive Behavioral Therapy

Both SP and CBT involve a focus on the present and an active therapist stance, and as a result, they share many interventions and approaches. Some of these shared interventions include:

- Focus on the here and now
- Behavioral activation
- Relaxation/mindfulness techniques
- Cognitive restructuring
- Use of structured sessions
- Homework
- Role-play

The implementation of CBT and its distinct features and associated techniques will be more fully discussed in Chapter 6.

5

Interventions/Approaches Shared by Supportive Psychotherapy and Psychodynamic Psychotherapy

Along the supportive-expressive continuum, there will be interventions and approaches that are shared by SP and psychodynamic psychotherapy. These include:

- Commenting on patterns of relationships
- Promoting the use of healthier psychological defenses
- Discussing how the past impacts the present
- Managing the transference relationship

A note here on transference in supportive versus psychodynamic psychotherapy. You will learn more about transference and countertransference in Chapter 7. However, a simple definition of "transference" would include the unconscious feelings, attitudes, and expectations that the patient has toward the therapist. Individuals undergoing SP may have extreme transference responses based on their childhood and past experiences in treatment. Patients will tend to recreate past relationships with the therapist playing a variety of roles. This is often a major focus of exploration and interpretation in psychodynamic psychotherapy. In SP, transference is handled differently. You will want to recognize and manage transference but not necessarily discuss or even comment on it. Extremes of either positive or negative transference must be dealt with expeditiously, but they are often adjusted without interpretation. Management of negative transference may require that you openly discuss what you are doing and why you are doing it.[66] For example, patients with an extremely negative attitude can be reassured that you are concerned about them and are working in their interest. This can be made in a matter-of-fact fashion without any reference to the early childhood origins of the transference.[64] Patients with an overly positive transference can be supportively reminded of the boundaries and limitations of the therapeutic relationship. Transference and related interventions will be discussed more fully in Chapter 7.

Conclusion

SP focuses on improving functioning, minimizing distress, enhancing social support, and directly addressing stresses. SP techniques can be found in most forms of psychotherapy, and SP often borrows approaches and interventions from a variety of other therapies; nevertheless, SP stands as a distinct and valuable form of psychotherapy that can be conceptualized as a stand-alone treatment. Practitioners of SP can use their skills with a vast array of patients, from those suffering with the most severe of chronic mental illnesses to those who are experiencing a temporary setback due to medical illnesses or life circumstances. SP can be modified and used successfully in all clinical venues. For these reasons, competence in SP should be a goal for all mental health clinicians. Disparaged as the "Cinderella of psychotherapies" for decades, it is now time to give SP its proper recognition as an impactful and important form of psychotherapeutic treatment.

Self-Study Questions

1. Describe the HOPE model of supportive psychotherapy.

2. After completing question 1, list at least two strategies for each of the four components of the HOPE model of supportive psychotherapy.

3. Supportive psychotherapy is an efficacious therapy but often not cited as an empirically supported treatment option. Why is that?

4. Create an example of a SMART goal.

5. List at least two commonalities between supportive psychotherapy and either psychodynamic psychotherapy or CBT.

RESOURCES FOR FURTHER LEARNING

Brenner AM. Teaching supportive psychotherapy in the twenty-first century. *Harv Rev Psychiatry.* 2012;20:259-267.

Crocker EM. Supportive psychotherapy. In: Black DW, ed. *Scientific American Psychiatry* [online]. Hamilton, ON: Decker Intellectual Properties; 2017. Available at http://www.SciAmPsychiatry.com. Accessed March 31, 2018.

Dewald PA. Principles of supportive psychotherapy. *Am J Psychother.* 1994;48:505-518.

Novalis PN, Singer V, Peele R. *Clinical Manual of Supportive Psychotherapy.* 2nd ed. Washington, DC: American Psychiatric Association Publishing; 2020.

Winston A. Supportive psychotherapy. In: Hales RE, Yudofsky SC, Roberts LW, eds. *The American Psychiatric Publishing Textbook of Psychiatry.* 6th ed. Arlington, VA: American Psychiatric Publishing, Inc; 2014:1161-1188.

REFERENCES

1. Crocker EM. Supportive psychotherapy. In: Black DW, ed. *Scientific American Psychiatry* [online]. Hamilton, ON: Decker Intellectual Properties; 2017. Available at http://www.SciAmPsychiatry.com. Accessed March 31, 2018.
2. Sullivan PR. Learning theories and supportive psychotherapy. *Am J Psychiatry.* 1971;128(6):763-766.
3. Conte HR, Plutchik R. Controlled research in supportive psychotherapy. *Psychiatr Ann.* 1986;16(9):530-533.
4. Markowitz JC. What is supportive psychotherapy? *Focus.* 2014;12:285-289.
5. Winston A, Pinsker H, McCullough L. A review of supportive psychotherapy. *Hosp Community Psychiatry.* 1986;37(11):1105-1114.
6. Hellerstein DJ, Pinsker H, Rosenthal RN, Klee S. Supportive therapy as the treatment model of choice. *J Psychother Pract Res.* 1994;3(4):300.
7. Dewald PA. Principles of supportive psychotherapy. *Am J Psychother.* 1994;48:505-518.
8. Sudak DM, Goldberg DA. Trends in psychotherapy training: a national survey of psychiatry residency training. *Acad Psychiatry.* 2012;36(5):369-373.
9. Pinsker H. The role of theory in teaching supportive psychotherapy. *Am J Psychother.* 1994;48(4):530-542.
10. Rockland LH. A review of supportive psychotherapy, 1986-1992. *Psychiatr Serv.* 1993;44(11):1053-1060.
11. Hellerstein DJ, Markowitz JC. Developing supportive psychotherapy as evidence-based treatment. *Am J Psychiatry.* 2008;165(10):1355-1356.
12. Luborsky L, Diguer L, Seligman DA, et al. The researcher's own therapy allegiances: A "wild card" in comparisons of treatment efficacy. *Clin Psychol Sci Pract.* 1999;6(1):95-106.
13. Munder T, Bruetsch O, Leonhart R, Gerger H, Barth J. Researcher allegiance in psychotherapy outcome research: an overview of reviews. *Clin Psychol Rev.* 2013;33(4):501-511.
14. Budge S, Baardseth TP, Wampold BE, Flückiger C. Researcher allegiance and supportive therapy: pernicious affects on results of randomized clinical trials. *Eur J Psychother Couns.* 2010;12(1):23-39.
15. Shear MK, Pilkonis PA, Cloitre M, Leon AC. Cognitive behavioral treatment compared with nonprescriptive treatment of panic disorder. *Arch Gen Psychiatry.* 1994;51(5):395-401.
16. Zitrin CM, Klein DF, Woerner MG. Behavior therapy, supportive psychotherapy, imipramine, and phobias. *Arch Gen Psychiatry.* 1978;35(3):307-316.
17. Klein DF, Zitrin CM, Woerner MG, Ross DC. Treatment of phobias: II. Behavior therapy and supportive psychotherapy: are there any specific ingredients? *Arch Gen Psychiatry.* 1983;40(2):139-145.
18. Lipsitz JD, Gur M, Vermes D, et al. A randomized trial of interpersonal therapy versus supportive therapy for social anxiety disorder. *Depress Anxiety.* 2008;25(6):542-553.
19. Cuijpers P, Driessen E, Hollon SD, van Oppen P, Barth J, Andersson G. The efficacy of non-directive supportive therapy for adult depression: a meta-analysis. *Clin Psychol Rev.* 2012;32(4):280-291.
20. Maina G, Forner F, Bogetto F. Randomized controlled trial comparing brief dynamic and supportive therapy with waiting list condition in minor depressive disorders. *Psychother Psychosom.* 2005;74(1):43-50.
21. Markowitz JC, Kocsis JH, Bleiberg KL, Christos PJ, Sacks M. A comparative trial of psychotherapy and pharmacotherapy for "pure" dysthymic patients. *J Affect Disord.* 2005;89(1-3):167-175.
22. Ashman T, Cantor JB, Tsaousides T, Spielman L, Gordon W. Comparison of cognitive behavioral therapy and supportive psychotherapy for the treatment of depression following traumatic brain injury: a randomized controlled trial. *J Head Trauma Rehabil.* 2014;29(6):467-478.
23. Gunderson JG, Frank AF, Katz HM, Vannicelli ML, Frosch JP, Knapp PH. Effects of psychotherapy in schizophrenia: II. Comparative outcome of two forms of treatment. *Schizophr Bull.* 1984;10(4):564-598.
24. Rosenbaum B, Harder S, Knudsen P, et al. Supportive psychodynamic psychotherapy versus treatment as usual for first-episode psychosis: two-year outcome. *Psychiatry.* 2012;75(4):331-341.
25. Hellerstein DJ, Rosenthal RN, Pinsker H, Samstag LW, Muran JC, Winston A. A randomized prospective study comparing supportive and dynamic therapies: outcome and alliance. *J Psychother Pract Res.* 1998;7(4):261.
26. Wallerstein RS. The psychotherapy research project of the Menninger Foundation: an overview. *J Consult Clin Psychol.* 1989;57:195-205.
27. Clarkin JF, Levy KN, Lenzenweger MF, Kernberg OF. Evaluating three treatments for borderline personality disorder: a multiwave study. *Am J Psychiatry.* 2007;164(6):922-928.
28. Jørgensen CR, Freund C, Bøye R, Jordet H, Andersen D, Kjølbye M. Outcome of mentalization-based and supportive psychotherapy in patients with borderline personality disorder: a randomized trial. *Acta Psychiatr Scand.* 2013;127(4):305-317.
29. Piper WE, Joyce AS, McCallum M, Azim HF. Interpretive and supportive forms of psychotherapy and patient personality variables. *J Consult Clin Psychol.* 1998;66(3):558.

30. McIntosh VV, Jordan J, Carter FA, et al. Three psychotherapies for anorexia nervosa: a randomized, controlled trial. *Am J Psychiatry.* 2005;162(4):741-747.
31. Markowitz JC, Kocsis JH, Christos P, Bleiberg K, Carlin A. Pilot study of interpersonal psychotherapy versus supportive psychotherapy for dysthymic patients with secondary alcohol abuse or dependence. *J Nerv Ment Dis.* 2008;196(6):468-474.
32. O'Malley SS, Jaffe AJ, Chang G, Schottenfeld RS, Meyer RE, Rounsaville B. Naltrexone and coping skills therapy for alcohol dependence: a controlled study. *Arch Gen Psychiatry.* 1992;49(11):881-887.
33. Luborsky L, McLellan AT, Woody GE, O'Brien CP, Auerbach A. Therapist success and its determinants. *Arch Gen Psychiatry.* 1985;42(6):602-611.
34. Najavits LM, Weiss RD. Variations in therapist effectiveness in the treatment of patients with substance use disorders: an empirical review. *Addiction.* 1994;89(6):679-688.
35. Block S. Supportive psychotherapy. *Br J Hosp Med.* 1977;18:63-67.
36. Conte HR, Karasu TB. Psychotherapy for medically ill patients: review and critique of controlled studies. *Psychosomatics.* 1981;22:285-315.
37. Williamson PS. Psychotherapy by family physicians. *Prim Care.* 1987;14(4):803-816.
38. Mohl PC. Brief supportive psychotherapy by the primary care physician. *Tex Med.* 1988;84(9):28.
39. Rockland LH. Advances in supportive psychotherapy. *Curr Opin Psychiatry.* 1995;8(3):150-153.
40. Schindler BA, Shook J, Schwartz GM. Beneficial effects of psychiatric intervention on recovery after coronary artery bypass graft surgery. *Gen Hosp Psychiatry.* 1989;11(5):358-364.
41. Salzmann S, Euteneuer F, Laferton JA, et al. Effects of preoperative psychological interventions on catecholamine and cortisol levels after surgery in coronary artery bypass graft patients: the randomized controlled PSY-HEART trial. *Psychosom Med.* 2017;79(7):806-814.
42. Sjödin I, Svedlund J, Ottosson JO, Dotevall G. Controlled study of psychotherapy in chronic peptic ulcer disease. *Psychosomatics.* 1986;27(3):187-200.
43. Svedlund J. Psychotherapy in irritable bowel syndrome: a controlled outcome study. *Acta Psychiatr Scand.* 1983;67:1-86.
44. Taylor CB, Zlutnick SI, Corley MJ, Flora J. The effects of detoxification, relaxation, and brief supportive therapy on chronic pain. *Pain.* 1980;8(3):319-329.
45. Rutledge T, Atkinson JH, Chircop-Rollick T, et al. Randomized controlled trial of telephone-delivered cognitive behavioral therapy versus supportive care for chronic back pain. *Clin J Pain.* 2018;34(4):322-327.
46. Spiegel D, Bloom JR, Yalom I. Group support for patients with metastatic cancer: a randomized prospective outcome study. *Arch Gen Psychiatry.* 1981;38(5):527-533.
47. Spiegel D, Bloom JR. Group therapy and hypnosis reduce metastatic breast carcinoma pain. *Psychosom Med.* 1983;45(4):333-339.
48. Mukherjee A, Mazumder K, Kaushal V, Ghoshal S. Effect of supportive psychotherapy on mental health status and quality of life of female cancer patients receiving chemotherapy for recurrent disease. *Indian J Palliat Care.* 2017;23(4):399-402.
49. Blanco C, Markowitz JC, Hellerstein DJ, et al. A randomized trial of interpersonal psychotherapy, problem solving therapy, and supportive therapy for major depressive disorder in women with breast cancer. *Breast Cancer Res Treat.* 2019;173(2):353-364.
50. Ruchiwit M. The effect of the one-to-one interaction process with group supportive psychotherapy on the levels of hope, anxiety and self-care practice for patients that have experienced organ loss: an alternative nursing care model. *Int J Nurs Pract.* 2012;18(4):363-372.
51. Ditzen B, Heinrichs M. Psychobiology of social support: the social dimension of stress buffering. *Restor Neurol Neurosci.* 2014;32(1):149-162.
52. Uchino BN, Garvey TS. The availability of social support reduces cardiovascular reactivity to acute psychological stress. *J Behav Med.* 1997;20(1):15-27.
53. Eisenberger NI, Taylor SE, Gable SL, Hilmert CJ, Lieberman MD. Neural pathways link social support to attenuated neuroendocrine stress responses. *Neuroimage.* 2007;35:1601-1612.
54. Roberts MH, Klatzkin RR, Mechlin B. Social support attenuates physiological stress responses and experimental pain sensitivity to cold pressor pain. *Ann Behav Med.* 2015;49(4):557-569.
55. Brown JL, Sheffield D, Leary MR, Robinson ME. Social support and experimental pain. *Psychosom Med.* 2003;65:276-283.
56. Uchino BN, Uno D, Holt-Lunstad J. Social support, physiological processes, and health. *Curr Dir Psychol Sci.* 1999;8(5):145-148.
57. Glaser R, Rice J, Sheridan J, et al. Stress-related immune suppression: health implications. *Brain Behav Immun.* 1987;1:7-20.
58. Berkman LF. The relationship of social networks and social support to morbidity and mortality. In: Cohen S, Syme SL, eds. *Social Support and Health.* San Diego, CA: Academic Press, Inc; 1985:241-262.
59. House JS, Landis KR, Umberson D. Social relationships and health. *Science.* 1988;24:540-545.

5

60. Plakun EM, Sudak DM, Goldberg D. The Y model: an integrated, evidence-based approach to teaching psychotherapy competencies. *J Psychiatr Pract*. 2009;15:5-11.

61. Lambert MJ, Barley DE. Research summary on the therapeutic relationship and psychotherapy outcome. *Psychotherapy*. 2001;38:357-361.

62. Wampold BE. How important are the common factors in psychotherapy? An update. *World Psychiatry*. 2015;14:270-277.

63. Halpern J. What is clinical empathy. *J Gen Intern Med*. 2003;18:670-674.

64. Novalis PN, Rojcewicz SJ, Peele R. *Clinical Manual of Supportive Psychotherapy*. Washington, DC: American Psychiatric Press, Inc; 1993.

65. Bordin ES. The generalizability of the psychoanalytic concept of the working alliance. *Psychotherapy*. 1979;16:252-260.

66. Misch DA. Basic strategies of dynamic supportive therapy. *J Psychother Pract Res*. 2000;9:173-189.

67. Brenner AM. Teaching supportive psychotherapy in the twenty-first century. *Harv Rev Psychiatry*. 2012;20:259-267.

68. Douglas CJ. Teaching supportive psychotherapy to psychiatric residents. *Am J Psychiatry*. 2008;165:445-452.

69. Holmes J. Supportive psychotherapy: the search for positive meanings. *Br J Psychiatry*. 1995;167:439-445.

70. Welton R, Roman B. Mood disorders: evidence-based integrated biopsychosocial treatment of bipolar disorder. In: Muse M, ed. *Cognitive Behavioral Psychopharmacology*. Hoboken, NJ: John Wiley and Sons; 2018.

71. Carr A. Michael White's narrative therapy. *Contemp Fam Ther*. 1998;20:485-503.

72. Stanley B, Brown GK. Safety planning intervention: a brief intervention to mitigate suicide risk. *Cogn Behav Pract*. 2012;19:256-264.

73. Fonagy R. *Attachment Theory and Psychoanalysis*. New York, NY: Other Press; 2001.

74. Winston A. Supportive psychotherapy. In: Hales RE, Yudofsky SC, Roberts LW, eds. *The American Psychiatric Publishing Textbook of Psychiatry*. 6th ed. Arlington, VA: American Psychiatric Publishing, Inc; 2014:1161-1188.

75. Gentile JP, Niemann P. Supportive Psychotherapy for a patient with psychosis: schizophreniform disorder. *Psychiatry*. 2006;3:56-61.

76. Kazantzis N, Whittington C, Dattilio F. Meta-analysis of homework effects in cognitive and behavioral therapy: a replication and extension. *Clin Psychol Sci Pract*. 2010;17(2):144-156.

77. Beck JS. *Cognitive Behavior Therapy: Basics and Beyond*. 2nd ed. New York, NY: The Guilford Press; 2011.

78. Wright JH, Sudak DM, Turkinton D, Thase ME. *High-yield Cognitive-Behavior Therapy for Brief Sessions: An Illustrated Guide*. Washington, DC: American Psychiatric Publishing, Inc; 2010.

79. Barber JP, Stratt R, Halperin G, Connolly MB. Supportive techniques: are they found in different therapies? *J Psychother Pract Res*. 2001;10:165-172.

80. Beck JS. *Cognitive Therapy for Challenging Problems: What to Do When the Basics Don't Work*. New York, NY: The Guilford Press; 2011.

81. Gabbard GO. *Psychodynamic Psychiatry in Clinical Practice*. 5th ed. Washington, DC: American Psychiatric Publishing, Inc; 2014.

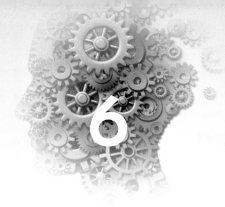

Cognitive Behavioral Therapy

DONNA M. SUDAK, MD AND PRASAD R. JOSHI, MD, PhD

Case Study: Steve—A Patient With Depression and Anxiety

Steve is a 26-year-old who grew up in a small suburban area and now lives in a large city. He is employed as an assistant chef in an upscale restaurant. Steve came for treatment for worsening depression and anxiety. He was dressed in sweats and slumped in his chair. He appeared anxious, shaking his legs, and wringing his hands. He said that he just could not seem to stop worrying about "everything in my life, my life is going nowhere" and ruminating about his lack of career progress, "I am still working as an assistant chef. I should be doing so much better by now." He finds it difficult to focus and concentrate, leading to mistakes at work. When coworkers point out his mistakes, he is easily irritated. His boss expressed concern about Steve's work performance last week. Ever since, Steve has been worrying "constantly" about termination, saying "I know my boss now hates me completely." He has initial insomnia and stays awake worrying about work, paying bills, and his relationship with his girlfriend. "She has been avoiding me lately; I know she does not really like me anymore; everything is going downhill."

About a month ago, while preparing for dinner service, he suddenly experienced chest pain, sweating, intense anxiety, palpitations, and dizziness and thought he was going to "have a heart attack." Steve went to a nearby emergency room and was told he had a panic attack. He has had panic attacks every 2 to 3 days since that time and leaves the room if he is with others until it passes. He feels "sad and low" most days over the last 2 months, with "no energy in the morning." He thinks his situation is hopeless, and he wants to "just give up," with occasions of wanting to not wake up, though he denies thoughts of suicide.

Steve reported that he previously had "long periods of gloom, especially in the winter, ever since I was a teenager," but handled these episodes on his own. He believes the onset of his first depression was when he was 16, after his family home was destroyed by fire. His family survived this calamity, but his beloved pet dog died in the fire. As Steve is an only child, this loss was particularly hard on him. He experienced recurrent nightmares about the fire "for years," though he denies current nightmares or flashbacks. Two years after the fire, Steve's parents divorced. He remembers starting to "worry a lot" at that time. "I did not know who I could count on and whether I would be able to go to college." He always wanted to be a chef and went to culinary school but was "always stressed." Steve is generally healthy with the exception of having asthma, which was "much worse" during childhood, now only worse during times of "stressful" events. His girlfriend and his aunt are described as his current closest supports, despite the fact that both parents live nearby.

INTRODUCTION

Cognitive behavioral therapy (CBT) is an action-oriented, empirically supported form of psychotherapy, which provides patients with skills that convey durable recovery from many psychiatric illnesses. It has broad applications and utility and is easily combined with pharmacological interventions. In addition, the principles of CBT are ideally suited for individuals who must cope with chronic medical problems. As the name indicates, CBT comprises an integrated approach to understanding and modifying thoughts (cognitive) and behaviors (behavioral) underlying common psychiatric conditions such as major depression and generalized anxiety. Although conceptualized as a seamlessly integrated therapy at present, the behavioral and cognitive streams of CBT initially developed separately.

We also need to dispel a bit of rumor and myth surrounding CBT as a treatment approach. Although CBT was manualized as a treatment in order to evaluate its efficacy in research studies, it is neither mechanistic nor unconcerned with emotional responses. Instead, CBT is a collaborative and principle-driven therapy that is creative and requires a strong therapeutic bond between the therapist and patient.

THEORETICAL FOUNDATIONS AND HISTORY OF CBT

The origins of the behavioral elements of CBT may be traced back to the early 20th century, beginning with the rise of behaviorism. Behaviorism, a framework to explain human behavior and motivation, originated in academic psychology and was based on evidence from laboratory studies of animal behavior. Strict behaviorists contended that the mind and its thoughts could not be measured directly and could not be quantified. Instead, behaviorists empirically investigated the effect of events or stimuli on particular behaviors; both of which can be observed and studied. This paradigm was in contrast to psychoanalysis, with its emphasis on material from clinical case studies and abstract concepts such as structures of the mind and defense mechanisms—phenomena that cannot be observed or quantified directly. Behaviorism was heavily influenced by learning theory, beginning with Pavlov and his now famous experiments. Pavlov's early work proved that humans (similar to lab animals) learned by associating one stimulus with another and that learning generalizes. Although controversial, as the experiment involved human subjects, the development marked an important step in application of principles of behaviorism to modify psychological and behavioral states in humans.

Thorndike and, later, Skinner were influential in promoting the development of methods to modify human behaviors. Skinner showed that animals increase or decrease behavior based on responses (operants) from the environment. When a behavior is followed by a reward (eg, completing homework is followed by being given a piece of candy), the behavior is strengthened (called reinforcement). On the other hand, if a behavior is followed by an aversive experience (called punishment), the behavior is weakened (eg, adding extra chores when failing to do homework). An early therapeutic application of behavioral principles was in anxiety and panic disorders, conditions marked by clearly delineated somatic and behavioral components accompanying aversive emotional states. **Behavioral experiments** showed that a specific fear or phobia can be effectively reduced by imagined or actual exposure to the feared situation.[1] These and other such principles led to the development of several behavioral therapies, including assertiveness training, progressive relaxation, systematic desensitization, and social **skills training**, which treated a variety of clinical conditions including phobias, social anxiety, generalized anxiety, bedwetting, insomnia, and stuttering. Such interventions in their contemporary form are a core part of a number of treatment protocols in CBT.

The central principle of CBT holds that our emotional and behavioral reactions to events are influenced not by the events themselves but by how we perceive them. This idea has its roots in stoicism, a Greek philosophy. CBT also incorporates ideas from existentialism and Buddhism.[2] CBT holds that cognitive patterns (thoughts) about events, and not the actual events, define how we perceive reality, and that in psychopathological states, those thoughts tend to be more extreme and inaccurate.

In the 1950s, an early precursor to CBT was developed by George Kelly, who wrote a two-volume work "*A Psychology of Personal Constructs.*" Kelly proposed a theory that covered a broad range of psychopathology entirely based on styles of cognitive processing (personal constructs).[3] He suggested that a person uses "constructs" to build a personal version of reality, influencing both "normal" functioning and psychopathological states. Kelly also proposed "constructive alternativism" whereby one could construct alternatives to counter preexisting maladaptive constructs. This therapeutic approach continues to exist in the modern version of CBT as the core of cognitive restructuring. In the 1960s, Albert Ellis developed rational emotive behavioral therapy (REBT), which integrated cognitive and behavioral approaches at a conceptual level. While developing this approach, Ellis used ideas from stoicism, including the idea that beliefs about a situation determine emotional responses and difficult life circumstances require coping efforts and, when necessary, acceptance.

Another major influence on the development of cognitive therapy was the "cognitive revolution," in the 1960s and 1970s. These decades saw an increasing congruence of theories in academic psychology, evolutionary biology, learning theory, behavioral science, neuroscience, and computer science, collectively known as the cognitive revolution. The cognitive revolution sought to establish the primacy of conscious mental operations to explain how animals (including humans) learn, form memories, develop behavioral plans, interact with the environment, and employ behavioral strategies. The *International Encyclopedia of the Social & Behavioral Sciences* (2001, pp. 9691-9695) describes the cognitive revolution as follows:

> The cognitive revolution was predicated on the possibility that brains—both human and animal—are process control computers contrived by evolution through natural selection. They assess their environment through sensory or perceptual processes; they symbolize the results of these assessments by values stored in memory; they manipulate those values by means of the relevant mental operations (the operations of perception and thought); and they use the results (percepts, inferences, and deductions) to control behavior.

In the 1960s and 1970s, Aaron T. Beck developed cognitive therapy, now more commonly known as cognitive behavioral therapy. Beck was a trained psychoanalyst, whose early career was focused on establishing an empirical basis for psychoanalytic theories of depression. While conducting his clinical studies, Beck noted that people with depression experience dreams with negative themes. Beck postulated the cognitive theory of depression—that a depressed person typically holds negative views of self, the world, and the future. This trifecta is referred to as Beck's cognitive triad. He further postulated that if these negative views were challenged by engaging in a Socratic method of questioning and a more realistic view was adopted, depressive symptoms can be ameliorated.[4,5] Beck's cognitive model postulated that distorted negative views contribute to negative behavioral outcomes (eg, lack of motivation, avoidance, and social isolation), leading to the integration of behavioral strategies in cognitive therapy. Beck also applied scientific rigor to the study of psychotherapeutic treatments.

Treatments Emerging From the CBT Framework

In the past 40 years, a number of new CBT treatment approaches were developed using the broad framework of CBT. One such approach, dialectical behavioral therapy (DBT), was developed by Marsha Linehan[6] to treat borderline personality disorder (BPD). DBT combines elements from CBT (such as exposure and response prevention, skills training, and cognitive restructuring) along with unique elements including mindfulness and behavioral translations of Buddhist practices taught as mindfulness skills. DBT was one of the first approaches collectively termed as "third-wave" cognitive behavioral therapies (strictly behavioral therapies were termed "first wave," and cognitive therapies including Beckian CBT were termed "second wave"). The "third wave" includes acceptance and commitment therapy (ACT) developed by Steven Hayes,[7] cognitive behavioral analysis system of psychotherapy (CBASP) developed by James P. McCullough Jr, metacognitive therapy developed by Adrian Wells, mindfulness-based cognitive therapy developed by Zindel Segal and Mark Williams, and schema therapy developed by Jeffrey E. Young, as reviewed by Hayes and Hofmann.[8] Each of these forms of therapy extends the original paradigm of CBT and integrates particular theoretical constructs that extend the reach of the treatment.

RESEARCH SUPPORTING THE USE OF CBT

A defining characteristic of CBT is a focus on empirical research to identify mechanisms of action as well as to determine efficacy. Cognitive behavioral therapies are typically manual-based and comprise a limited number of sessions *when empirically tested*. However, this manualized method of employing the treatment was not the original intent regarding clinical practice, where individual case conceptualization and treatment planning determine the length of treatment.

CBT is especially well studied for major depression and for the full range of anxiety disorders. However, CBT techniques have also been applied to a fairly diverse group of mental disorders that range from body dysmorphic disorder to personality disorders. A large number of meta-analytic studies, based on results from individual clinical trials, have confirmed the efficacy of CBT in diverse clinical populations for a number of psychiatric diagnoses.[9] Accordingly, available evidence indicates that CBT for depression is more effective than waiting list or no treatment, with a medium effect size, and comparable to pharmacotherapy. The addition of pharmacotherapy to CBT produces additional benefits in depression. CBT is more effective at prolonging time-to-relapse than medication. When compared with other psychotherapy approaches for depression, it is unclear if CBT holds an advantage. Few head-to-head randomized controlled trials of psychotherapy exist relative to comparing medication to therapy or therapy to placebo or waiting-list controls. Another deficiency in the literature exists in terms of a lack of matching studies, which would help us to be more prescriptive about types of therapy or whether combined therapy and medication would be indicated for a particular patient.

The strongest support for the efficacy of CBT approaches exists for anxiety disorders, somatic symptom disorders or "somatoform" disorders, bulimia, anger control problems, and general stress. CBT is considered a first-line treatment for a substantial number of anxiety disorders. The effect sizes range from medium to large. The gains achieved following treatment continue or, in some cases, even improve, during the follow-up period. CBT is superior to pharmacological treatment and produces more durable results. This has obvious public health implications when one considers the cost of untreated anxiety and the lifetime cost of treatment with medication.

CBT and exposure and response prevention (ExRP; a form of behavioral therapy) are both equally efficacious for obsessive compulsive disorder (OCD), with both showing large effect sizes. CBT and pharmacotherapy produce comparable results for OCD. CBT approaches (collectively known as trauma-focused CBT or TF-CBT; see text box below) are effective in treating posttraumatic stress disorder (PTSD) and are considered first-line treatment. These approaches include predominantly cognitive (cognitive processing therapy, CPT, or cognitive therapy for PTSD, CT-PTSD) and behavioral (prolonged exposure or PE therapy).

CBT-Informed Trauma Treatments

Trauma-informed CBT treatments have considerable evidence in all types of trauma. Each requires specific training in the approach. Below is a list of the most common contemporary approaches.

1. Prolonged exposure (PE): PE, developed by Edna Foa and her colleagues,[15] is based on emotional processing theory, which posits that traumatic events are not processed emotionally at the time of a traumatic event. PE focuses on reactivating memories associated with the traumatic event and reinterpreting emotions (eg, fear) in the light of new information.

2. Cognitive processing therapy: According to CPT, developed by Patricia Resick,[16] a traumatic event is followed by inability to adequately process trauma memories and additionally that certain distorted cognitions about self, the world, and the future are common and must be addressed in therapy.

3. Trauma-focused CBT (TF-CBT): TF-CBT, developed by Mannarino, Cohen, and Deblinger,[17] combines both cognitive and behavioral elements, eg, exposure with cognitive restructuring.

4. CT-PTSD, as developed by Ehlers and Clark,[18] combines both exposure-based interventions along with correcting distorted cognitions, integrating new information about the trauma into the trauma memory, and reclaiming prior-valued life pursuits.

CBT approaches have also been applied to a large number of other conditions as well, though the results are less robust. These conditions include, though are not limited to, substance use disorders, insomnia, eating disorders (excluding bulimia nervosa), psychotic disorders including schizophrenia and bipolar disorder, and personality disorders. In addition, CBT is ineffective for antisocial personality disorder, and there are few studies regarding the effectiveness of CBT for personality disorders in general, with the exception of schema therapy and DBT for BPD. DBT is particularly effective in the treatment of BPD and may have other applications for individuals with mood disorders and other conditions that involve dysregulation, such as comorbid substance use disorders. CBT is also not effective in situations where learning is impaired (as in dementia), although in neurocognitive disorders, behavioral activation (BA) is often quite helpful in the early stages of the illness and can be quite helpful for caregivers.

CLINICAL LIMITATIONS OF CBT

CBT is less suitable for patients who have difficulty learning or remembering. Certain conditions have limited or no evidence regarding its use. Individuals who have difficulty forming relationships or trusting care providers require modification of the treatment, particularly as regards enhancing motivation, goal setting, and out-of-session practice. Patients with mania and psychosis may benefit from interventions after the acute symptoms are managed with medication. As with all other therapies, including pharmacotherapy, practitioners must keep a close eye on **measuring progress** with validated instruments and manage lack of progress by discussing and choosing alternative forms of evidence-supported interventions with the patient.

WHERE DO YOU START?

Before beginning, prepare carefully...

Cicero

As noted at the beginning of this chapter, CBT is an action-oriented, empirically supported psychotherapy based on the cognitive behavioral model and learning theory. It seeks to understand and modify the unhelpful thinking and behavior that are associated with common psychiatric conditions. Before reviewing the specific cognitive and behavioral concepts and techniques common to CBT, we must first review the general structure and broad components of this treatment approaches that will help you get started. This includes making a solid assessment, building a therapeutic alliance, collaborative treatment planning, and goal setting.

6

Assessment

All good therapy starts with a good diagnostic assessment, performed while capably attending to the therapeutic alliance and followed by forming a treatment agreement with the patient. In CBT, attention is paid to particular aspects of the history that will determine the course of treatment. These include listening for patterns of typical negative **automatic thoughts** (although not highlighting those during the assessment), evaluating the patient's ability to form a trusting relationship, determining the degree of severity of the patient's diagnosis and the number of comorbid conditions, and whether behavioral deficits or excesses require an initial focus in treatment. The patient's prior experiences in therapy (if any) are assessed, and their ideas about what therapy will entail are elicited. You mentally prioritize a hierarchy of treatment targets as the assessment proceeds, particularly those involving life-threatening behaviors, interpersonal problems that will make therapy more challenging (eg, personality issues or interpersonal chaos in the patient's life), and life circumstances that may become emergencies if not rectified (eg, a college student who is severely depressed and likely to be expelled without an intervention with the Dean's office).

The Therapeutic Alliance

Warmth, genuineness, activity, and shared responsibility are the hallmarks of the **therapeutic alliance** in CBT. Relationship building can be more challenging in patients with more severe problems or in those patients with a history of poor interpersonal functioning. One critical component that facilitates alliance formation is to elicit **feedback** throughout the session. Such feedback makes certain that the patient understands interventions planned and rationale for their use.

Providing assistance with **problem-solving** can often enhance the therapy bond. Many patients enter therapy with a myriad of real-life problems and think that they are incapable of generating solutions. When the therapist helps the patient to slow down the process and implement steps to find and deploy solutions, two things may occur. First, the patient will be relieved and develop a connection to therapy and the therapist. Second, the therapist will develop an understanding of the roadblocks that exist that prevent the patient from solving problems independently. Such information informs the treatment plan for the future work to be made.

In patients who have more problems with relationships, in addition to the general practice of deliberately obtaining feedback at the end of the session, you should specifically inquire about any negative reactions the patient is having to you or the treatment. Patient nonverbal communication and lack of adherence to therapy tasks and limits are conceptualized with the history in mind and directly and sensitively addressed. Any breach in the relationship is attended to in a matter-of-fact way, with both curiosity and empathy, as a way of **managing alliance ruptures**. Problems with trust may affect the speed with which therapeutic interventions may be deployed. There is a real tension here since when therapy is effective, the alliance improves. Engagement strategies from motivational interviewing, validation, or a slower pace are vital with reluctant patients.

CBT Case Conceptualization

The role of individualized **case conceptualization** makes CBT a treatment that is individualized to a particular patient's needs, vulnerabilities, and strengths. The therapist identifies the central themes and developmental origins that alter the patient's perceptions in day-to-day life and identifies skill and motivational problems that affect the patient's ability to manage stress and interpersonal relationships. The conceptualization is a working hypothesis that is constantly revised as more information is obtained. It should predict obstacles in treatment and help the therapist plan treatment more efficiently.

The conceptualization is a synthesis of the patient's personal and developmental history and the cognitive model for a particular disorder. For example, in an individual with social anxiety disorder, the therapist would be looking for themes regarding fear of negative evaluation and the avoidance of any situation that would invite scrutiny. Thereafter, the therapist would be evaluating what developmental influences, biological and genetic vulnerabilities, and interpersonal and social interactions may have had a bearing on the patient developing such thinking and behavior. This process should include as wide an array of influences in the biopsychosocial history as germane to the patient.

One way of thinking about case conceptualization is that we obtain information for it by considering the patient's formative influences and current interpersonal environment and the problematic thoughts, emotions, and behaviors that the patient has in day-to-day life. We are interested in what the patient thinks at times of trouble as well as how did they learn to think that way about the world. We are also interested in how thoughts and behaviors perpetuate the problem that the patient is having and what strengths have assisted them in coping with setbacks. Thus, we use a combination of information about the patient's current patterns of thinking and behaving at times of negative emotion to get a typical picture of the way the patient reacts to difficult events, combined with a good developmental history and knowledge about particular patterns of thinking and behavior that underlie psychological problems that have been identified by CBT research.

Several questions help us consider the problems a patient is having. First, we might list the problems in the patient's life and ask ourselves what has kept the patient from solving these on their own? We may consider whether any common behavior problems (ie, avoidance) underlie many of the problems. We will look for skill deficits that have a bearing on the patient's lack of effective coping. Another useful question at this point is, "How did this patient learn to think this way about the world?"

There exist diagrammatic and written formats to organize thinking about case conceptualization (the books listed in "Where to Learn More" are a source for such materials and an expanded view of how to conceptualize patients). We suggest writing out case formulations to help clarify and expand thinking about the patient and plan treatment further.

6

Case Study—Preliminary CBT Case Conceptualization

The following is the preliminary case conceptualization that Steve's therapist wrote after the second visit.

Diagnosis: On clinical presentation, major depressive disorder, R/O generalized anxiety disorder, and panic disorder.

Precipitant: Worsening work-related stress. This is superimposed on the background of recent interpersonal stressors and stress related to the recent move to a new city.

Activating situations include most social interactions including with coworkers, friends and girlfriend, and work-related concerns.

A cross-sectional view of current cognitions and behaviors: Steve presents with an overwhelmingly negative view of himself, the world, and the future. Steve's thinking shows evidence of several cognitive errors related to his depression including mental filtering (magnifying negative details and filtering out positive aspects), polarized or black and white thinking ("my life is going nowhere"), overgeneralization ("my boss now hates me"), and catastrophizing. He compensates for these negative views by avoidance of social contact and has followed his lack of motivation by decreased engagement in pleasurable activities. This has worsened his mood. Steve's negative world view is also contributing to thinking he is helpless and he is overwhelmed by his symptoms and a sense that he cannot solve his problems. Steve is also experiencing anxiety and associated panic attacks, with symptoms of anxiety compounding his depressive symptomatology and hypervigilance regarding physical sensations associated with anxiety.

A longitudinal view of cognitions and behaviors: Steve has a history of previous episodes of depressed mood as well as persistent anxiety; both of which were untreated. When he lost his home and his dog in the fire at age 16 years, followed by his parents' divorce (and lack of availability), he began to have a world view that he was "unlucky" and that "things will not work out for me." He has seen setbacks in his current circumstances through this lens and has lost the ability to counterbalance this view with data about his successes. Steve has a history of asthma in the past, which likely exacerbated (and still influences) his anxiety/panic.

Steve's strengths/assets: Include being intelligent, financially independent, and motivated for treatment. He also has been able to sustain good relationships with friends, a girlfriend, and his aunt and uncle.

Steve's problem list: (1) Depressed mood with accompanying lack of motivation and anhedonia and (2) anxiety with accompanying panic attacks.

Treatment goals: (1) Reduction of his depressive symptomatology and (2) to reduce symptoms of anxiety/panic. Antidepressant use may be warranted depending on symptom severity and individual preference.

Preliminary Treatment Planning and Goal Setting

Ideally, at the end of the assessment, you discuss a preliminary treatment plan. The plan should include a description of the diagnosis, types of treatment available, and why you recommend CBT—basically, you provide informed consent for therapy. Further, you should describe the nature of CBT treatment and whether combined treatment with medication is advisable. Although a specific number of sessions is not always specified, a range is generally discussed that is consistent with the present-focused, problem-oriented nature of the treatment. A mutual agreement about entering into the relationship should then occur, and if time permits, some preliminary **goal setting** follows. Depending on the patient, other early interventions may include readings about CBT, **structuring** a typical CBT session, reviewing beliefs the patient holds about therapy and correcting any misconceptions, and/or determining the patient's willingness to participate. Your intention is to help the patient understand that a partnership with you will help them learn new skills to manage situations differently and lead to a better life.

Goal setting should be an early focus of attention for every patient, either started with the patient at the end of the assessment and continued as an initial homework assignment or delayed until the subsequent session. Setting goals early in treatment increases the patient's motivation and sets a road map for change. Goals should be specific and targeted toward elements of the patient's day-to-day life that would be different if conditions improved. For example, you can ask Steve when therapy is over, if he accomplished all that he wanted, how would his daily life be different? What would he do/feel/think more or less if therapy was successful? This inquiry helps you to identify small steps that have a high probability to change things for the better. Often goal setting is facilitated by asking the patient to recount a typical day now (hour by hour) and then describe a day in similar detail prior to the onset of the illness. Patients can also use prompts to look at domains of valued activities (such as work, friendship, health, etc.) and what they would aspire to in each of these areas. Finding something that the patient has strong inclinations to want to accomplish is highly desirable.

It is important to recognize that sometimes patients avoid activities that may be important for them and substitute other activities instead. For example, patients may spend leisure time watching television and identify this as an enjoyable activity, when, in fact, it produces little pleasure and has replaced seeing friends or exercising. Patients who have a task to accomplish that does not seem particularly rewarding (such as studying or writing a paper) will often substitute another "acceptable" activity like cleaning or shopping even if it is not related to the more important goal at hand. Such patterns become part of the conceptualization and treatment plan.

Goal setting engages the patient in imagining a more hopeful future. As with all interventions, goal setting may help you assess roadblocks (such as negative cognitions or skill deficits) that contribute to the patient's problems. For example, if a patient has ideas like "If I try something, I am sure to fail" or "Someone must help me or I will fall apart," setting goals will present a problem and often stall the process. In this instance, you would ask Steve about what thoughts he has when you ask him to identify something that he wants to change in therapy. Once you have elicited these automatic thoughts, you can begin to help the patient evaluate them and experiment with alternative ways of thinking and behaving. At such a moment, the therapist may use evidence gathering and Socratic questioning, which will be described in a later section, to help the patient move forward, knowing that the process of teaching the patient to examine automatic thoughts himself remains to be accomplished.

Goals must also be continually revised as therapy continues. You may provide suggestions for goals that the patient may not have considered but which need attention (such as tackling specific areas of avoidance). If the patient is reluctant to consider a goal that you believe is critical for recovery (such as refusing to prioritize substance use when it clearly relates to her symptoms and problems), you use **psychoeducation**, nonjudgmental questioning, and evaluate the advantages and disadvantages of avoiding this goal for now and in the future.

Case Study—Goal Setting

Goal setting occurred at the end of Steve's first session. After discussing the potential advisability of combined treatment for his condition, he wanted more information regarding medication, so the therapist provided written information about antidepressants. She then turned her attention to a preliminary discussion of treatment goals.

Therapist: I'm wondering if we could spend some time talking about what targets the two of us should work toward in trying to make things better for you.

Steve: I can't imagine anything changing. I don't even know where to start.

> **Therapist:** That makes total sense. When people are depressed, they often feel overwhelmed by the number of things that seem to be off-kilter and think that change is impossible. Perhaps we could start out by talking about what your day is like right now. Just walk me through hour by hour like we were watching a movie about you.
>
> The two of them go through the activities that comprise Steve's day, which is generally completely dominated by work, with little to no social contacts except at work, and no hobbies, exercise, or pleasant activities. This was a stark contrast to his life prior to his depression. Steve was able to recognize that there were significant areas in his life that had "gone downhill." His therapist normalized this as typical in depression and likened his situation to rehabilitating from a significant orthopedic injury, which resonated with Steve. They set a goal for Steve to exercise one time after work in the next week and to call one of his good friends.

WHAT DO YOU DO NEXT: TREATMENT PLANNING AND THE "ORDER OF OPERATIONS"

A goal without a plan is just a wish...

Antoine de Saint-Exupéry

A specific aim of the CBT practitioner is to plan treatment both during a specific session and across treatment sessions, to maximize efficiency and target the most pressing problems of the patient. Consistent effort is made to alleviate distress by choosing a salient issue to work on at each session. You balance the needs of the patient in the moment and the underlying strategy that has the most promise to help the patient. Generally, these are woven together such that you work with the patient on a current problem in a way that illustrates a concept that can further help the patient. For example, if the patient is having difficulty with task completion, you might use activity scheduling (discussed in further detail later in this chapter) to help the patient and explain that this tool may be used to help with scheduling pleasurable activities, which may improve the patient's mood. If the problem also involves negative automatic thoughts, you may elect to teach the patient what these are and begin the process of testing and changing them.

Create Overarching Plans for Treatment

The plan for treatment is determined by the patient conceptualization, current life circumstances, and particular interventions that are known to effectively alleviate symptoms. Therapists who employ CBT must spend time and effort between sessions considering what might be a good strategy to employ in the next treatment session.

One effective method for beginning therapists to learn about treatment planning is to consult treatment manuals that present validated sequences of therapeutic interventions for a particular diagnosis, such as social anxiety disorder. This will help you develop a strategy that incorporates the patient's conceptualization and which follows a design with a high likelihood of success. In patients who present with comorbid disorders, it may be necessary to devise a treatment plan based on your clinical judgment and the patient's history. In addition, it is important to keep abreast of current psychotherapy research, particularly when more commonly used interventions are ineffective or when the problem is more complex.

For example, in Steve's case, there is a pressing need to increase his engagement with valued and pleasurable activities, alongside a need to manage his anxiety. The order in which this would occur would be determined by a collaboration between the patient and therapist and by the therapist's knowledge about treatment plans for particular conditions. Sometimes, progress is derailed by an issue that was not in the initial treatment plan. Although *manualized* CBT had a predetermined number of sessions, there is no "hard-and-fast" rule regarding such a number in actual clinical practice. The guiding principle is that treatment is present-focused and the patient is taught skills to use independently after the goals of treatment are met.

Treatment plans in CBT generally follow a similar overarching order, with the particular components varying based on the patient's diagnosis and severity. Engagement follows assessment and is generally characterized by psychoeducation about the illness, the therapy, and its interventions, setting goals and inspiring a sense of hope about the future. You often review the initial case conceptualization with the patient during this time, which can help the patient understand their illness and the role of thoughts and behaviors in their life. In addition, employing **capsule summaries** during sessions also improves patient engagement and treatment adherence. Subsequently, you address behavioral issues. Such work may take the form of behavioral activation if the problem is depression or some form of exposure-based intervention if the problem is anxiety related. Addressing behavioral issues may need to be delayed if there are life-threatening issues (such as substantial hopelessness or suicidal ideas or behaviors) or there is a need to spend extra time relationship-building or directly problem-solving to avoid psychosocial crises. Next, the patient would be taught principles of automatic thought recording and cognitive restructuring. Cognitive restructuring would be tailored to target specific thoughts and themes related to core ideas that may leave the patient vulnerable to future recurrence, as we describe in a later section.

Finally, the patient prepares for termination and engages in a slow taper of sessions with the purpose of reinforcing learning that has occurred in therapy. During termination, there are active efforts to help the patient prepare to manage situations that have caused problems in the past with new tools and skills learned in therapy (see section Termination and Relapse Prevention).

What to Treat First

Deciding what to treat first requires determining which of the patient's problems is most likely to derail progress toward a goal. If Steve's panic attacks are so severe that he will not go out with his friends, his anxiety will need to be treated first for behavioral activation to be effective. Combined treatment with medication and psychotherapy may allow patients with comorbid diagnoses to make more rapid progress but should be implemented with an eye on the evidence that exists regarding single or combined treatment (see Sudak, 2011, for a review of such literature). In addition, time is often of the essence. By the time many patients have reached your office, they may be at a crisis point at work, in relationships, or in their financial life. These problems must be directly addressed early in treatment. Many times, mood or anxiety disorders incur such a toll on work, finances, and relationships that the burden of these losses increases the difficulty of therapy and lessens the chance for a durable recovery.

The "order of operations" is also influenced by patient acuity. Dialectical behavior therapy, a type of CBT for borderline personality, prioritizes treatment targets that are useful to keep in mind in treating any patient. Any behaviors that threaten the patient's life are the top priority, followed by any threats to the therapeutic alliance. Lastly, problems related to the patient's quality of life are considered. This rubric keeps you and the patient focused on the most critical issues. Enlisting the patient's agreement to work on these issues as a priority prior to starting treatment may decrease the chaotic nature of treatment, which may occur in patients with high levels of acuity.

Common Roadblocks Early in Treatment

An iterative process occurs as you work to solve the patient's current life problems while simultaneously engaging in activities that alleviate the patient's psychiatric condition. Roadblocks generally emerge and necessitate an evolution of the treatment plan and conceptualization. A very important part of the conceptualization involves classifying the root cause of the patient's inability to effectively manage obstacles independently. To do so, you determine if the patient has skill deficits or motivational deficits and target them accordingly. Skill deficits comprise particular psychological tools that the patient has yet to acquire. Everyone functions more effectively when equipped with skills to manage time, be assertive, name and regulate emotions, just to name a few. Skill deficits may be developmental (eg, a late adolescent may not be particularly good at perspective taking) or acquired (eg, if the family you grew up in flung dishes to manage interpersonal conflict, you might have some deficiencies in this area).

Motivational deficits—when the patient has a skill and does not use it—must also be conceptualized and managed accordingly. They may come from internal (thoughts, emotions) or external (interpersonal reinforcement) sources. For example, if a patient was able to be assertive in prior relationships and now has an abusive partner and never directly states her needs, that lack of self-assertion clearly relates to the understandable fear that this might be dangerous, not a lack of skill. Beliefs are often the origin of motivational deficits. If you have persistent and unrecognized thoughts like "If I try, I will fail" each time that you have a new challenge, you are unlikely to engage in behavior that will help you to effectively face the challenge.

Case Study—Roadblocks and Motivational Deficits

A good example of motivational deficits occurred in Steve's treatment after he set a goal to go exercise after work and then call two of his friends. Motivational deficits prevented him from taking either of these actions. When he went to pack his clothes and leave for the gym, he was overwhelmed by a sense of heaviness in his chest, a feeling of low energy, and thought he should put the gym off until he felt physically more energetic and motivated. He sat down by the television and put aside the plan, and then proceeded to feel sadder, thinking "I will never get back to my old self." The next day, he had planned to call his friends. When he looked at his activity plan, he thought "I'm such a failure. I couldn't even go exercise yesterday. Why should I bother to try and call? This is useless. I'll never get better."

Both instances of Steve's derailed plans represent motivational deficits. Steve regularly exercised prior to his illness and often engaged in social activities. Both the physical sensations associated with his depression (lack of energy, heaviness in his chest) and his lack of ability to counter his thoughts regarding the need for motivation before he went to exercise led to avoidance. You would work diligently in the next session to counter this pattern (see section Behavioral Interventions). Following his failed attempt to exercise, Steve had thoughts that sapped his motivation and led him to jettison his plan to call his friends. This illustrates how lack of activity may be interpreted by the patient as evidence he is a failure, incurring further damage to his self-regard, which leads to the vicious cycle of inactivity and mood disturbance. Steve's therapist would highlight and help him to change such deactivating cognitions (see section Cognitive Interventions).

6

BEHAVIORAL INTERVENTIONS

Actions speak louder than words.

Teaching patients to record and observe behaviors may by itself effect change. Patients are often unaware of patterns of behavior and the relationship between behavior and mood or anxiety. At least two of the commonly used behavioral interventions employed in CBT are potent, stand-alone treatments: behavioral activation and exposure. Although this section is focused on **behavioral techniques** within CBT, it is important to recognize that cognitive restructuring (discussed later in this chapter) is frequently necessary in some form to enlist the patient's involvement in these activities. For example, you may engage the patient about a particular way of thinking in order to help them engage in new behaviors. Such questions may produce change in a single instance and are often used for thoughts that are hopeless or thoughts that may prevent the patient from engaging in behavioral techniques. For example, if a patient says "I can't go out if I do not feel like it," testing that thought in the session may produce the willingness to try, despite the lack of motivation. Engaging in new behaviors also may provide alternate data and experiences and cause the patient to draw different conclusions without engaging in formal cognitive restructuring.

Behavioral Activation Defined

Behavioral activation is of substantial importance in CBT for depression and is known to be effective as a durable, stand-alone treatment for some patients. It is also commonly intertwined with a CBT approach in other diagnoses, as many of the principles of BA help patients with procrastination and assist with task completion. The core techniques of BA involve behavioral monitoring and scheduling activities, with the therapeutic relationship as the initial reinforcement to motivate the patient to engage in previously avoided activities. Lewinsohn[10] was an early proponent of behavioral activation and determined that an increase in contact with pleasurable activity is effective in making positive changes in mood. Since that time, the model has been expanded to include assigning valued and important activities and to specifically target avoidance of certain activities. Beck contributed the idea of **graded task assignment**[11]—that is, breaking tasks that seem overwhelming into manageable pieces and assigning a small amount at a time in order to help a depressed person complete an important activity.

Doing Behavioral Activation

You often begin BA by explaining the relationship between mood and activity. Understanding the rationale for any intervention you suggest makes it more likely that a patient will participate and helps the patient learn the principle behind the intervention, so that the patient will use the tool at times of future vulnerability. Fundamentally, when a person is depressed, it makes sense to do less—avoiding responsibilities and enjoyable activities when predicting that one will fail or be disappointed is logical. However, the very act of avoidance leads to more sadness, and the patient may draw more helpless and hopeless conclusions. Life circumstances also deteriorate. Thus, increasing contact with pleasurable and important activity improves mood and functioning.

Once this rationale makes sense to the patient, you determine what the patient does with his or her time and note connections between mood state and current activity. The link between mood and activity is generally established by asking the patient to contemporaneously note hourly activities for a day (and a weekend day if the patient's schedule is different), each with an associated mood rating. Next, a hierarchy of avoided activities is constructed (including novel ideas that could produce even small positive changes). Lists of possible pleasurable activities (such as the Pleasant Events Schedule[12]) may serve as a tool to assist in determining activities associated with positive feelings, especially when the patient is unable to recall prior sources of pleasure. You emphasize that engaging in such activities may not produce joy, but that at this stage, any shift in mood in a positive direction is a plus.

The next step is to assign three to five activities to attempt in the next week. This assignment must be made quite deliberately. You explicitly assign when the activity will occur, with whom the activity will occur and so forth, and predict and problem-solve obstacles to the completion of the activity with the patient. You must repeatedly emphasize an appreciation for the lack of energy and motivation that the patient feels but simultaneously emphasize the fact that action does not require motivation and has a high likelihood of improving the patient's condition. The therapy session is highly oriented toward assigning, troubleshooting, and assessing the outcome of the assigned activities. In depression, this phase of treatment typically precedes work with cognitions and continues until the patient regularly engages in previously valued day-to-day pursuits without the therapist's intervention. Ideally, the patient will learn the core principle that maintaining an active and engaged life is a protection against mood problems.

Case Study—Introducing Behavioral Activation

An example of an initial attempt at behavioral activation occurred in Steve's treatment. Steve agreed to call a friend or two and to go to the gym as initial steps he could take to improve his mood. This initial attempt was unsuccessful, so his therapist decided to take a more structured approach to increasing his activity. She put activity scheduling on the **agenda** as part of **agenda setting**.

Therapist: Steve, I wonder if you ever thought about what the relationship was between depression and activity?

Steve: Not really. All I know is that I've got no interest in doing anything. It feels like I can barely drag myself through the day.

Therapist: That's exactly right—when we're depressed the natural tendency is for us to want to do less. It makes total sense that you want to do less, but I wonder if you thought about the consequences of that.

Steve: Not really.

Therapist: Well, being involved in fewer pleasurable activities likely increases your sad mood. Not exercising or eating well saps your energy and could affect your sleep. When you didn't go to the gym last week, you actually thought even more negatively about yourself. What do you think about that?

Steve: It's true. When I don't do something I have planned I think I am a real loser. I'm always exhausted—I can't imagine feeling any worse.

Therapist: I'm wondering if we might consider doing an experiment to see if your mood could change by trying one or two things that might improve it even by a small amount. I'll help you to find ways to avoid the trap of "I just don't feel like it" and together we can see if this will help you.

The therapist works with Steve to identify two previously enjoyed activities that he agrees could positively impact his mood: seeing his friend Mike and watching a football game with his aunt and uncle. These activities are of a size and difficulty that Steve agrees he can manage. Instead of just suggesting that Steve try this out, the therapist very specifically delineates a time when each activity will occur and asks Steve to carefully consider what obstacles could interfere with his participation. Steve says that he does not foresee any obstacles, not recognizing that his own lack of motivation is often what leads him to postpone activities that have the potential to improve his mood.

Therapist: Okay, one of the things you haven't mentioned that would keep you from trying this experiment is the possibility that you could be stopped by a lack of motivation. How could you handle it if suddenly you're thinking about leaving the house, and then feel like you're just too tired and don't feel like going?

Steve: I'd be likely to cancel.

Therapist: What could you do to make that less likely?

Steve: I guess I could tell my aunt and uncle I was coming. Once I knew they expected me, I'd go.

Therapist: I think that's a fine idea! Some of my patients find it's helpful for them to remind themselves that depression may cause them to want to avoid activities, but that acting according to a plan will help them out of the depression. It's almost like taking an anti-depressant; these "activity prescriptions" are one way you can help yourself get well.

The therapist and Steve develop a written action plan incorporating these activities. She will focus the next therapy session on the result of the plan, further emphasizing its importance. As Steve notices the positive benefits of his actions, he should begin to be more active with less and less reminding, although he may find the scheduling of important activities a helpful tool to keep using throughout his life.

Exposure Techniques Defined

The second important behavioral intervention used in CBT is exposure. The definition of exposure is to deliberately contact non-life-threatening stimuli that are associated with an unpleasant emotional state and to stay in contact with such stimuli long enough for habituation and new learning to occur. Exposure is a powerful intervention and may be used as a stand-alone treatment for many anxiety disorders. Often, however, patients are reluctant to engage in it, and on-the-spot cognitive restructuring will be required to help the patient increase courage and motivation. Exposure works because it teaches patients that anxiety is time-limited and manageable, that they habituate to the stimulus, and they learn new things about the actual danger of the feared stimulus. It provides patients with a sense of mastery and self-efficacy.

Three types of exposure are used in CBT. Imaginal exposure is generally used in situations that are difficult for the patient to contact or in circumstances where it would be too dangerous for the patient to be in contact with the stimulus, such as in PTSD. Imaginal exposure may also be used in circumstances where the patient is so reluctant about actual exposure to the cue that one needs to start more slowly. In vivo exposure (exposure to the actual feared situation) is the cornerstone of effective exposure treatment. Interoceptive exposure is a particular kind of in vivo exposure, comprising exposure to feared body sensations. Most individuals with anxiety are exquisitely sensitive to the physical sensations associated with anxiety. Panic disorder is characterized by a catastrophic misinterpretation of such sensations. Exposing the patient to body sensations helps them to recognize them as safe. Interoceptive exposure may be done easily in the office. One can reproduce feared body sensations by having the patient run in place or hyperventilate in session, then focus on these sensations and develop an increased tolerance. There are certain circumstances (chronic obstructive pulmonary disease [COPD], for example) where consultation with the patient's healthcare provider is needed before attempting interoceptive exposure or when it may be inadvisable because of health concerns. Many novice therapists are understandably concerned about increasing anxiety in their patients with such procedures. We provide an introduction to the key principles of exposure here and suggest further reading and supervision to guide you in working with this highly effective intervention.

Doing Basic Exposure

As with all CBT interventions, you must provide a rationale, explain the procedure, and get patient buy-in. This emphasis on teaching the rationale is a core tenet of CBT, both to bolster patient engagement and to increase the likelihood of the patient's "ownership" of the tool and its future use. A good way to introduce the rationale for exposure is to ask a question about how a common phobia would be cured. For example, how would someone become less afraid of dogs or spiders? Most people are aware that it would require engagement with a dog or spider in order to reduce the fear. Teaching patients that learned dangers are recorded strongly in our memory as a protective mechanism and that unlearning takes considerable effort helps them understand the need for repeated practice. In addition, patients should understand that each time they avoid the feared stimulus, they are actually teaching themselves that the stimulus is extremely dangerous. This helps to explain why the urge to avoid the stimulus is so strong—most of the time the patient has avoided the stimulus a countless number of times.

Next, a **fear hierarchy** is constructed with the patient. A common tool is to teach the patient the SUDS (**Subjective Units of Distress Scale**). This is when patients place on a scale of 0 (meaning nearly asleep) to 100 (meaning absolutely terrified) all the things that they avoid associated with a particular fear. You should provide particular anchor points on the scale—"awake but calm" at a SUDS level of 15 or 20. Discussion helps the patient generate examples below the "90" level when even thinking about the feared stimulus is avoided. More subtle forms of avoidance (ie, safety-seeking behaviors) may be listed as steps in the hierarchy when everything associated with the stimulus appears to terrify the patient. For example, if a patient cannot imagine going food shopping, you might consider adding in steps like going and standing in front of the grocery store with her sister, going two steps into the store with her sister, walking down a single aisle with her sister standing in the doorway, and so forth.

After the hierarchy is constructed, the next task is to identify, plan, and implement exposure assignments. Such assignments may be performed with or without you. The initial assignment should be conducted with a stimulus predicted to evoke a small amount of anxiety (SUDS of 30 or 40). The patient should be informed that when they begin, the experiment anxiety may be quite high, even when choosing a less challenging item. At this point, there is often the urge to avoid. When possible, you should conduct the initial exposure with the patient to help the patient manage this urge. If you are not doing so, you must carefully discuss with the patient what they will say to themself at the moment of fear to motivate them to continue with the exposure. Patients should predict how anxious they believe they will be during the procedure before it begins so they can compare this with what actually happens. During exposure, the patient must pay attention to the cue and attend to anxious sensations. Ideally, the patient stays in the presence of the cue until such time as anxiety decreases by about half. Above all, the goal is to resist the urge to avoid. After exposure, the patient rates anxiety once again and debriefs about what is learned. The patient must practice the same exposure repeatedly until rapid diminishment of anxiety occurs and then gradually move up the hierarchy. Repeating the exposure constitutes the "action plan" for the patient in the subsequent week.

Case Study—Basic Exposure Intervention

Steve and his therapist have started to explore what he has been avoiding since he has developed panic attacks. As they discuss the situation, she determines that some of his concern about returning to the gym is because he is worried about experiencing the sensation of his heart beating faster. She knows that Steve had a thorough physical evaluation when he was seen in the emergency room. She decides to try some informal interoceptive exposure.

Steve: I know it is silly, but every time I sense my heart beating faster I am just terrified. The doctor said I am fine and there is nothing wrong with me but I still feel so scared.

Therapist: You know, that is not at all unusual. The very first time you had a panic episode, I am sure it was a terribly frightening experience. We know fear memories are "sticky." Once we learn something is dangerous it is hard to unlearn. It's almost like you have developed a phobia of noticing your heartbeat.

Steve: That is it exactly.

Therapist: Well, if you had a friend who had a phobia, what would you tell him to do to help that get better?

Steve: I guess to learn to tolerate it.

Therapist: Well, that is sort of it. Actually, we think two things happen. First, your body adapts to the feeling you are having, since nothing terrible occurs. Think for a minute about getting into a cold swimming pool in the summer. What does that feel like at first? And what happens after a few minutes?? It's like that. Second, you learn that the thing you are afraid of is not actually going to hurt you. If we taught you to do this gradually about getting your heart rate up, it might help. What do you think?

They plan for Steve to climb one flight of the stairs in his apartment building rapidly and pay attention to his heartbeat, with the goal of increasing his tolerance of these sensations. Of note is the very small increment of sensation they discuss, as well as the collaborative nature of the assignment.

The assessment must accurately identify the consequence of exposure to a feared stimulus in order to adequately plan exposure. For example, a person who washes hands repeatedly may not be afraid solely about germs but of contaminating the family's food causing their illness or death. The exposure required for this fear would be quite different than if the fear was only about germs on her hands. A critical requirement of exposure is consistent practice both during and after therapy. Exposure must occur in multiple different contexts and performed over a substantial period of time to be durable. Generally, anxious patients practice avoidance of feared stimuli for decades, so substantial practice is needed to unlearn this response.

Relaxation and Controlled Breathing

Two other behavioral techniques are employed routinely in CBT. Progressive muscle relaxation (PMR), as described by Jacobsen,[13] is a demonstrably effective way to reduce anxiety. It also is quite helpful for insomnia. There are a number of tutorials available on the internet and on many relaxation and mental health websites that can be used with a patient to promote the regular practice of PMR. The basic premise is that by systematically tensing and then releasing muscle groups the patient can cue a relaxation response. Regular and consistent use, initially when calm, will give patients a tool that allows them to feel more in control. PMR is also helpful for insomnia and lowers the general tension level in patients with generalized anxiety disorder.

Controlled breathing is another tool that helps patients cope with anxiety and fore-stall panic. Patients must be taught that controlled breathing will help them to cope with anxiety but is actually unnecessary, since anxiety is not dangerous. Controlled breathing involves counting or using a second hand of a timepiece to slow breathing to about 15 times per minute. It is not "deep breathing" but *slow* breathing that we are after. Patients can be taught to think of each breath as a slow inhale, then wait, then slowly exhale, then wait and then repeat the cycle. As with PMR, patients must learn and practice this technique when calm to easily deploy it when anxious. This intervention, if taught, must not be used during exposure itself, since, as we describe, the goal is to experience anxiety in a controlled fashion.

6

COGNITIVE INTERVENTIONS

Nothing either good or bad, but thinking makes it so…

Shakespeare

The theoretical underpinning of CBT is the **cognitive behavioral model**. This model, most simply stated, is that our interpretation of events may significantly influence our emotional state and our behavior. CBT places a unique emphasis on explicitly identifying erroneous and maladaptive cognitions in session and then educating and training patients to do so independently. The ability to correct distorted cognitions conveys a lifetime of protection against the negative effects of such thinking. These cognitions are classified into three categories—automatic thoughts, intermediate beliefs, and core beliefs—based in part on the ease with which they are identified and changed. Automatic thoughts (ATs) are defined as conscious thoughts that spontaneously arise in response to a change in the environment. Intermediate beliefs are classified as rules that guide a person's behavior, which often are derived from development and culture. Core beliefs are defined as central beliefs that people hold about themselves, others, and the world. Core beliefs are also called **schemas** in some CBT writings. Schemas are defined as hypothesized mental structures that contain rules, emotions, beliefs, and memories about a particular topic, which can be activated simultaneously with particular stimuli. A core belief is one part of this constellation as we define it. Schemas are hypothesized as fundamental to efficient function in the world, but the beliefs within them are an area that may be targeted in treatment, specifically when they are highly charged and negative.

Educating the Patient

The application of **cognitive techniques** in CBT involves a seamless integration of psychoeducation and altering maladaptive cognitions. As before, the goal is to teach the patient how to employ these tools for a lifetime. Psychoeducation teaches the patient "to think about thinking." Altering maladaptive cognitions involves learning to identify and critically evaluate automatic thoughts as well as developing alternative ways of thinking in similar circumstances in the future. Cognitive techniques have the goal to diminish or eliminate debilitating negative cognitions, with an attendant change in the emotions and maladaptive behaviors that often accompany negative cognitions and emotions. In the setting of depression and anxiety, a patient has pervasive thoughts that their situation is hopeless or overwhelming. You educate the patient in easy-to-understand language about the basic principles of CBT and impart not only a sense of purpose but hope for positive change.

Case Study—Educating the Patient on Cognitions

The following is an example of how Steve and his therapist began the process of educating him about the role of thinking early in his treatment.

Therapist: I am wondering if you have noticed any changes in how you think as you have become more depressed.

Steve: I feel terrible. I just don't see anything good about my life.

Therapist: You have been having a really tough time. Depression does affect thinking so that you have an excessively negative view of yourself, the world and your future. It's like you have glasses on that change the way you view everything. Have you noticed that?

Then you can begin to illustrate the **basic cognitive model**—that humans are capable of viewing situations in ways that may be inaccurate or exaggerated, especially when depressed or anxious, resulting in emotional distress and problem behaviors. Finally, you point to the fact that the highly negative thoughts common to depression and anxiety may be reevaluated and changed, resulting in improved mood and function.

Identifying Automatic Thoughts

Working with automatic thoughts (ATs) forms the core of CBT with many patients. ATs are "stream of consciousness" cognitions that are experienced throughout the day when we are not consciously directing our thoughts. In conditions like depression, they are likely to be biased and negative. Patients are generally unaware of ATs, but they are easily accessible to identification because they are generally associated with a negative mood shift. More importantly, ATs are habitual and reflect underlying intermediate and core beliefs, which, along with the patient's developmental history, help you refine the case conceptualization and point you and patient toward the salient cognitions that require modification.

You may employ several techniques to teach the patient about ATs. In session, an emotionally charged example from the recent past may elicit ATs associated with that event. Thus, you demonstrate in situ how ATs are recognized. You guide the patient to recount an event in a way designed to stimulate emotion and then ask for the patient's thoughts when their mood shifts. This teaches the patient how to elicit ATs by noticing mood shifts, as this example illustrates.

Case Study—Identifying Automatic Thoughts

Therapist: I am sorry to hear that your last few days have been rough. I am wondering if we can talk about a specific event that you found to be particularly troubling.

Steve: Last Friday, I had a really bad time at work…

Therapist: What happened?

Steve: I mixed up my orders and sent out the wrong entrée. My boss was pretty upset with me. He came into the kitchen and told me to fix it ASAP.

Therapist: Ok, that does sound pretty difficult. If we can travel back in time in your mind and examine the whole event as if in slow motion, would that be okay?

Steve: Yes.

6

In this instance, the therapist uses the technique of **guided discovery**. This is a method of questioning designed to stimulate emotion and uncover patterns of thinking about which the patient is unaware, so that the pair may investigate them for accuracy to generate new or more functional perspectives. In other words, you guide the patient's attention to a particular part of the narrative, and the patient discovers that there are patterns to thinking about the self and the world that relate to mood and behavior. Using this process, you help the patient reflect on the way they process information (thinking about thinking).

Case Study—Guided Discovery

Therapist: When you found out that you had mixed up your orders, what thoughts went through your mind?

Steve: I felt terrible; I wanted to run away….

Therapist: That must have been awful for you. But I would like to get a clearer picture of exactly what was happening. Let's try and slow things down. Can you picture where you were in the kitchen?

Steve: Yes. By the order stand.

Therapist: And what did your body feel like at the moment you recognized that you had not handled the orders correctly?

Steve: I felt like I would explode with embarrassment.

Therapist: What was going through your mind?

> **Steve:** That my life is over…I am no good for anything…things will never ever get better for me.
>
> **Therapist:** What were your emotions?
>
> **Steve:** Just so very sad.
>
> **Therapist:** Any other thoughts?
>
> **Steve:** Why do these things happen only to me? I am born with bad luck…

The therapist used several common techniques in order to elicit Steve's ATs (*my life is over, I am no good for anything, things will never get better*). The therapist chose a situation that was emotionally charged. She asked Steve to describe it in some detail, and as he became more emotional while thinking about it, Steve's attention was drawn to a number of thoughts he experienced. The therapist also distinguished feelings (emotions) from thoughts (cognitions), as this is a distinction most patients initially struggle to make. She focused on the relevant part of the event and kept probing until several ATs were elicited.

A further method of helping patients identify and modify ATs includes the use of **thought records**, where the patient keeps a written record of situations, emotions, and ATs. Many such instruments in the public domain are available via an online search or in the references provided at the end of this chapter. A thought record is typically assigned to the patient to record ATs after he learns how to elicit these in session. When the patient has difficulty identifying ATs, using a checklist of categories of typical automatic thoughts can be useful. A common activity in session is for you and the patient to review thought records together. This recording device often has prompts to help elicit previously neglected evidence and record conclusions that may be drawn from this wider, more rational view, and then record subsequent emotional and behavioral outcomes. They typically include columns to record the situation, automatic thought, emotion, and behavior; subsequent columns record evidence gathered about the thought, an alternative perspective considering the evidence, and the emotions and potential consequences of such a new perspective.

Once the patient understands the basic cognitive model and recognizes ATs, you teach the patient strategies to evaluate thoughts and increase their accuracy. One of the most powerful techniques to do this is **Socratic questioning**, which is a collaborative style of questioning intended to promote curiosity and inquisitiveness, and assumes that, because we are human, biases will occur. Instead of asking leading questions or telling the patient what to think, Socratic questioning helps the patient develop alternatives to repetitive perceptions by including a wider array of facts. Discovering new information with a process of collaborative inquiry increases the believability of alternative ideas. Socratic questioning is also an extension of the principle of **collaborative empiricism** ("let's examine this together"). Several methods may be employed to teach and practice evidence-based thinking. One useful method is to make a "for and against" list where the patient is encouraged to list actual evidence supportive or against particular ATs. For example, Steve could list the evidence for and against the AT, "things will never get better" and then draw a conclusion based on the actual evidence. By the very nature of this exercise, Steve learns that there are multiple ways to think about a situation. Identifying types of **cognitive errors** is another strategy that helps patients widen their view. Cognitive errors are categories of types of faulty logic or errors in reasoning, for example, absolutistic thinking, which help patients recognize these errors in their own thoughts.

Other strategies to help the patient consider alternative ways of thinking include **role-playing** (where the therapist takes on the role of a significant person in patient's life; see glossary in Appendix), brainstorming, moving out of the current time frame (ie, to a different time frame where the patient was much more successful and experienced positive emotions), and asking others for opinions. Decatastrophizing, where the patient estimates the likelihood or envisions coping with a feared situation, is a helpful tool to employ when the patient is anxious. Therapeutic benefits are derived from identifying and correcting erroneous cognitions with a resultant change in both emotions and behaviors. Cognitive techniques may be challenging but form the core of CBT for many patients. Practice, both in session and at home, is crucial.

Case Study—Identifying and Correcting Thinking Errors

Steve and his therapist worked with one such situation.

Steve: I made another mistake in the kitchen. I'm sure to get fired. That will be the end of me.

Therapist: You do seem very worried about being fired. I'm wondering what you mean when you say that being fired will be the end of you.

Steve: My life will be over…I will be a total failure.

Therapist: It would indeed be stressful to lose your job. However, I'm wondering if you have looked at the evidence that suggests that you will be fired for this mistake? How often do the other line cooks send out the wrong order?

Over the next few minutes, the therapist and Steve establish that although sending out the wrong order is not optimal, it is not generally a cause for dismissal.

Therapist: OK, if we really want to help you worry less about this, we also need to consider what you would do in the worst-case scenario. What would you really do if suddenly you found yourself without a job?

Steve: It would be awful, but I guess my life wouldn't be completely over. I would look for another job. I do have a good education and experience and I have some money saved.

6

As therapy advances, the task becomes helping the patient to be able to employ the tools to change thinking to be more accurate outside the session. Since our thinking patterns are often habitual, patients are taught **cognitive rehearsal** whereby they mentally rehearse ways to change cognitions and behaviors in anticipation of typical problematic situations in the future. **Coping cards**, where the patient prepares digital or actual index cards with written instructions about what to do or alternative thoughts to consider when a typical difficult situation arises, can also be a helpful reminder of skills learned in therapy. These tools make what happen in the session more easily transferable to the patient's day-to-day life.

Beyond Automatic Thoughts

Working to change automatic thoughts is a challenging task, and a full description of such work within CBT is beyond the scope of a single chapter. Beginning therapists should read further about this in some of the excellent texts listed in the references. However, it is important to note that CBT often goes beyond the techniques listed above and, with time, takes a deeper look at the underlying patterns to a patient's ATs and concurrent emotions and behaviors. As therapy proceeds, you generally identify underlying patterns in the patient's ATs. These underlying patterns relate to rules the patient has about himself and others, and how he should operate in the world. Such rules are classified as **core beliefs** and **intermediate beliefs**. These are deeply held internal constructs that are generally formed throughout a patient's development and reinforced by behavior and information gathered over a lifetime. For example, in Steve's case, one such rule he expresses is *"I should be doing much better by now."* This implies that he has standards about his life that he applies without considering context. If Steve rigidly applied this idea to his station in life—whether his current living situation, his employment, or his relationships—he would be constantly disappointed and have a recurring sense of failure. Furthermore, Steve has not really defined what he means by "much better." Thus, therapy may help Steve identify, examine, and modify the underlying belief.

Not all core and intermediate beliefs are maladaptive. Humans have a mixture of beliefs that help us make sense of and navigate the world. In some patients, there may be a preponderance of negative, maladaptive beliefs that cause them to have considerable difficulty with everyday stressors (as in personality disorders). In other patients, particular stressful situations may activate maladaptive schemas that begin to operate to process information and influence behavior in a negative way. This stress-diathesis hypothesis is central to how CBT considers problems. This hypothesis posits that an interaction between a psychological vulnerability and life stressor results in symptom formation. It can thus be helpful to both identify and modify these maladaptive beliefs.

The first step in this process is to educate the patient about the nature of schemas or core beliefs—often by reviewing the conceptualization and your hypothesis about the patient's beliefs. Another approach to uncover underlying beliefs is to employ the **downward arrow technique**. In this approach, you sequentially uncover negative ATs and probe further for what the thought would mean about the patient if it were true. This technique must be performed sensitively and with care; the patient must know that you do not believe that the thought is true. Instead, you are asking to look for underlying personal meanings the thought may have. Yet another technique that may help uncover beliefs is called the **life history review**.[14] As the name suggests, this technique involves asking the patient about formative influences and situations that might have influenced the development of core beliefs. An attempt is made to uncover details about relationships, parental influences, traumatic experiences, and any cultural aspects of development.

Although similar tools are used to modify beliefs as with automatic thoughts, a significant investment of time and effort is required to make a change in these deeply ingrained ideas. Patients need to be aware that this is a process that will take some time. The patient must develop sufficient insight and work diligently to change such mental habits. Socratic questioning, guided by a consistently revised case conceptualization, is targeted toward uncovering contradictions in the patients thinking. Examining the evidence helps break through the internal set of maladaptive beliefs and starts to open a world of other possibilities.

One example is to collaborate with the patient to list the evidence for and against a particular belief and maintain the stance of a coinvestigator. Listing advantages and disadvantages of having a belief may assist the patient with anxiety that is engendered by the thought of relinquishing a rule that is seen to be protective (ie, "I must always be perfect"). The patient generally has little difficulty identifying advantages but may never have considered disadvantages in retaining a particular belief. By using tools like the cognitive continuum (a method of evaluating how one compares to others on a continuum of standards—such as between good and evil), you can help the patient recognize that core beliefs can be malleable, rather than absolute. As the patient becomes comfortable with idea of alternate ways of thinking, alternative schema must be developed. Thereafter, the patient must engage in a process of evidence gathering over a significant period of time to strengthen this new belief.

6

THE ROLE OF PRACTICE IN CBT

Knowledge is of no value unless you put it into practice…

Chekov

One of the central tenets of CBT is that patients learn new ways to think and behave that replace habitual patterns associated with problems in interpersonal relationships and in goal attainment. New skills may be taught, such as problem-solving, interpersonal effectiveness, distress tolerance, and emotion regulation. In order for such interventions to be enduring, patients must practice them not just in the office but in day-to-day life. In addition, the patient must employ these tools under situations akin to those associated with emotional distress in the past. Implementing the powerful interventions of therapy only when in a therapy session is not very useful.

Patients are given particular out-of-session activities that broaden, deepen, and reinforce new learning as a routine part of CBT. Assigning out-of-session practice ("**homework**" or "action plans") may be challenging. First, patients have a considerable amount of distress when initially in treatment. If assignments are not made both tactfully and collaboratively, the patient may feel both demoralized and upset by them. One must consider the patient's response to prior education—for many the idea of "homework" is associated with bad experiences, and tasks are more readily approached when called action plans or experiments. For example, phrases such as "How could we find out more about this next week?" or "How could you practice some of what we learned today?" may be much more inviting. Activities should be assigned in amounts that make it likely the patient will succeed. Assignments should be provided in written form, or they will not be remembered, and obstacles to completion should be discussed and rectified prior to the patient leaving the session. Finally, homework must be discussed in the next session.

A variety of types of activities may be assigned for homework—these include reading, small assignments in behavioral activation, recording behaviors, exposure experiences, automatic thought records, or some aspect of problem-solving that leads the patient toward a goal. You ideally determine something that naturally follows from the session that can be continued by the patient in the week to follow.

You must employ empathy and motivate the patient to try new behaviors and keep in mind the patient's current stressors and demands. For example, a college student facing final exams is unlikely to readily participate in extensive exposure experiences. Accurate optimism, genuineness, and specific feedback all help the patient muster sufficient morale to tackle the extremely challenging work of change. An excellent method for therapists to learn about how realistic an assignment is is to try the activities themselves. Refer back to the section on behavioral activation to review how action plans are implemented most effectively.

TERMINATION AND RELAPSE PREVENTION

Since CBT is predicated upon learning new skills, the process of termination involves the review of what was learned in therapy as well as when such skills will be deployed. **Relapse prevention** is a fundamental tool in CBT. Relapse prevention occurs when the patient mentally identifies particular areas of vulnerability, imagines situations that could produce problems, and rehearses the use of CBT interventions at times of prior vulnerability. This activity ensures that important interventions are well rehearsed and able to be used when they are needed most. First, the patient must identify trouble spots that may occur in the future. Second, the patient must recall interventions learned in therapy that would be useful at such times of distress or vulnerability and mentally rehearse the employment of these interventions. Imaginal practice teaches the patient alternative responses and actual practice increases confidence.

Booster sessions are the rule in CBT. These are sessions that are staggered at increasing intervals as therapy is coming to an end. The patient is instructed to collect problems that have occurred between sessions and to describe what tools he used to manage these. The session troubleshoots any difficulty that the patient has had in recalling or implementing the tools learned in therapy. These booster sessions occur for several months. In addition, the patient and therapist discuss the very real issues involved in terminating the relationship itself.

Finally, an underlying principle in CBT is the value of tolerating discomfort. Discomfort is necessary for growth in most life endeavors—problem-solving obstacles to tolerating discomfort in the service of a goal and enhancing this capacity (eg, by giving rewards) often facilitates new behavior and goal attainment. Although termination can be uncomfortable, learning to tolerate this is a necessary part of this therapeutic approach.

Conclusion

This brief chapter provides an introduction to CBT. CBT is a well-researched, empirically supported form of psychotherapy based on learning theory and the cognitive behavioral model of psychopathology. It entails engaging in an active and collaborative therapeutic alliance, developing a case formulation, and then using cognitive and behavioral strategies that are employed based on an individualized treatment plan. The patient is taught skills that can be used at times of future stress in the hope that this will convey a durable and sustained recovery.

In this chapter, we reviewed the key features of the therapeutic relationship in CBT, including the establishment of an active, collaborative alliance, structuring and planning treatment, and developing a case conceptualization to guide therapy. We described several important techniques for managing depressed and anxious patients, including behavioral activation, exposure, and cognitive restructuring. These are tools to help patients think more accurately and behave more effectively in their lives, with the goal of ameliorating distress and improving functioning.

There are many excellent books, videos, websites, and in-person training opportunities for further learning, some of which are listed below. An important teaching strategy that CBT employs is the use of role-play to train novice therapists. Such practice is key to increasing confidence and facility in implementing treatment. Supervision that involves role-play and review of taped material from patient sessions also plays a major role in the development of therapist competence.

6

Self-Study Questions

1. Find a colleague who is also interested in learning CBT. Take turns role-playing explaining the cognitive behavioral model and particular elements of a session to a patient.

2. Think of a task that you are struggling to accomplish. Break it into component parts and use activity scheduling to assign yourself these parts of the task. Notice the obstacles that get in the way.

3. Find a PMR recording and practice it.

4. Track negative mood shifts for yourself for a week and jot down your automatic thoughts. Notice the types of common cognitive distortions that are present.

5. Choose a patient you have recently seen or observed and write a cognitive case conceptualization.

RESOURCES FOR FURTHER LEARNING

Organizations

Association for Behavioral and Cognitive Therapies (ABCT)—www.abct.org
Academy of Cognitive and Behavioral Therapies (ACT)—www.academyofct.org
Behavioral Tech (A Linehan Training Institute)—www.behavioraltech.org
Centre for Clinical Interventions—https://www.cci.health.wa.gov.au/
Oxford Centre for Cognitive Therapy—www.oxcadatresources.com
The Beck Institute—www.beckinstitute.org

Readings

Beck JS. *Cognitive Therapy: Basics and Beyond.* 2nd ed. New York, NY: Guilford Press; 2011.
Greenberger D, Padesky CA. *Mind Over Mood.* 2nd ed. New York, NY: Guilford Press; 2015.
Linehan MM. *Cognitive-Behavioral Treatment of Borderline Personality Disorder.* New York, NY: Guilford Press; 1993.
Sudak DM. *Cognitive Behavior Therapy for Clinicians.* Philadelphia, PA: LWW, Inc; 2006.
Sudak DM. *Combining CBT and Medication: An Evidence-Based Approach.* Hoboken, NJ: John Wiley and Sons; 2011.
Wright JH, Brown GK, Thase ME, Basco MR. *Learning Cognitive-Behavior Therapy: An Illustrated Guide.* 2nd ed. Arlington, VA: American Psychiatric Publishing; 2016.
Wright JH, Turkington D, Kingdon D, Basco MR. *Cognitive-Behavior Therapy for Severe Mental Illness.* Washington, DC: APPI Press; 2009.
Wright JH, Sudak DM, Turkington D, Thase M. *High-Yield Cognitive-Behavior Therapy for Brief Sessions: An Illustrated Guide.* Washington, DC: APPI Press; 2010.

APPENDIX—GLOSSARY OF COMMON TERMINOLOGY AND INTERVENTIONS

Common Terminology

Agenda	The agreed upon tasks set by you and the patient for each therapy session. Agenda items are individualized based on the primary treatment goal, though certain elements are common to all CBT sessions. Agendas typically include a symptom check, review of homework assignments, and creating a plan of action for the session. This process enhances efficiency and learning.
Automatic thought and automatic thought record	Thoughts that are not consciously directed that occur in response to a situation and are sometimes associated with an emotional response or problem behavior. These thoughts are not volitional, arise quickly, and may remain at the periphery of consciousness. In psychopathological states, these thoughts are often inaccurate, remain unexamined, and are associated with negative emotion and dysfunctional behavior.
Booster sessions	Sessions designed to reinforce concepts learned and tools use, scheduled at increasing intervals at the end of treatment. Booster sessions are used to monitor progress, emphasize gains, and troubleshoot any problems as they arise.
Cognitive behavioral model	The central principle of CBT states that rather than situations, our interpretation of events may significantly influence our emotional state and our behavior.
Cognitive errors	Initially described by Beck, these are errors in logic that lead to faulty information processing. Six types of cognitive errors have been described: selective abstraction, arbitrary inference, overgeneralization, magnification and minimization, personalization, absolutistic or "all or nothing" thinking.
Collaborative empiricism	A process whereby you and the patient work together as a team (collaborate) to evaluate thoughts and behaviors for accuracy or usefulness and modify them according to the evidence.
Core belief	Global, absolute rules that stem from early life experiences and modeling of significant others. For example, "I am incompetent," "the world is unsafe." These rules influence behavior, interpersonal rules, and the automatic thoughts that occur in response to particular situations. Some CBT writers refer to this as a "schema."
Graded task assignment	A method for making complex or seemingly unmanageable tasks manageable by breaking them down into multiple smaller simple tasks more easily achieved.
Guided discovery	This technique utilizes Socratic questioning designed to stimulate emotion, uncover patterns of thinking about which the patient is unaware, and then investigate them for accuracy to generate new or more functional perspectives.
Intermediate belief	Another category of thinking that describes rules that guide a person's behavior. Conditional, "if-then" rules, eg, "if I disagree with others, then they won't like me," "musts," "should" often comprise such beliefs.

6

Relapse prevention	A CBT approach originally developed to treat patients with alcohol use disorder. The principles of RP have now been incorporated into all CBT work so that patients approach termination anticipating challenges and rehearsing skill use.
Schema	A hypothesized mental structure that contains rules, emotions, beliefs, and memories about a particular topic that can be activated simultaneously with particular stimuli. Often is used as a synonym for core belief although it is more complex.
Socratic questioning	A collaborative style of questioning intended to promote curiosity and inquisitiveness. You engage the patient with a series of questions that helps the patient evaluate thoughts empirically and correct errors in logic, leading to improvement in emotional and behavioral regulation.

Common Interventions

Agenda setting	You and the patient collaboratively agree on a plan for the session and decide how much time to allot to each agenda item.
Behavioral experiments	Powerful methods designed to bring about change in patient's functioning by testing negative automatic thoughts and beliefs with actual experiments.
Behavioral techniques	Specific interventions designed to reverse maladaptive patterns of behavior; common examples include behavioral activation in depression and exposure and response prevention in OCD.
Capsule summary	Periodic summaries that "encapsulate" and reemphasize salient points discovered in the session.
Case conceptualization	Synthesizing the patient's developmental and current interpersonal history along with the cognitive model for a particular disorder to develop an explanation for the patient's current situation and an individualized treatment plan.
Cognitive rehearsal	The patient imagines a problematic situation that elicits negative emotions and behavior and envisions new ways of thinking or rehearses more adaptive cognitive and behavioral strategies to increase the likelihood that this will occur outside of session.
Cognitive techniques	The application of the scientific method to thinking.
Coping cards	Coping cards can be paper or digital reminders of important points learned in a session. They facilitate the use of new thinking and skills in day-to-day life.
Downward arrow	Otherwise known as vertical descent, this technique is designed to uncover underlying rules and assumptions that give rise to automatic thoughts. It consists of asking the patient if an automatic thought was true, what would it mean to or about the patient. It requires the therapist to clearly inform the patient that he/she knows that the thought is not true but is merely exploring further to find underlying ideas that increase the patient's distress.

Fear hierarchy	The therapist and patient work together to identify as many ways that the patient may encounter a feared stimulus as possible and place them on a list ordered from least to most anxiety provoking using the Subjective Units of Distress Scale.
Feedback	Bidirectional feedback is essential to strengthen the therapeutic alliance as well as to make certain that key concepts are understood.
Forming a therapeutic alliance	The therapeutic alliance in CBT is fostered by the shared vision of treatment goals, Socratic questioning (collaborative empiricism), empathy, genuineness, and seeking frequent feedback from the patient.
Goal setting	Setting specific and measurable targets for change. Goals are set jointly and incrementally through therapy.
Guided discovery	Guided discovery is a teaching strategy. It utilizes Socratic questioning to uncover patterns of thinking and then to evaluate this thinking with Socratic questioning to develop new insights.
Homework	Also called "action plans" or "practicing outside of session." Patients need to practice new ways of thinking and behavior in their daily life and under conditions where emotions are high. Small increments of practice help the patient make the skills learned in therapy a new habit and insure durability.
Life history review	A technique by which the patient is assigned to review their personal history to identify life events that had significance in forming key belief systems and learned behaviors.
Managing alliance ruptures	Therapists actively seek patient feedback about each session and monitor nonverbal behavior that could indicate that a patient is having an emotional response to something in the session. Should such a response be negative, you use CBT tools to evaluate the thoughts the patient has and seeks to collaborate to preserve the relationship and correct any misunderstandings.
Measuring progress	Symptom inventories are regularly performed and discussed with the patient to make certain that there is progress and, if not, the treatment plan or reason reassessed.
Problem-solving	Using cognitive and behavioral techniques to solve specific problems by generating alternatives, identifying the advantages and disadvantages of each, choosing and implementing an action plan, and then evaluating the results.
Psychoeducation	A key aspect of CBT: providing information, guidance, and direct advice to the patient. Includes educating the patient about basic concepts of the CBT model, the diagnosis, prognosis, and treatment options.
Role-play	A technique used to elicit and evaluate automatic thoughts or rehearse coping strategies "in vivo." Role-playing involves you taking on the role of a significant person in the patient's life, as it relates to goals of therapy. Roles can also be reversed with you taking on the role of the patient to demonstrate alternative strategies or manage distressing situations and emotions.

6

Skill training	Teaching psychological skills that the patient lacks.
Structuring	Structuring is a distinct feature of CBT. A typical CBT session, agreed to in collaboration with the patient, would include agenda setting, review homework, symptom check, working on the agenda items, periodic feedback and summaries, and homework assignment.
Subjective Units of Distress Scale (SUDS)	SUDS is a tool used in exposure. The patient and therapist work together to assign a value from 0 to 100 of the degree of arousal/anxiety associated with encountering a particular stimulus. 0 is equal to asleep, 15 with barely awake, 30 with just noticing anxiety, and 100 with terror.

CBT, cognitive behavioral therapy; OCD, obsessive compulsive disorder.

REFERENCES

1. Wolpe J. *The Practice of Behavior Therapy.* 4th ed. New York, NY: Pergamon Press; 1990:xvi, 421.
2. Leahy RL. *Cognitive Therapy: Basic Principles and Applications.* Northvale, NJ: J. Aronson; 1996:xi, 250.
3. Winter DA. Still radical after all these years: George Kelly's the psychology of personal constructs. *Clin Child Psychol Psychiatry.* 2013;18(2):276-283.
4. Beck AT. A 60-year evolution of cognitive theory and therapy. *Perspect Psychol Sci.* 2019;14(1):16-20.
5. Kovacs M, Beck AT. Maladaptive cognitive structures in depression. *Am J Psychiatry.* 1978;135(5):525-533.
6. Shearin EN, Linehan MM. Dialectical behavior therapy for borderline personality disorder: theoretical and empirical foundations. *Acta Psychiatr Scand Suppl.* 1994;379:61-68.
7. Hayes SC, Strosahl K. *A Practical Guide to Acceptance and Commitment Therapy.* New York, NY: Springer; 2004:xvi, 395.
8. Hayes SC, Hofmann SG. The third wave of cognitive behavioral therapy and the rise of process-based care. *World Psychiatry.* 2017;16(3):245-246.
9. Hofmann SG, Asnaani A, Vonk IJ, Sawyer AT, Fang A. The efficacy of cognitive behavioral therapy: a review of meta-analyses. *Cognit Ther Res.* 2012;36(5):427-440.
10. Lewinsohn PM. A behavioral approach to depression. In: Friedman RM, Katz MM, eds. *The Psychology of Depression: Contemporary Theory and Research.* New York, NY: Wiley; 1974:157-185.
11. Rush AJ, Beck AT. Cognitive therapy of depression and suicide. *Am J Psychother.* 1978;32(2):201-219.
12. MacPhillamy DJ, Lewinsohn PM. The pleasant events schedule: studies on reliability, validity, and scale intercorrelation. *J Consult Clin Psychol.* 1982;50(3):363-380.
13. Jacobson E. Progressive relaxation. *Am J Psychol.* 1987;100(3/4):522-537.
14. Wright JH, Brown GK, Thase ME, Basco MR. *Learning Cognitive-Behavior Therapy: An Illustrated Guide.* 2nd ed. Arlington, VA: American Psychiatric Association Publishing; 2017:xviii, 321, 196-197.
15. Foa E, Hembree E, Rothbaum BO. *Prolonged Exposure Therapy for PTSD: Emotional Processing of Traumatic Experiences Therapist Guide.* New York, NY: Oxford University Press; 2007.
16. Resick PA, Monson CM, Chard KM. *Cognitive Processing Therapy for PTSD: A Comprehensive Manual.* New York, NY: Guilford Publications; 2016.
17. Cohen JA, Mannarino AP, Deblinger E, eds. *Trauma-focused CBT for Children and Adolescents: Treatment Applications.* New York, NY. Guilford Press; 2012.
18. Ehlers A, Clark DM, Hackmann A, McManus F, Fennell M. Cognitive therapy for PTSD: development and evaluation. *Behav Res Ther.* 2005;43:413-431.

6

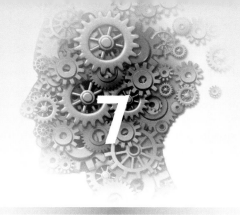

Psychodynamic Therapy

LARRY THORNTON, MD

Case Study

Mr. B, a man in his mid-30s, came to therapy because he was depressed. He and his wife had recently moved to the community and were expecting their first child. He described feeling out of place everywhere and not truly at home anywhere in his present life. Near the end of a session he said, "I've got to stop early today. My wife is having a repeat sonogram. The first one looked like it might be Down syndrome."

"Oh. I'm sorry to hear that. What is your reaction to that possibility?"

He looked perplexed. "Uh, nothing, really."

I thought a moment, perplexed now myself. "Really? That's…remarkable."

He shrugged and left.

At his next session he said, "I told my friend what you said. He said it wasn't remarkable that I didn't have a reaction to the sonogram. He said it was pretty damn weird! I thought about what he said, and I guess he's right. I guess it was a little weird. I'm not sure why I didn't react."

I responded, "Well, where do your thoughts go when you think about it?"

INTRODUCTION—A MICROCOSM, A MAP, AND A METAPHOR: THREE WAYS OF THINKING ABOUT PSYCHODYNAMIC THERAPY

Psychodynamic Psychotherapy as a Microcosm

This brief interaction represents psychodynamic therapy in a microcosm. Two people are talking and something important comes up. A question is asked about an experience, then attention is focused on some salient aspect of that experience. This leads, ideally, to a period of self-reflection. The therapist then joins the patient in wondering. This process of learning to reflect and wonder is central to the benefits of psychodynamic psychotherapy because they are associated with changes in self-awareness.

As the above story shows, psychodynamic therapy is not abstract or vague. It involves the active exploration of experiences as they happen. It is about important things like birth and death and the health of those we love. It is about wondering why we are reacting the way we are.

The goal of this chapter is to help you learn how to do psychodynamic therapy. Basic dynamic concepts and interventions will be presented in a language that is relatively free of technical jargon, except when it genuinely increases our understanding of the patient, helps suggest what to say or do, or facilitates communication with other professionals. We will focus on paying attention to the direct experience of talking with patients and keeping speculation about unconscious mental states at a minimum. Such speculation can be helpful at times, but it needs to be grounded in what the patient actually says and does.

The Map of Psychodynamic Psychotherapy

So what exactly is psychodynamic therapy? How does it work and who is it for? How do you listen and think about your patient? How do you decide when to speak and what in the world do you say?

Here is where the map comes in. When entering any new territory, some place we have never been before, a map is very useful. A map gives a quick view of the landscape's main features. It gives a sense of where we are headed and what we are likely to meet along the way. The map may be only a rough representation of the actual terrain, and it may oversimplify things quite a bit, but it shows the main landmarks and roads. Without it, it is easy to get lost. The map helps us find our way.[1]

Psychodynamic therapy can also have a simple map, with a beginning, a pathway, and goal. We begin with the therapist and the patient talking. Eventually, they talk about what is most important to the patient. Talking and listening with growing attentiveness becomes the pathway. The therapist, by paying meticulous attention to the patient's talk, helps the patient develop an increasingly fine-grained awareness of their own experience. Regarding goals, psychodynamic therapy has two related and fundamental aims that can be stated quite simply. The first is to be able to talk clearly about what really matters to the patient. The second is to learn to be increasingly attentive to the realities of the patient's experience. *All the theoretical descriptions and jargon should not obscure these fundamental aims.*

Now that we know the beginning and the end on this map, let us further discuss the "pathway" of talk. Psychodynamic therapy is, at its heart, just two people talking. It is conversation and dialogue and communication. It is something that is deeply familiar, something you have grown up with, something you already have some ability to do. You listen and respond. It is in this listening and responding that dynamic therapy* happens. Helping the patient pay more attention to their own experience is the pathway of psychodynamic therapy.

---

*Note: Throughout this chapter, the terms "psychodynamic" and "dynamic" are used interchangeably.

Attentiveness to what is happening in the room as it happens is a central feature of psychodynamic therapy. There is a focused attentiveness to the other person's expression of feelings, to the flow of their stories, to their descriptions of people and events in their lives, to the atmosphere and music of their speech. It is also based on a similar attentiveness to your own emotions and trains of thought, to the tensions in your body, and to the times that your attention wanders.

Why is attentiveness to talk itself so important? For our purposes, *a person's talk is their mind made manifest.* Talk, even when it is evasive and concealing, is available for inspection and clarification. Talk may indicate and suggest depths that will always remain elusive, but our talk is a way we bridge the gaps between each other. Talk is a fundamental way we reveal who we are.

Now by talk, I mean, primarily, the actual words the patient uses. This is the most basic and most important aspect. But I also mean the tone and rhythm of a person's speech, their cadences, speed, and pauses. This is supplemented by the patient's behavior, their actions, their posture and gestures, as well as displays of feeling. Sometimes, silences and omissions, too, can convey or alter meaning. They all contribute to the feeling of the other person's presence in the room.

However, what we primarily work with in dynamic therapy is concrete speech, especially the patient's stories and their commentaries on them. As we explore these stories with the patient, more stories and feelings come, story after story, some recurring in different contexts with new variations, regularly accompanied by more intense feelings. From this perspective, psychodynamic therapy takes place in the open between people when they talk aloud, and not hidden inside the patient's unobservable mind.

Recall that the second aim of psychodynamic psychotherapy is to be increasingly attentive to the patient's experience. For example, the experience of Mr. B on the way to his wife's sonogram was that he had no feelings about it. After my observation and his conversation with a friend, he began to question this absence of feelings. It became clear over time that this lack of feelings where they otherwise might be expected was a long-term pattern for him. It showed up time and again. Eventually, we began to actually feel the anxiety and grief in his life as we talked. So, his experience of himself had broadened to include things he was not aware of before.

These types of experience are key. They suggest that we are not always aware of the implications of what we are saying. By becoming more aware of these implications, the self changes and grows. This is a way of thinking about the **unconscious** in psychodynamic therapy. The term "unconscious" refers to those aspects of ourselves that, while influencing our actions and awareness, are unknown to us. Again—one aim of dynamic therapy is to make known what is not yet known.

A Metaphor of Psychodynamic Psychotherapy

I will now shift to the metaphor I mentioned at the beginning of this section. It will give you a taste of what psychodynamic work is like and help prepare us for another way of thinking about our goal.

In *Titus Groan*, Mervyn Peake's[2] masterpiece of gothic fantasy, the daughter of the castle has a stairway behind her bed that leads to a secret attic. When she is upset, she goes there. Climbing the staircase, she trembles with love: "It is the love of a man or a woman for their world. For the world of their center where their lives burn genuinely and with a free flame."

Where this genuine, free flame burns is where you will truly find your patients. It is where you will find what really matters to them, what moves them and drives them, and what wakes them up at night. It is where they are most truly themselves. It is the therapist's job to follow the patient up their private staircase to the attic where they really are. This happens in listening and responding.

Let us continue to follow the daughter of the castle, up her staircase. The first room in the attic is filled with broken instruments, forgotten toys, and dusty paintings of dead ancestors. She crawls through these "incongruous relics of a past," toward her true destination: the immense and empty second attic room. Standing at the precipice of this room, she trembles again. This second room is her "attic of make believe," the place where she comes to dream. All the characters from her imagination play together here as if on an enormous stage.

This scene captures some of the thrill of following a patient through a labyrinth of stories of the past into a theater where what is most cherished and most feared come to act and speak and play. By attending and responding, the therapist helps bring this theater and these dramas into clearer view.

What bears emphasizing in this metaphor is this: *dynamic therapy happens when, by our attentiveness to the patient's speech, what matters most comes into the open.* The dynamic therapist engages with the artifacts, the memories, the past hurts and triumphs, and the stories and ideas about who the patient is. But what is of paramount importance is the living play of the patient's thoughts and feelings.

It is in this living play that discovery happens. It is here that previously unrecognized forces begin to show themselves. Our patient will begin to say things that surprise herself. She will see things she had not seen before and think things that do not fit with her old ideas about herself and others. Something she had not been aware of is working in her. That is also what we mean by the unconscious. It is not some place or some goal to reach; it is a way to think about these forces acting in our lives that we had not been aware of before.

This metaphor assumes patients have relatively easy initial access to their inner world and the expectation that something good will come from talking. However, some patients may not be as immediately in touch with their inner world but could still benefit from psychodynamic therapy. The first task is to help them become more aware of their thoughts and feelings and to be able to put them into words.

Mr. B is a good example of the latter type of patients—the ones who are not as immediately in touch with their inner world. Initially, he was not aware of any feelings about important things, both in his present and his past. Much of our early work involved helping him begin to look inward, to recognize situations where he might expect to have feelings, to notice when he was pushing feelings away, and to gradually let them in.

The most common way to interest a person in their inner life is by being interested in it ourselves. We ask questions about their experiences, pay attention to answers, then ask more questions in line with what we have heard. It is very rare to be listened to this closely. It is even more rare to be listened to with no other goal than to understand. This is very powerful. With time, most people in psychodynamic psychotherapy begin to talk more freely and to bring their inner world to the fore.

Now doing all this is not so easy. When attempting to talk clearly about what matters and to attend to the play of forces in ourselves, we run into many obstacles, both in the patient and ourselves. Noticing these obstacles, noticing them when they occur, and noticing how they work constitute the central practical actions of psychodynamic work.

Case Study—Example of an Obstacle in Therapy

During the early weeks of treatment with Mr. B, the therapist forgot a session scheduled over the lunch hour. He remembered it while eating, but it was, of course, too late. Mr. B had gone. In the next session, the patient did not bring up the therapist's absence.

"You haven't mentioned that I missed our session," the therapist stated.

Mr. B replied, "Oh, I figured it was an emergency. I know doctors get emergencies."

The therapist had a decision to make here. He had made a mistake in forgetting the session and felt foolish and a bit ashamed. This was a problem he had created and one so early in the treatment! It was tempting to let the patient's convenient excuse for him stand, but that felt like an evasion. He decided it was best to address his reaction.

The therapist responded, "It sounds like it's ok as long as it was an emergency."

After a long silence, Mr. B said between tight lips, "It sure as hell better have been."

Another decision for the therapist, who responded, "Well, what if it wasn't?"

Teeth now clenched, Mr. B stated, "We're not going to talk about that possibility right now."

This was a tough moment. The therapist now decided to let it drop. It was early in treatment, and Mr. B's feelings were intense. The therapist thought that to push the matter would be disruptive. But, he kept this scene in mind. In that moment, all that the therapist knew was that he was in the face of something very powerful, that this meant a lot to the patient, and that the two of them could not yet find words to talk about it.

7

Tying Together the Microcosm, Map, and Metaphor

Let us return to our map. Psychodynamic therapy starts with two people talking, one helping the other speak about what is most important to them, helping them notice more clearly their own experience as it happens. But where is all this leading to? What is the destination? By becoming more attentive to their experience and by wondering about the unnoticed forces that may be influencing their thoughts, feelings, and actions, patients in dynamic psychotherapy learn a new frame of mind. In this mode, the mind pays attention to its own workings and becomes curious about itself.

Learning this frame of mind leads to a number of very good things: greater self-acceptance, a tolerance of painful feelings, compassion and forbearance for others, and thoughtfulness in the face of stress or strong emotions. Old ways of reacting shift, and old patterns of behavior alter. These arise naturally from the new frame of mind that begins to notice and wonder.

The following pages will give detailed examples of what this all means in practice. We will begin with the patient's first visit. What sorts of problems can dynamic therapy help with? What patient characteristics suggest a good candidate for dynamic therapy and what suggest otherwise? What does a dynamic therapist listen for in the first session?

As we proceed, try to keep in mind our map and metaphor: *Psychodynamic therapy is talk between two people that aims at speaking clearly about what truly matters. It is going up the staircase to the attic where what is most important to the patient comes out to play.*

THE DSM AND PSYCHODYNAMIC PSYCHOTHERAPY

There are many systems for categorizing suffering. The model you are probably most familiar with currently is the Diagnostic and Statistical Manual of Mental Disorders (DSM).[3] Let me first talk about the DSM and psychodynamics before moving to various psychodynamic ways of thinking about suffering.

The current version of the DSM takes a symptom-oriented approach that places patient symptoms in discrete diagnostic categories. As you have experienced, it can be a very powerful tool for guiding treatment. But as with any model, the DSM views people from a particular perspective. Psychodynamic therapy is an additional perspective, one that is more attentive to the patient's subjective experience, her relationships with herself and others, and how she finds meaning in her world.

DSM and psychodynamics are not mutually exclusive—they are simply different ways of organizing what the patient is telling us. Both are useful and may be used together to help our patients. As you grow as a clinician, you will incorporate these and other perspectives and be able to move comfortably from one to another as the situation demands. Let me give you an example of how the DSM and psychodynamics can be intertwined in a specific case.

Example—DSM and Psychodynamics

A psychiatrist was treating a woman, Ms. C, with severe recurrent depression. When ill, she was suicidal, unable to concentrate, and spent extended time in bed. She eventually found a complex regimen of medication that helped her achieve remission. She began seeing a therapist to work on chronic feelings of self-hatred and feeling rejected. Over time, she developed a greater understanding of how her relationship with her parents had influenced her feelings about herself. She had interpreted their unhappiness as her fault and their criticisms as the truth of who she was. This recognition helped her when her mood would dip. She could see when these dips were due to some hurt she had experienced. She was able to make this connection, think through her reactions and interpretations, and regain a stable mood through psychotherapy.

Unfortunately, she began to react strongly to a criticism for an error at work. She was sure she was going to be fired, even though the mistake had been minor. She drew upon her insights in therapy, but her mood continued to deteriorate, and she became increasingly hostile in her thoughts about herself.

She soon developed another major depressive episode. My colleague made some medication adjustments, and she was back in remission within a few weeks. As she improved, she was able to draw upon her insights from therapy, and her self-image and her interpretation of recent events shifted, even before she was fully well again.

It appears that, sometimes, a psychological hurt could drive her into an episode of major depression requiring medication adjustments. The next time she had a relapse, she knew she was misinterpreting slights as gross rejections and did not react as strongly. As therapy progressed, she was still subject to periodic relapses of depression, but her life between was much richer, she developed better relationships, and was able to regain remission more quickly.

At other times, she might experience an apparently unprovoked relapse and, as part of it, be very sensitive to slights and be prone to self-hatred. Sometimes, the major depressive disorder seemed to be driving her negative self-image; at other times, her negative self-image seemed to drive her into a major depressive episode. Clinically, it was important to keep both these perspectives in mind because sometimes she needed a medication change and, at others, she needed to focus on therapy. It was not always immediately clear which was which. As a result, the psychiatrist and the therapist needed to keep an open mind, in that DSM symptoms and diagnoses informed psychotherapy, and progress in psychotherapy informed symptom remission.

WHAT IS THE EVIDENCE FOR PSYCHODYNAMIC THERAPY?

Psychodynamic therapy is essentially an individualized therapy. It is about what is most important to the unique person you are working with. Understanding ourselves better tends to make for a richer life and more satisfying relationships, but people often come to us with symptoms of specific psychiatric disorders such as depression and anxiety. Can such an individualized approach like psychodynamic therapy be helpful for the common symptomatic presentations of these disorders?

There is, in fact, substantial empiric evidence demonstrating the efficacy of psychodynamic therapy in a wide range of mental disorders. Leichsenring and Klein[4] performed meta-analyses of 47 randomized controlled trials of psychodynamic therapy in the treatment of specific psychiatric diagnoses. They reported that psychodynamic therapy is effective in the treatment of depressive disorders, anxiety disorders, somatoform disorders, personality disorders, eating disorders, complicated grief, and posttraumatic stress disorder. Obsessive compulsive disorder, though, does not typically respond to psychodynamic therapy.

Psychodynamic therapy is contraindicated for some disorders. For example, the process of intensive self-observation and reflection can lead to increasingly disorganized thinking in patients with psychosis. Some patients with paranoia and more primitive defenses (we will discuss these in detail later) may show a tendency to become more unstable in psychodynamic therapy. If a patient becomes unstable during the course of psychodynamic therapy, especially in the early sessions, it could be a sign that the treatment is not right for them, and consultation is needed in such situations.

PSYCHODYNAMIC THEORY

Psychoanalytic theory is the foundation for psychodynamic therapy. The theory was developed to account for observed clinical phenomena. Some familiarity with its core concepts will help you listen better to your patients, help you organize what you hear, and guide you in what to say.

Classic psychoanalytic theory[5] has a small set of core ideas of great importance to psychodynamic psychotherapy:

1. The presence of unconscious internal conflict,

2. The use of psychological defenses against unpleasant feelings,

3. The abiding impact of early relationships on later life, and

4. The concept of psychological development.

From a classic psychoanalytic perspective, *psychological difficulties arise from internal conflict*. Internal conflict arises because we have competing needs, wishes, and fears that do not always fit well together. For example, I may really want something but be ashamed to ask for it. My wishes may also come into conflict with others. Someone else may want what I want badly enough to fight. Classic psychoanalytic theory pictures us navigating through these conflicting feelings, finding compromises that bring us a blend of satisfaction and safety.

The concept of defenses is a fundamental psychodynamic idea, one of the most central. These compromises are motivated by anxiety, stated simply as *anxiety motivates defense*. This means that when we perceive a dangerous situation, fear mobilizes protective measures to protect us from the danger. Imagine you are walking down the street. Suddenly, you see someone you really do not want to meet. You duck into a shop until they pass. Defenses are like that, except they protect us from meeting dangerous thoughts and feelings in the mind. They tend to function without much conscious awareness. Recognizing defenses is a key skill for a psychodynamic therapist. We will address this in detail later.

Another fundamental psychoanalytic idea is that *our early relationships are critically important to who we are*. These early attachments influence what we care about, what we aspire to, how we react to loss and frustration, and how we develop later relationships. As therapists, we are therefore very interested in the nature of these early ties and the ways that they live on in later life. We are especially interested in what constitutes closeness and feeling loved.

A final key idea is that *we develop over time.* The mind of a 5-year-old differs from a 10-year-old. Different periods of life are associated with particular developmental challenges and different ways of managing thoughts and feelings. Inner conflicts and ways of relating may arise during specific developmental stage, influencing the person's tendency to react to current situations as if they were replays of the past.

Several text boxes in this section will help explain additional models and theories relevant to psychodynamic psychotherapy, for further learning and consideration.

Erikson's Model—Common Conflicts Across Life Stages

Another way of thinking about psychological conflict and danger is from a developmental perspective. Erik Erikson's model is very helpful in this regard. For Erikson, human development took place in a series of stages, each of which is characterized by a specific conflict.[6] Instead of the conflict being thought of as between two distinct parts of the mind, Erikson imagined the child being pulled between two different states of mind. The task for the person in each stage is to come to some adjustment to this conflict. How a given person manages each stage has a defining impact on their later personality. Erikson thought that each family and culture promoted certain solutions to each of these basic conflicts.

This developmental schema is useful to therapists as a set of basic scenarios that help capture recurrent aspects of human experience. The schema reminds us that different times of life bring their own set of demands. Development does not stop with childhood, and later life conflicts do not simply replay childhood dramas, even when these earlier issues are stirred again.

Erikson's model provides terms that draw out the core emotional issues of life and help organize a seemingly disparate group of phenomena. These terms are helpful to keep in mind while listening to your patients.

The stages in this model are as follows, with rough ages in which they are thought to be most predominant:

Basic Trust Versus Mistrust (0-18 months). Will I expect good things from other people, or will I expect to be hurt?

Autonomy Versus Shame and Doubt (18 months-3 years). Will I be able to do things myself, or will I be hampered by self-doubt?

Initiative Versus Guilt (3-5 years). Will I be able to make something new, or will I feel I've done something terribly wrong?

Industry Versus Inferiority (5-13 years). Will I be able to work and be persistent, or will I forever be less than everyone else?

Identity Versus Role Diffusion (13-21 years). Will I be able to find a relatively stable sense of who I am and what matters to me, or will I continue to wonder what really matters?

Intimacy Versus Isolation (21-39 years). Will I be able to be genuinely close to someone, or will I feel cut-off and alone?

Generativity Versus Stagnation (40-65 years). Will I be able to contribute and grow, or will I feel stuck and empty?

Ego Integrity Versus Despair (65+ years). Will I be able to develop an abiding sense of who I am and what life has meant, or will I fall prey to nihilism?

A Closer Look at the Structural Model of Psychoanalysis

The psychoanalytic theory that developed to account for internal conflict and defenses is called **structural theory**.[7] Structure here refers to the classic tripartite set of mental functions whose terms you are likely familiar with: the ego, the id, and the super ego. It is unfortunate that the early translators of Freud saddled us with these Latinate words. Freud's German terms were das Ich, das Es, and das Uber-Ich. These might be better translated as the "I," the "It," and the "Over-I." These terms are much closer to the lived experience Freud was trying to account for.

The **id** refers to the mental representation of our desires and biological drives. Freud's term the "It" captures the autonomous and somewhat alien quality of our desires. We want what we want, often without clear reasons. We can feel driven by something internal that feels like it is not fully under our control.

The **super ego** has at least two major faces. On one side, it incorporates the prohibitions we have been taught by our family and culture and is represented by feelings of guilt when we transgress or think about transgressing. Freud's "Over-I" gets at this feeling we have of being observed and judged, even within our own minds. This feeling of self-observation is built upon societal or family norms but may be strict beyond anything we actually experienced externally.

The other face of the super ego is our ideals. These are our aspirations to do what we think we should do, as well as be what we think we ought or would most like to be. The feelings of pride and satisfaction we get from coming close to our ideals are an aspect of super ego functioning in this model.

The **ego** (the "I") sits between the id, the super ego, and the outer world. Its role is to mediate between the demands of our biological drives, the prohibitions we have developed, the ideals we aim for, and the realities of the world we live in, with all its possibilities, necessities, and barriers. The ego synthesizes and makes compromises between all these factors. In psychoanalytic theory, the ego is responsible for the defenses we talked about earlier. When the ego perceives threats, either from internal or external sources, it institutes measures ("defenses") to avoid or diminish pain or distress.

Kohut's Self-Psychology and Personality

Heinz Kohut created self-psychology as a modification of psychoanalytic theory to better account for patients who presented with problems such as narcissism, internal emptiness, and poor self-esteem.[5,9,10] Kohut argued that conflicts around sexual or aggressive wishes were important, but they were not the primary problem. He thought that such conflicts arose in the course of development as a secondary problem stemming from core deficits in the sense of self.

In self-psychology, a child is understood to develop their sense of self through internalizing the empathic mirroring they receive from the parent. When the parent fulfills this profound need, Kohut referred to them as being a "self-object." The self further develops through building up a set of ideals and aspirations, often also internalized from perceptions of the parents, along with other cultural inputs.

A Closer Look at Common Fears

As we mentioned, a fundamental psychodynamic idea is that anxiety motivates defense. Anxiety arises in response to inner dangerous thoughts, dangerous feelings, or dangerous memories. There are various ways to classify the typical psychological danger situations we face in life and in therapy. In psychoanalytic theory, there are traditionally *five crucial psychological dangers* (one of which, "castration anxiety," is notoriously controversial). These five are based on Freud's original four dangers, augmented by an appreciation that blows to one's sense of self carry their own specific threat:[8,9]

1. Loss of an important person

2. Loss of the important person's love

3. Physical damage or mutilation

4. Guilt

5. Shame

Loss of an important person is typically accompanied by intense fears of abandonment and panicky anxiety. The other person is felt to be absolutely gone, and the patient frantically wants them back. Similarly, when an important person's love is lost, the other person still exists, but they no longer care for you anymore. We all know what this feels like.

The fear of physical harm or bodily mutilation is universal. Early psychoanalytic theory, however, focused particularly on castration anxiety and thought it was crucial for both boys and girls. Contemporary psychodynamic thinkers believe that represented a profound error in understanding female psychology, yet there are some male patients who do have a focus on this specific fear.

The fear of guilt is present when we do not do something because we know we will feel bad afterward. The feeling of guilt seems to be primarily attached to specific acts of wrongdoing. Shame, on the other hand, is more global and is a feeling that one's entire being is wrong, laughable, or contemptible. Often associated with intense shame is intense envy, a feeling of not having something highly valued.

It is a useful exercise to listen to your patients with this simple list of five common threats in mind. You will be surprised by how much of human anxiety fits under this short set of fears. Sometimes, things are not as complicated as we make them out to be.

But what about depression? Whereas anxiety is the fear that one of the dangerous situations is going to happen, depression is the feeling that the danger has *already* happened and nothing can be done to reverse it. In this situation, the person feels doomed to be alone, doomed to being unloved, and doomed to perpetual guilt or shame. Pointing out this feeling of being doomed can be a helpful technique in focusing on this particular reaction.

7

Lacanian Model—Suffering Results From Indoctrination and Alienation

Another example of ways of organizing what the patient is suffering from is the work of Jacques Lacan, a French psychoanalyst who died in 1981.[5,11] At the risk of oversimplification, for Lacan, a major task we all face is integration into what he calls the symbolic order. This order involves the representations of all the values and meanings that exist within the particular family, culture, and historical time we are born into. Examples are the language we are born into, the values that we are offered, what is presented as desirable or prohibited, what is considered bad and undesirable, etc.

For Lacan, we all, as children, must necessarily conform to this order, and therefore our wishes and ways of thinking about them are not really fully our own. An aspect of therapy from this perspective would be uncovering the history of this indoctrination and alienation from oneself and discovering what the patient really wants.

One simple but effective way to use this Lacanian perspective in an initial meeting is to ask the patient how they got their name or how they chose the names of their children. Names are a key way of placing a child within the meaningful order of things as the parent sees them. The child has a place within the world of the parents before she is even born, and some of those meanings will be reflected in the choice of her name.

An Alternative Perspective—The Buddhist Model of Suffering

Let me offer another model of suffering from a different tradition. It is an old and simple way to categorize suffering that complements the dynamic models we have been exploring. From a Buddhist point of view, suffering is thought to arise from a limited set of situations.[12] First, there are existential issues: being born, getting sick, getting old, and dying. Then, there are what we might think of as psychological issues: being separated from those you love, being forced to be with those you do not like, and not getting what you want. As an exercise, listen to your patient with this Buddhist set of categories in mind. You might be surprised how much falls within these simple groups.

Applying Psychodynamic Theory to the Case Study

Let us return to the case of Mr. B. As the work progressed, the therapist learned more about Mr. B's development and family dynamics:

Mr. B, who had no feelings about the sonogram, described his father as intelligent and ambitious. He seemed completely preoccupied with his career. To the patient, he was without emotion, never needing anyone, and capable of doing anything. His mother, who was just as smart and educated, seemed more fragile and needy. She wilted in the face of conflict or strong emotions. His father was contemptuous of this "weakness." Mr. B knew both of them loved him, but he felt distant from his father and a bit contemptuous, too, of his mother.

Mr. B was sent to boarding school soon after the sudden death of his younger sister when he was a young teen. He said his family never talked about her death or showed much feeling about it. His mother seemed to withdraw, and his father divorced her and left the state to start on a new career. They both wanted him to "carry on." After college, Mr. B traveled around the world alone, often to dangerous places, but then had trouble keeping a job. He would lose interest, immerse himself in research about some subject, then become disenchanted and depressed. He had trouble feeling close to others because "there is really not much to me."

We can develop some initial hypotheses about the impact of early experiences on Mr. B using the core aspects of psychodynamic theory we have described above. These and other specific models (described in various text boxes in this chapter) give us ways of thinking about his current difficulties, as well as cues for things to pay attention to as the treatment goes forward.

Mr. B described his father as being without emotion. This sounds similar to his lack of reaction to the sonogram and suggests that Mr. B wanted to be like his father. Recall the core features of most psychodynamic approaches: (1) the presence of unconscious inner conflict, (2) the use of psychological defenses against unpleasant feelings, (3) the abiding impact of early relationships on later life, and (4) the concept of psychological development.

It is already clear from our first two interactions that Mr. B is not entirely conscious of his remarkable "lack" of feelings about important and emotional events in his life. Theory also suggests he has been strongly impacted by early relationships in his life, even now.

Maybe he developed contempt for his own feelings, similar to the contempt he thought his father had for his mother's emotions during his childhood. The silence of important others regarding his sister's death reinforces the idea that feelings are dangerous, especially those related to relationships and loss. He carries on (just like his father) leaving those with feelings behind, yet exhibits anxiety when they arise. Mr. B's eagerness for travel and study shows that some things do truly matter to him, that he does, in fact, have passionate feelings. It also demonstrates how he grows and develops across the lifespan as a person, with unique interests and life story beyond his childhood. But, his recurrent disenchantment may indicate some internal inhibition against caring too deeply, some difficulty letting things matter too much and exposing him to loss. Put in another way, we can imagine Mr. B longing for closeness but afraid of loss, defending himself against feelings by repressing them (a form of psychological defense to be discussed later). However, self-protection comes at a price—he often feels isolated and empty and is unsure why.

There is another way of thinking about this brief biography of Mr. B. Maybe early in life he was very close to his mother. Maybe he had strong feelings and expressed them openly at one time, but perhaps the death of his sister showed him that those with feelings get despised and left behind. As a result, he may have learned it is better to become unfeeling and carry on.

Both of these hypotheses lead us to pay close attention when Mr. B shows that something matters to him. We would want him to talk more about this, watching for signs of defenses against feelings or emotional closeness to others. We would pay close attention to his reaction to any real or threatened losses. We would be very interested in who he sees as his heroes. Are they stoics like his father? How does he react to the therapist in session? Does he see him as a cold intellectual or does he fear he will lure him into the dangerous and contemptible arena of experiencing and expressing feelings and prevent him from being able to use his typical defenses? Maybe he even imagines the therapist will leave him if he gets too needy?

As you can tell, these different hypotheses are not mutually exclusive. They each suggest different perspectives on Mr. B's experience, helping us listen for different things. Each view might better speak to aspects of the patient's experience at different times. It is important not to become too attached to a given model or way of thinking about your patient. Patients will always be more than the sum of all our models and always more than we can understand or say. The therapist's goal is to become familiar enough with a variety of dynamic models so that multiple ways of organizing our understanding of our patients can occur.[13]

PSYCHODYNAMIC THERAPY IN ACTION—IMPORTANT FIRST STEPS

Is Psychodynamic Psychotherapy Appropriate?

How do we decide if psychodynamic therapy is likely to be of help? If this particular person at this particular point in her life develops a deeper understanding of what is going on in her mind and her relationships, if she is able to pursue a further exploration of thoughts and feelings so that these come into greater awareness, will this lead to something good?

This depends on important considerations about the patient, as addressed in Chapter 3 of this book on selecting a therapy modality. From our perspective, the most important criteria for selecting a patient for dynamic therapy are as follows: *Does the person have an ability to reflect upon their own mental processes, to wonder about them, and, most critically, can they accept some degree of responsibility for them?*

How do you assess this capacity? A history of long-standing relationships or other commitments, either academic, personal, or professional, indicates some stability of wishes and an ability to adapt to adversity. Long-standing interests or hobbies suggest an ability to find meaning and pleasure in things, some ability to direct energies in gratifying ways. Asking the patient in the first meeting what she makes of her reactions and feelings can give you some sense if she takes responsibility for them. For example, consider again Ms. C who reacted so strongly to criticism from her boss at work. In the early sessions, she commented, "I think I was hurt" and "I'm not really sure, but it bothers me I got so mad." This suggests an ability to stand outside an immediate experience and think about it. These comments have a different sense than if she said, "My boss made me so mad. If he would just understand, I wouldn't get so angry" or "My boss is such a jerk. How can he expect me to do what he says?" This ability to wonder and take responsibility for oneself is not absolute. Dynamic therapy can help to develop or bring out these abilities.[14,15] And although these abilities continue to grow during treatment, some rudimentary capacity at the outset is necessary.

Sometimes it only becomes clear with repeated experience that a patient has great trouble in their ability to reflect and wonder, and that dynamic therapy is not suited to help them. Assessing these abilities is an ongoing task for therapists. You will sometimes see patients who seem "psychologically minded," in that they can talk extensively about their feelings, speculate about motivations, and make connections between their early life experiences and their current reactions. But with time, they do not change. Their insights do not lead to increased responsibility, and their explanations seem more and more like justifications. Being able to talk about one's inner life is not necessarily the same as having a sense of personal agency and responsibility. This resistance to true responsibility would then become the focus for therapy.

The First Meeting

The first session is a beginning, a chance to start getting to know the other person, to get a sense for how they speak about themselves and their world and to find the rhythm of their conversation. It is also a chance to find out why they are there. For the most part, patients come to us because they are suffering. Even when someone else has insisted the patient come, the patient is suffering in some way. The therapist's job in the first session is to develop an initial understanding of this suffering and to share this understanding with the patient.

The first meeting is also when the patient begins to develop *transference reactions*. From the first moment they thought about therapy, the patient is developing an idea about who you might be. From the first session, you are keeping yourself relatively anonymous so that the patient can use you to reflect upon their inner world. Simply defined, **transference** occurs when we take ways of relating to some important person from the past and place them on someone in the present.[16] Transference is fundamental to psychodynamic psychotherapy, and we will discuss it in detail later in the chapter. For now, it is important to recognize that *psychodynamic therapy is set up to facilitate the development of transference*. Keeping this in mind will help you understand why therapy is started the way it is, and why expectations, framework, and boundaries are addressed in specific ways in psychodynamic therapy from the very beginning.

So if our goal is to understand the other person's suffering, how do we do this? The simple answer is that we listen. The patient will tell us what is troubling them. But, we will listen better if we have some ways of organizing what we hear. In developing our understanding, it is best to begin with what the patient thinks the problem is. The patient who had no feelings about the sonogram primarily felt out of place and could not feel at home in his present life. Another patient could not ever get really close to anyone, while another was never really sure what she wanted to do. Still another could not deal with the loss of a child.

It is important for the therapist to reflect back at some point in the first session to what they are hearing. This helps establish the alliance with the patient. This initial understanding does not need to be complex. It can be as simple as, "It seems like you are struggling with how to feel closer to your husband" or "Your mother's death has been hard for you." You will be surprised at how these kinds of straightforward statements help and provide a sense of clarity. To say to Mr. B, "It sounds like

7

you've had a hard time feeling at home since you moved here," may seem obvious, but it may clarify something for the patient that had not been quite so clear before.

This is a good place to remind you that you cannot know more than you know at this point. A common worry of many beginning therapists is that they should be able to have deep insight into a patient very quickly. They also tend to think that patients expect this of them. It is helpful to let this burden go. There is so much you do not know about the patient at this point and things that may shift your entire perspective on them. You may have an initial sense of what they are dealing with now, some feeling for their personality and ways of thinking, but it is important not to imagine that you can derive too much from this. Experience as a psychodynamic therapist gives you the ability to ask helpful kinds of questions and to listen more closely to their answers so that the other person may come to a better understanding of themselves. However, experience does not make you a mind reader.

This may be a helpful example for what I am talking about. A patient of mine had what she considered to be a very helpful course of therapy. A year after ending treatment, she wrote me a letter that stated, "I thought you would listen for a while, then offer me deep interpretations. But, you didn't. You were consistently underwhelming. But, you provided a space in which I could understand myself. For that, I am very grateful." It is a good aspiration for a dynamic therapist to be consistently underwhelming.

Explaining Recommendations for Psychodynamic Treatment

Once you determine psychodynamic psychotherapy will be helpful at this particular time for this patient, how do you communicate this to them? You might say something as straightforward as, "I think talking more about your marriage will be of help to you" or "Understanding more about the impact your parents' divorce had on your relationships could be helpful to you." This is usually sufficient.

It is important to use clear, direct language here. This is a good approach to always keep in mind. Our comments as therapists are usually most helpful if they are relatively short, direct, and concrete. Elaborate, abstract formulations generally promote intellectualization and avoidance rather than genuine engagement with thoughts and feelings.

Some patients, though, will ask how dynamic therapy works. This will be a question you can answer better as you get more experience. You could say something like, "Therapy can help you better see the recurring patterns in your relationships that are causing you problems, so you can change them" or "Therapy can help you understand yourself better and how you came to be the way you are. This will help you with your current problems." You will need to flesh out this general form of answer with specifics from the patient's history to make these statements meaningful. For example, we could say to Mr. B, "I think helping to understand the impact the loss of your sister had on you will help you feel closer to your children."

Recognizing Patient Expectations and Giving Basic Instructions

Knowing what the patient expects from the therapist is also important. Asking the patient about any previous experience in therapy and what they expect from you is a good practice. Some patients want a lot of feedback, some want advice, and some fear that the therapist will only listen and not offer any understanding. Some want to be friends with the therapist and hope that the therapist will share aspects of life with them. Some, on the other hand, already know something about boundaries in therapy and may use this as a reason not to ask questions or reveal fantasies about the therapist (see Chapter 4 of this book for additional information on boundaries across all therapy types). Be aware that patients present with a host of expectations and that setting the frame for psychodynamic therapy early on is necessary (further discussed in the next section).

Once therapy begins, it is helpful to begin by giving the patient some basic instructions about how to do psychodynamic therapy. I usually say something like, "It's best for you to say whatever is on your mind. It can be something you've been thinking about, something that comes to mind on the way here or in the waiting room or something that comes up in the moment. It can be about anything, a dream, a memory, something that happened that day, some feeling you are having, or some thought or feeling about me. If we go with what is most on your mind, we'll usually end up where we need to be." Saying whatever is on one's mind, with as little editing as possible, is called **free association**. The interaction that occurs when the therapist and patient pay attention to these associations is called the **dynamic process**. (That is why detailed notes of psychodynamic psychotherapy sessions are called **process notes**.)

Setting the Frame—Time and Fees

The **frame** in psychodynamic therapy is the set of rules that help create the space in which the exploration and revelation of the patient's inner life can happen.[15] It consists of regularities of time and place, a set of boundaries and expectations for each party in the relationship, and a set of processes by which the work proceeds. Simply put, the patient and therapist dedicate themselves to regular meetings that begin and end at a certain time. The therapist's role is to listen and to help the patient better understand herself. The patient's role is to talk about whatever comes to mind, attempting as much as possible to avoid censoring herself.

One of the most important regularities is the appointment time. It is best to have a set day and time to meet, rather than make a new appointment at each visit, though this is not always possible, especially when you are in training. The ritualization and regularity of therapy sessions are valuable for creating a reliable and safe place to speak freely. I do not typically talk about how important not missing appointments is unless this becomes a problem, but other dynamic therapists may feel differently.

We also set the fee during the first session. Money has many meanings for people, and much gets lived out around paying. Being comfortable talking about money is an important skill for a therapist. The fee is a moment of real interchange between the therapist and patient, a place for emotions to get played out. It is easy to avoid money, especially in training when you may not be dependent for your livelihood on collecting the fee or when a staff member deals with fee transactions before sessions.

Example—Avoidance of Fees

I was seeing a woman during my residency whose husband had lost his job after a head injury. She did not pay for a couple of months and I neglected bringing it up, thinking that I was being compassionate about her situation. At some point, she mentioned not being able to pay a bill, and I finally brought up our unpaid balance. She began to weep and stated, "I feel so guilty about not paying. I don't feel like I deserve to get any benefit from this since I'm not paying. But, I don't want to have to stop coming." We discussed her feelings and her situation and were able to renegotiate a fee that worked for her. I had thought I was being kind by not bringing up the bill, but both the patient and I had in fact been avoiding a painful group of feelings.

Roles and Boundaries

The psychodynamic therapist's role, as we have seen, is to listen, to understand, and to share this understanding in ways that will deepen the patient's ability to understand himself. *We are there for the patient; we are not there for ourselves.* Any other needs and wishes we feel beyond the wish to better understand the patient must not be acted on. To do so betrays the fundamental trust upon which therapy proceeds.

We may have a whole host of feelings toward our patients. This is normal and unavoidable. We are going to like some patients, identify with some, feel irritated or angry toward some, or even feel romantic or erotic longings toward some patients. We may want to take care of some patients or have wishes that they would leave an unhappy marriage or find another job. We cannot help but feel these things, and we need to be aware of them. But, we need to be very careful not to let them interfere with our role (see later sections on transference and countertransference).

The patient's role is to talk. To talk about what is important, to talk about what comes to mind, to talk about not wanting to talk, and to talk about feelings, memories and dreams, about relationships and frustrations, and about grief. Everything and anything can be talked about. This may include feelings and wishes that are about the patient's relationship with you. But, none of these wishes will be acted on. She can talk about wishing you could meet her for coffee, but you will not do that. He can talk about how he would like you to talk with his boss, but you will not do that.

For example, a wealthy patient I was seeing for medications came in with his wife. He was hypomanic and wanted to let me buy in on a stock option that he was sure would be an enormous winner. His wife said, "He can't accept that, dear." The patient said, "I can ask." I responded, "You're both right." *You want the patient to be able to talk about their wishes, but you cannot act on their wishes.*

One of the most common situations in which patients touch upon the therapist's boundaries and role is by asking personal questions. These include personal questions such as if we have children, what religion we are, or why we went into this kind of work. This almost always makes beginning therapists anxious (and experienced ones, too). Having a comfortable response is important for the psychodynamic psychotherapist, in terms of maintaining the frame. You can say something like, "It's most helpful to our work to understand what led you to ask the question and what ideas you have about how I might answer. It would be more helpful to explore these things than it is for me to answer your questions." You are making clear that not answering is in the service of better understanding the patient, not protecting yourself. This may sound formulaic to you. In addition, not answering questions may feel socially awkward or stereotypical. However, this response is based on the truth, and eventually these types of responses will seem natural. It is no more artificial than a surgeon gloving and gowning before surgery. These are both techniques aimed at creating a safe environment in psychodynamic psychotherapy so that certain ends can be accomplished.

By not revealing much about ourselves in psychodynamic psychotherapy, we achieve what can be called **relative anonymity**.[17] This relative anonymity of the psychodynamic therapist is very important. First, it speaks to something I said before but will repeat because it is of such fundamental and absolute importance—*the therapist's personal needs are kept in abeyance during treatment.* Our only agenda is for the therapy to proceed, for the dialogue to continue, and for understanding to deepen. Being smart, in control, in the know, respected, and loved—none of these matter for the psychodynamic therapist. They may come up as feelings and are worth examining in a separate setting, as we will get to in our discussion of countertransference, but these wishes do not need to be satisfied in the treatment or by the patient. This relative anonymity also allows for the transference to develop. We will continue to discuss the importance of transference later, but it is very important to keep in mind. This is a unique kind of relationship, one not really found much elsewhere, and transference is key to psychodynamic effectiveness.

Also, I have been saying relative anonymity (instead of a "blank slate"), because the boundaries are not absolute by any means. Our office decor, the way we dress, our speech, what we pay attention to in the sessions, the fact that we are therapists at all—these are all very revealing about who we are. Patients get to know us, in some ways, very well. They know how our therapist minds work. In fact, some patients may be hesitant to recognize how much they know about us.

Example—Self-Disclosure

A patient asked near the end of treatment if I had any children. I wondered with her why she asked. "We've talked about my daughter a lot, and what you've said has been very helpful. But, you never mentioned if you had kids yourself. I had a therapist once who helped me during my divorce. Eventually, she told me about her divorce. After a while, she spent a lot of our session telling me about her experiences, but it wasn't really helpful. Thank you for not ever mentioning if you had kids."

It is helpful to realize that by focusing on understanding the patient and keeping your own needs to a minimum, you are giving the other person a rare gift. You are not simply withholding out of some tired convention of therapy. *Relative anonymity and abstention are critical tools in creating a psychodynamic therapeutic relationship.*

ESSENTIAL SKILLS IN PSYCHODYNAMIC THERAPY

Listening

Our primary task as therapists is to listen. Our ability to understand and ultimately to help is based upon this skill.[18] As we have stressed in earlier chapters, you already know how to do this. Psychodynamic listening is built on this basic human skill. Training and experience will help you become quicker and more sophisticated in your ability to listen, but you already have the fundamental ability. Two exercises can help you begin to sharpen your skill at listening.

Labeling Exercise. As you listen, pay attention to the natural shifts in the patient's speech. When we talk, we pause, shift topics, move off on new tangents, show a new affect, or change the tone or rhythm of our speech. Whenever one of these shifts occurs, give yourself a label for the patient's previous section of speech, the simpler the better. Often a single word will suffice.[19]

This exercise will help you develop a number of important skills. First, it will help you learn to step back periodically from the flow of the patient's speech and reflect upon what is happening. This is critical to being able to simultaneously participate in the relationship and then think about it as it happens. It will also help you remember the flow of the session and eventually guide you in what you want to say. Noticing shifts and learning to name them will help you notice themes in the patient's speech and patterns in how the patient's feelings or thoughts interact.

Example—Applying the Labeling Exercise

Let us return to the example of Ms. C, now later in her therapy. The depression has recurred, now brought on by grief over her brother's recent death. Her therapist has asked her to pay attention to when her brother comes to mind. She starts the following session by recounting a number of instances over the past week when she recalled him. In great detail, she talks about specific times when she has missed him. She pauses. Here, at this pause, we can do our internal exercise in labeling. We could mentally label this section many things. "Brother," "Sadness," "Noticing," or "Missing."

She then talks about her fears that this grief will never end. She wants to move on, but she does not want to forget him. As she starts to recount a specific memory, we have another opportunity to label a section of the session. Again, there are many choices. "Don't forget," "Never get better," or "Ambivalent."

At her brother's funeral, people told so many funny stories. There were things she had never heard of. She smiled as she remembered games they made up together, a secret code they had for talking through the walls at night, and when she had found an old letter after he had died. Reading it, she could hear his voice. This shift to warmth and smiling offer another time to mentally label what we have heard, such as "Good memories," "Presence," and "Life."

The therapist said, "Your brother was present in that note. He seems so vibrant."

She smiled and responded, "That's a good word for him. He really was vibrant. That's how I want to remember him, not like at the end. He wasn't himself then."

She thought a while, then commented, "Maybe I should start writing about him." Another shift. We might label it "Writing," "Memory," or "Preservation."

The therapist said, "Tell me about writing."

"I took a history class in college. I interviewed some Vietnam War vets. They told me some really terrible stories, things they'd never told anyone. Afterwards, their wives thanked me for helping them talk." She looked up at the therapist, further commenting, "I really worked to make sure I got their stories right. I wanted to make sure I put them together in the right way. It felt like a big responsibility. I had to get it right." Another natural pause in her talk. How would you summarize it? "Stories told to someone," "Sharing," "Putting it together right?"

Linking our possible labels and amplifying them a bit, we can tie together "Grief for my brother," "I don't want to forget," "Warm presence in stories and presence in a letter," "Maybe I should write," and "Writing powerful stories and getting them right helps." Hearing this flow of thought led the therapist to emphasize the brother's presence in the letter and to ask a question about writing, which led to a story about the healing effect of sharing a painful story.

7

We can see here how mentally labeling or summarizing the sections of the session helps the therapist see the flow of topics as meaningful. Having a schematic flow of the session in mind then helps the therapist reflect as the session is happening, and seeing this flow naturally suggests helpful things to say. It is important to see in this example that what was said by the therapist was clearly based on what the patient had just said. This practice of noticing natural shifts in the session and mentally labeling them will sharpen your awareness of the dynamic process in the session and will be useful throughout your career.

Metaphor Exercise. The second exercise is a natural extension of labeling and summarizing. It involves noticing or inventing metaphors that capture important aspects of your patient's experience. By metaphor I mean an image or scenario that represents an important issue or feeling for a person. Such metaphors have a concreteness that helps us grasp what is at the heart of what the patient has been telling us. Metaphors can also help us see when a situation is being repeated. They have both a vividness and an ambiguity that encourage further exploration, helping us see implications in what the patient has been telling that may not have been clear.

Example—Applying the Metaphor Exercise

When Ms. C spoke about the note from her brother, it suggested to the therapist someone warm and alive, something very different from the stories of his depression and death. The therapist thought of the word "vibrant" while listening, a metaphoric term implying something moving rapidly and something vibrating and alive. This word caught something warm in her memories of her brother, something that could be caught (another metaphor) in stories.

When Ms. C spoke about writing the veteran's stories, she said she wanted to "put them together in the right way." This is an evocative phrase vividly suggesting the construction of a physical object, like a model or puzzle. It suggests getting the proper parts, putting them in the correct position, and leaving out what is unnecessary or ugly or wrong. For stories, it means, in part, what to include and what to leave out. This metaphor of construction becomes a powerful way to think with Ms. C about her brother's death. It leads us to wonder what pieces she will use, and what she will toss away in building his story. This opens up a clear path for us to attend to in therapy and to help the patient better understand through our questions and our listening.

Storytelling

Stories, as Ms. C shows, are an important way we organize, remember, and share experience. To have an experience, in fact, often means having a story to tell about something. Much of our everyday conversations involve sharing stories about what happened that day, about some past event, an episode from a book or movie, maybe a dream we had last night, or a hope we have for the future.

It is helpful for psychodynamic therapists to be aware of how stories are put together, how they function, and the various forms they take.[20] Such awareness helps us listen more acutely. The form of a story has a great impact on what it is able to say.[21] To help appreciate this impact, let us look at different ways of presenting Mr. B's story. We can use these variations to begin thinking about stories as stories, as different ways of organizing and presenting information, rather than simply as content.

One form of story we are all very familiar with is the history of present illness (or the HPI):

> Mr. B is a married White male in his mid-30s with a history of depression. He presents with a 12-week history of low mood, decreased energy, poor concentration, and low appetite. There has been passive suicidal ideation, but no plans or intent. He has been on sertraline 100 mg for 4 weeks without any improvement.

Physicians will immediately recognize this style of story. It starts with a character who is defined by age, marital status, ethnicity, and medical history. The story is about his symptoms, and it is derived from a meeting with a mental health professional aiming at helping him with a specific problem, defined as a set of symptoms. The language, such as "history of" and "reports" and "passive suicidal ideation," immediately identifies the story's origin within the mental health professions.

Now imagine this story told from the point of view of Mr. B talking to his wife:

> I think it's happening again. I just feel terrible all the time. I can't get up in the morning. I don't want to eat. I can't keep my mind on anything. I'm falling behind at work. I'm afraid they're going to fire me. I wish I wouldn't wake up in the morning. I'm sorry I said that. Don't worry. I'm not going to kill myself. The medicine's not helping.

These are essentially the same facts about how Mr. B feels, but they are now told from a first-person perspective, using language more suited to regular speech than to a medical chart. The incidents are the same, but the feel is very different. "I wish I wouldn't wake up" is more personal, closer to lived experience, than "passive suicidal ideation." "I don't want to eat" is more vivid than "low appetite."

Each of these stories is constructed to achieve different ends. This is the first key thing to remember about stories. They are always told to someone else with a purpose in mind. This purpose influences what things are chosen to be told, the order in which they are told, and the words used to tell them. The HPI aims to convince the reader that the diagnosis of depression is correct based on shared ideas about symptoms and their meaning. It urges us to increase his sertraline. The patient's account conveys fear and a plea for help. It urges the listener to feel concern for his suffering and to offer comfort. This difference between the facts and how they are presented is crucial.

Imagine now another way of telling this story. Here Mr. B's wife describes the situation:

> It's awful seeing him like this. He's not eating. He's not getting out of bed. I think he's getting in trouble at work. I'm afraid of what he might do, he feels so bad. I was afraid this would happen after we moved. It's just like last time. He loses his old friends and feels so alone. It has always been hard for him to make new friends.

This version is told from another point of view. The speaker is worried. In addition to some of the same facts about symptoms and history, we now have a new piece of information: there has been a loss. This version names this loss as the cause for the depression. In a very important way, Mr. B's story has now changed.

Now imagine Mr. B sometime later in therapy. He is now able to reflect on the meaning of his childhood experiences:

> Our family wasn't the same after my sister died. My dad moved off and I was sent to school, and they both remarried when I was gone. I never really had a home to go back to after boarding school. I remember just sitting alone in a strange room staring at the wall. I have that same reaction when there are big changes in my life now, like the recent move or the baby. I just get paralyzed.

This reflection on the past changes the current story significantly. We now are presented with a version that links the current depression with a meaningful series of events from long ago. It is helpful sometimes to imagine your patient's story told from another point of view or told in a different way. This will help free you from the confines of the story as presented and help you realize how much the way it is told colors a story. When the point of view changes, when the events are told in different ways, or when new events are added, the meaning of the story shifts, sometimes in dramatic ways.

It can also be helpful to think about the people your patients tell you about as being characters in stories rather than actual people. This allows you to talk directly about the way the patient experiences and perceives these figures in their stories without making comments about how these other people actually might be.

For example, two characters who recurred regularly in Mr. B's stories were his parents. He talked about his father with words like "cold" and "controlled." With his mother, he used words like "helpless" and "incapable." Using this approach, you could focus on his use of these words. You might say to him, "The way you talk about your father, it's as if he had no feelings." Or you might say, "The way your mother comes across in your stories, it's as if she couldn't do anything for herself."

Again, this emphasized to Mr. B that he is the one creating these particular stories and these particular versions of his parents. They are his characters, and they play out their roles in his inner drama. Seeing this more clearly helped him realize over time that these images of his parents were, in fact, caricatures. They were not exactly false, but they were exaggerated and lopsided. The more he was able to appreciate this, the more compassionate he was to their suffering, and his relationships with them improved.

The Value of Reading Fiction

One of the best ways for young therapists to learn how to listen more carefully to patients' stories is to read and discuss the storytelling in fiction. There is an advantage to working with written texts because we can slow down and reread. This makes it easier to notice how the narrative style influences the meaning of the story. First, we notice if the narrator is an actor in the story and what information they have access to. Then, we notice the vocabulary chosen and this directs our thoughts. We can then pay attention to the order in which episodes are presented and how they are juxtaposed. Our reaction to the text will be heavily influenced by this. We can also pay attention to the dominant images in the text. These often recur, either as variations on a central metaphor or as a cluster of related adjectives used to describe some character or scene. Through reading fiction, you will likely become more sensitive to the emotionally loaded words the patient uses that cue you to the dominant themes in each session. You will also get better at picking up on the helpful metaphors we talked about earlier.

These brief examples show the limitations of every story. Each picks out certain things and leaves out others to achieve its effect, like Ms. C, deciding which memories of her brother "got it right." By recognizing this aspect of stories, we can help our patients stand outside their stories and see the ways they can be trapped in the stories they create. They can come to realize there are other valid ways of telling their stories. There are other incidents and perspectives to include that may shift the meaning of things in unexpected ways. Gradually, their stories begin to change.

Ms. C began with a story of a brother who was dead; she ended with a story of a brother who had been vital and alive. With this shift, she regained hope and her mood lifted. As we realize how our stories about ourselves can change, we begin seeing ourselves in different, more open-ended ways. This is another powerful way to think about the path and goal of psychodynamic therapy.

Understanding Resistance and Defenses

As you develop your skills in listening, you will also become more attuned to noticing that some important things are *not* being said. Even though you have asked the patient to speak freely and they may fully intend to do so, you will notice that some important aspects of the patient and their story are not being given a voice. You are noticing that something in the patient is resisting expression, and you will find that people often do this in characteristic ways, which we call **defenses**.[22,23] We have already referenced the concept of defenses in this chapter, so let us look at this concept a bit more.

We will begin by looking at the clinical phenomena of **resistance**.[16,24] This term has some pejorative baggage (ie, "the patient is resisting the process of analysis"), but it does get at a common experience we all have. Imagine for a moment you have to tell your supervisor you made a mistake, a serious one that you should have known better than to make. You feel guilty and ashamed and are afraid of the consequences. Your supervisor can be harsh at times. But, you know you need to tell her. It is the right thing to do. As you think about it, you feel anxious and you try to think of ways to avoid the worst. Maybe there is a way to frame it that does not look so bad. Maybe if you fall on your sword she will realize you feel bad and not be too hard on you. As you start to speak, you feel an inner tension causing you to hesitate. This inner tension is resistance. So, how does this look on the surface to an observer? In the example above, you might stammer at first. Your voice might be quieter than usual. You might be vague. Such behaviors suggest that resistance is active.

But, in the above example, you are consciously aware of both the uncomfortable material and the resistance. This is often not the case. Imagine that the mistake came at the end of the therapy session and you find yourself having filled up the supervisory meeting with lots of detail and speculation about something earlier in the therapy session. When your supervisor says it is time for you to end, you are surprised that you lost track of time and realize that you had forgotten that you needed to talk about the mistake. In this case, your resistance to talking about the mistake had been working unconsciously.

Resistance is inevitable in any psychodynamic therapy.[19] We are asking the patient to tell us their most important stories, and we know that some of those stories have been kept silent because they are disturbing. The patient's mind will find ways to resist giving voice to the disturbing material. How does this unconscious resistance show up clinically? What are observable behaviors that suggest inner conflict and resistance? Here is a list of some of the more common ways resistance is manifested:

- Prolonged silence
- Missing sessions

- Chronic lateness to sessions

- Lack of feeling about what is being talked about

- Fixation on a time period (either only about the present or only about the past)

- Fixation on one particular feeling (for example, always anger but never sadness)

- Fixation on one particular person (for example, only talking about father and excluding mother)

- Talking in abstractions without concrete, current details

- Talking only in a chatty, conversational way and avoiding more weighted matters

The important thing for a therapist to know is that when there is resistance, there is meaning. When there is resistance, something that is important to that person is active and alive. Clinically, this is the most important point in this section. Let me stress this again because it is so important. *The presence of resistance indicates the presence of meaning.*

Over time, beginning during childhood, a person's ways of resisting the experience of painful or disturbing thoughts and feelings usually coalesces into some typical and characteristic patterns or defenses. None of us can live without using defenses, but the quality of one's life often hinges on how adaptive, or mature, these defenses are.

Recognizing defense can be aided by a quick overview of the most common types of defenses. It is a useful piece of knowledge for therapists. In clinical practice, defense takes on many forms, but they can be usefully grouped in terms of how severely they distort reality. These groupings are commonly labeled primitive (immature), neurotic (intermediate), and healthy (mature).

Primitive (Immature) Defenses

Projection means attributing one's own feelings to another. For example, "I'm not mad, you are." Instead of owning the disturbing feeling, the patient attributes personal anger and hostility to someone else. Feeling persecuted is not the best adaptive move—it still involves distress—but it allows the projector to feel innocent, and that they matter enough to have someone plotting to do them harm.

Splitting involves separating good feelings from the bad and attaching them to different people. Splitting is thought to arise when a person cannot tolerate having both good and bad feelings toward the same person. In more immature mental states, people fear that badness always overwhelms goodness, so they have to be kept apart. So, if the patient were to hate someone, they fear this hate would destroy all the potential for feeling love in that relationship.

Some patients will take their most unacceptable feelings and divert them into their body, resulting in **somatization** (experiencing vague symptoms in the body) or **hypochondriasis** (a preoccupation with worries about bodily illness or injury). By doing this, the patient can turn a psychic pain into a physical one. This can also have the benefits of garnering comfort and attention for being physically ill.

Denial means acting as if something were not so. In the extreme, this can become delusional, but usually people using denial can acknowledge the facts while dramatically minimizing the implications. For example, a person might know there has been some conflict at home but not realize that their marriage is about to end.

Acting out means taking disturbing feelings/thoughts and displacing them through impulsive action. This is different from directly expressing a concern. Acting out involves action that allows the person to not have to reflect on and experience feelings—for example, using substances, getting into fights, or driving dangerously.

Intermediate (Neurotic) Defenses

Repression means unconsciously forgetting some important matter. But although we can conceal it from ourselves, we cannot completely eradicate it. As a result of repression, a patient may feel troubled, have difficulty concentrating, or difficulty falling asleep that they cannot explain.

Fantasy sometimes is considered an immature defense, but really it is all a matter of degree. I have grouped it among the intermediate defenses, but there are times when it may be a mature solution as well. Some fantasy is not only acceptable, but it can be quite healthy and is involved in all our appreciation of the arts (both high and low brow), where we get to lose ourselves in a story, identify with a character, and refresh our spirits. Better to say that an *exclusive* retreat into fantasy would be the problem. However, fantasy becomes problematic when a person gets so absorbed in their fantasy life that it becomes the only place where they can experience either aggression/anger or intimacy/affection. In that case, it is no longer a completely adaptive solution and becomes a neurotic defense.

In **reaction formation**, a person takes all the energy of the negative or disturbing material and transforms it into its opposite. To be distinguished from hypocrisy or being two-faced, the person who uses reaction formation is honestly unaware that their intense positivity masks an underlying negative set of feelings. Reaction formation can fuel the zeal of a reformer or the piety of a believer, but they may seem brittle and uncompromising to those who must live or work with them.

Two related defenses that often are used together are **intellectualization** and **isolation of affect**. Intellectualization means taking something as an idea, not as a real, lived experience. Isolation of affect means removing the feelings from thoughts and things. When we use these defenses, we remain aware of the relevant thoughts but make them abstract and disconnected from feeling. One example of this is when Mr. B talks very starkly about the sonogram and is unaware of any feelings attached to the idea. The possibility of a fetal anomaly is treated as merely a thought, not as related to his actual child.

Displacement involves moving the feelings from one object to another. This can be the source of a phobia, for example, where a patient is unreasonably frightened or repelled by something because those feelings originally belonged to something or someone else entirely. This kind of distortion will still allow the disturbing feeling to be experienced, but the feeling is now aimed at something that is a safer target.

Healthy (Mature) Defenses

Suppression means consciously putting off experiencing something difficult until a later time. Unlike repression, suppression is at least partly conscious, or accessible to consciousness, and is a decision to temporarily dismiss or submerge unacceptable thoughts and feelings until a more optimal time.

Humor is often used to laugh at realities that cannot be changed, without denying their existence. This is to be distinguished from making fun of someone, which generally is a form of projection where we mock the other person for some quality that we are afraid we may have. Sarcasm is one form of humor that walks a fine line between humor (as defined above as a healthy defense) and overt hostility.

Sublimation means taking a wish for one thing that is not available and directing it to another. For example, "I wanted to save my little brother's life, but I couldn't stop his cancer. So, I've become an oncologist." People can use sublimation to take unacceptable impulses and channel them into a socially productive outlet. For example, a young man with a hot temper and a thrill-seeking temperament may channel them into a career as a firefighter. What is originally a socially disturbing impulse becomes instead a means to contribute to the world that is rightfully appreciated and rewarded. Another excellent route for sublimation is in creative endeavors and the arts. Many wonderful contributions to culture have been in part a solution to managing disturbing feelings and ideas.

There are other named defenses, but the important thing here is that they range in the degree to which they impair relationships and overall functioning. The idea of healthy defenses reminds us that we are regularly and repeatedly forced to deal with painful situations and feelings. The better we are able to do this, the better we are able to accept and adjust and get along with others or to decide to fight when things need to change.

Case Study—Identifying Defenses

Mr. B primarily used the defenses of intellectualization and isolation of affect. He remembered important events in his life, like the death of his sister and his parent's divorce, but the memories were typically devoid of any feelings. He would talk about these events in a neutral, matter-of-fact way. He would sometimes read books on psychological theory and question me on what I thought about various ideas. It was as if he wanted to have an intellectual discussion about his mind rather than a real experience of feelings. Given his description of his early life, we can imagine Mr. B using these defenses to ward off painful feelings of loss and vulnerability. Feelings were for the weak and helpless.

Mr. B also used repression. There were many details, especially about his sister's death, that he seemed to have pushed out of his awareness. When these emerged later in therapy, strong feelings came with them.

Another way of thinking about Mr. B's defenses brings us back to storytelling. When Mr. B spoke of his childhood, on the rare occasions that he would bring up his sister's death, his parents' divorce, or being sent away to boarding school, his stories felt drained of feeling, so much so that they were forgettable. In fact, I regularly forgot these critical events had even happened. Mr. B's use of isolation of affect and repression led to gaps in his story. Working on these defenses allowed other aspects of Mr. B to speak so that his story about himself became richer and more coherent.

Despite these gaps, Mr. B's defenses did not severely distort reality. He was able to have enough feelings to marry and have a child, and he could get quite excited by intellectual things. He also was able to laugh at himself, think about the well-being of his wife, and make genuine sacrifices for his children. In many ways, Mr. B showed mature defenses. As he gradually used less and less isolation of affect and intellectualization, he began to have more feelings, and he dealt with these with acceptance and, at times, real humor.

As with resistance, when we observe defense, we know we are near something important. We do not need to know what it is yet. We do not even need to know what the defense mechanism is called or how it came to be. What we need to know is that we are in the presence of meaning. Our job now is to explore this meaning.

Using Clarification and Confrontation to Explore Defenses

As we mentioned at the outset of this chapter, the goal of all this is to help the patient learn more about their own minds, to begin to notice things in a more fine-grained way, and to see for themselves the signs of defensiveness or evasion. We want to help the patient wonder, to become more curious, and to become a question to themselves. This is the frame of mind we hope they will learn because it is from this frame of mind that the good things from psychodynamic therapy flow.

We explore defenses by asking questions about the matter at hand. This is called **clarification** or **questioning**. It is essentially asking focused questions, based on our knowledge of defenses and the presence of meaning. We may find with our questioning that the defense is very strong and we do not learn much. This is common, and we file these moments in our memories that there is something important here, something highly defended.

Case Study—Clarification or Questioning

Let us go back to Mr. B, whose wife was having a repeat sonogram for possible Down syndrome. When he said he had no feelings about the possibility, this was a sign of defense. There was no time to explore further in that particular session, but if there had been we might have asked, "Tell me more about the sonogram" or "How is your wife reacting?" or "What if it is Down syndrome?" There are many options here, none of which is necessarily better than another. The point is that we know to ask questions here because the presence of defense indicates the presence of meaning.

A second technique, which often follows our clarifying questions, is to point out the defense or the behavior associated with the defense. This is commonly called **confrontation**. It does *not* mean being aggressive or strongly challenging the patient. It means simply pointing out something that you have observed in the room.

Case Study—Confrontation

For example, you might say to Mr. B in the opening vignette, "You don't have any feelings about possibly having a child with Down syndrome?" Or at other times you might say to him, "I've noticed you talk a lot about your father, but you never mention your mother."

The beauty of this approach is that it does not rely on speculation. It is based on observations made in the room at that moment. We are dealing with active meaning, not hypotheticals.

Most of the work of a psychodynamic therapist consists of using these techniques. The therapist is alert to the presence of active meaning, often signaled by the mobilization of defense. The therapist asks questions about this area. The patient may begin to answer, and their talk may become deeper with feeling and meaning, or we may run into further defense. This pattern of questions and confrontations, fueled by the therapist's desire to understand, moves dynamic therapy forward.

Such learning tends to lessen the use of more problematic defenses over time, to make their use less tenable. Having seen them over and over again for what they are, patients tend to catch themselves more quickly. Patients are freer to deal with what is actually happening within themselves and the world with less distortion. What we have outlined in this section is meant to help you focus your attention to where such questioning is most likely to lead to the identification of active meaning and how to induce a state of wonder about these things.

Exploring Dreams

Many beginning therapists feel challenged when patients bring up dreams. They feel pressured to "figure them out" and to have a quick answer for what it means, as if we had one of the handbooks of the ancient Greeks that offered ready interpretations for common images in dreams (thus, Caesar's dream of making love with his mother meant he was going to rule Rome). Some patients will, in fact, tell you a dream and wait for your interpretation. You can explain to the patient that it is in the flow of their thoughts *about the dream* that the meaning of the dream for them will become clear. That will usually suffice.

Talking about dreams can be a very good way to help patients explore the disturbing wishes, thoughts, and feelings that patients defend against. Many patients regularly bring up dreams in psychodynamic therapy. They may do so for many reasons. For some, it is an expected aspect of psychodynamic therapy, almost as a stereotype of what one talks about in therapy. For others, being in therapy itself seems to stimulate the recall of dreams and their loaded imagery presses for expression. As mentioned before, I tell patients at the beginning of therapy that dreams are part of dynamic therapy, so this may lead some patients to bring them up more often. We may also, at times of impasse, ask patients specifically if they have been dreaming. The reason for this will become clearer in the paragraphs below.

Freud's *The Interpretation of Dreams* was published in 1900.[25] It is a classic work and deserves to be read by all aspiring therapists, more for the frame of mind it illustrates than for the specific formulations. Freud famously referred to dreams as the royal road to the unconscious. He thought that dreams were wish fulfillments disguised by defenses. The therapist's job was to sort through these defenses to find the true aims and reveal them to the patient. He would ask the patient to let their thoughts roam freely to individual elements of the dream. In these "free associations," the patient's underlying wishes and fears would gradually be displayed.

Most psychodynamic therapists consider this too narrow an understanding of dreams. While some dreams may fulfill wishes, other dreams repeat trauma, and still other dreams seem to be ways to work on important problems in our life. Sometimes it is not possible to understand what the purpose of the dream is. Fortunately, we do not need a definitive theory about where dreams come from or what their function is. In dynamic therapy, we are using the strong images and feelings in dreams as a springboard for the patient's reactions.

When we listen to the patient's associations, we wonder with them about their current life and how it might be involved in the reactions to the dream. We wonder about the context of the session and of the treatment. Why bring up this dream now? What preceded it in the session, and/or what has been on the patient's mind over the past weeks? We can think of what came before as a sort of prelude to the dream.

So, what we have is the patient's account of the dream, something already removed from the actual dream, and their reactions in the session to their account. Our approach to dreams is fundamentally the same as with any other material a patient brings forward in session. We ask questions guided by our recognition of meaning and directed by the presence of feelings and defense. We try to help the patient wonder about what is going on, we watch for feelings and defense arising in response to our questions, and we point out what we observe.

The Meaning of Trauma and Grief in Psychodynamic Therapy

So far, we have been talking about painful and threatening thoughts and feelings and the way the patient's mind deals with them through defenses. But, sometimes people experience terrible things that are beyond their capacity to defend against and therefore overwhelm their defenses. This is what we mean by **trauma** in psychodynamic thinking.[26,27] In its common usage, trauma is a word that refers to many kinds of experiences. For example, there is the trauma of being shot in a war, injured in a car accident, sexually assaulted, or beaten as a child. But, the word "trauma" is also sometimes used to refer to the impact of chronic neglect, witnessing severe parental conflict, and/or stress over a long period of time. All these traumatic experiences have in common the following: that the mind's capacity to bear and integrate the experience is overwhelmed.

There are some key similarities in most traumatic reactions. First, the person regularly feels in peril in the aftermath of acute, severe trauma. Second, they regularly feel that the certainties of their former world have been ruptured and that they are living in a dangerous new reality that others do not understand. The trauma has revealed to them some new truth that has disrupted a previous reality.

As a result, the person who has been to war understands violence and sudden death in a new way. The person who has been raped knows the truth of what some people are capable of and what it is like to be utterly helpless. The person who has been hit by a car in a parking lot sees now how carelessly many people drive. The neglected child knows that those who claim to love you do not always mean it. In this sense, trauma functions like a kind of initiation into a new and fearful way of being that others cannot see or understand. This knowledge puts the traumatized person into a different world and into a kind of exile from their previous world and from those still living in it. The traumatized person also knows things that you do not necessarily know.

From this perspective, the psychodynamic therapist's job is not so much to understand because this is not fully possible. Most of us cannot truly know what it is like to have seen a friend vaporized by a bomb or to have been raped by their father. We may come to appreciate more and more of what our patients tell us, but there will always be a gap between our understanding and their experiences. What the therapist can do is to bear witness, listen to the stories, and acknowledge their gravity and impact, without reducing their experiences to some platitude or reassuring phrase. Such witnessing can be hard to bear at times for the therapist, but it regularly leads to the patient feeling a little less alone, a little more a part of the world the rest of us live in, and a little less exiled by what has happened.

Example—Trauma You Have Not Experienced

I was seeing a Korean War veteran during my residency. He had been a medic during a terrible winter campaign. He had seen steam coming from open bellies, and comrades had begged him to kill them with morphine. I never knew whether he had or had not, and I am not sure he was even certain himself. In the early weeks of therapy, before I knew any of these things, the therapy was not going well. He was becoming more and more silent and irritable. While sitting with him one day, the absurdity of the situation hit me. How could I pretend to help him? My experience was not remotely like his. What could I possibly say? I decided in that moment to share my thoughts, in the service of propelling therapy forward.

I said to him, "I wonder if you're thinking, 'How could a young, inexperienced guy like me could ever hope to understand what you've been through?'"

He thought a while, then smiled wryly. "I have been thinking that." There was a bit of challenge in his voice. I waited a moment.

"Well, at least we understand that together," I said.

He smiled quickly and more broadly. "I guess we do doc, I guess we do." He visibly relaxed in his chair.

Therapy started to get better after that, and over the next months he gradually told me more about what had happened to him and about some of the things he had done. He began to feel less isolated and his mood improved. I think that this moment in which I abandoned any claim to really understand, a moment in which we understood together that I could not really understand, helped create the interpersonal space that undid a little bit of his traumatic exile.

Working with trauma in dynamic therapy is similar to dealing with **grief**. With grief, the bereaved person has been confronted with the inescapable reality of loss and the rupture with the world of the past. The therapist listens and helps create a place where memory and sadness can be felt and the loss can be incorporated into the new world. Again, the therapist's role is not to explain away the loss, or to suggest some ideal way to deal with it, but to help the patient articulate and share the meaning of the loss. This, too, leads to a return from exile.

Example—The Importance of Sitting With Trauma

I once saw a man whose daughter had been murdered in a particularly atrocious way. Coming into the office each time, he looked as if he had been struck by lightning. After a few sessions, he brought in a large photograph of his daughter. We sat together for a long time looking at her picture. It was hard and sad and I wanted to look away. But it was important that I spend some time with that picture, to not look away too soon, so that we might sit together acknowledging the reality of this terrible loss.

Bearing witness like this can be very hard for therapists. The raw pain, the reality of terror and helplessness, and the agony of irremediable loss are difficult to face. It is tempting to avoid it or to offer up some words to shift attention away, before the feelings have run their course. It helps significantly to talk with your supervisor and colleagues about these cases. You will feel less alone, less exiled yourself. It will also remind you that there is comfort in having pain simply and directly acknowledged.[28]

TRANSFERENCE AND COUNTERTRANSFERENCE

What Is Transference?

We have already mentioned transference a few times in this chapter. This section is meant to focus more specifically on the role of this concept in psychodynamic psychotherapy. **Transference** is the redirection of feelings from one person to another. It is a common human phenomenon and most often happens without our being aware we are doing it. Transference most commonly involves redirecting feelings about our earliest caregivers into later relationships.[15,16] In dynamic therapy this means that the patient is likely to experience you as they experienced their parents or other important early figures. How does this happen?

We are born into a world that already exists. Those who are already in that world show us how to get along. They show us how to speak and how to manage and express our feelings. They show us what is important, what to do, what to avoid, and all the many rhythms of life. We can think of this as training in what it means to be a member of a family, in a certain part of the world, at a particular moment in time. We might say that parents are training their children to live in the world as they have come to see it.

A critical component of this training is how to relate to another person. From the start we are shown how to be with other people, typically our parents and any siblings first, then to a steadily wider group of other adults and children. We learn how to speak to one another, how to share or not share our thoughts and feelings, what to expect or not to expect from other people, how to show affection and anger, and, in short, how to be involved.

For the most part, this training goes pretty well. Most of us learn how to behave and to get along in most social situations. But when it comes to truly intimate relationships, things often go awry. In intimate relationships, our deepest wishes and vulnerabilities are at play, and we tend to feel conflicted about these. For example, we want something from our partner, yet feel ashamed to ask and fearful of rejection.

Under such circumstances, when our core conflicts (such as guilt and the fear of not being loved) are mobilized, anxiety and forms of defense arise. We often return to early, overlearned patterns of behavior that may or may not fit very well with the current situation. We begin responding to others, not as unique individuals, but as players in our old internal dramas. We may transfer the feelings and modes of relating from a past figure onto a new one. *This is what we mean by transference.*

We all have this unavoidable tendency to repeat the patterns of our relationships later in life. It is an essential aspect of our humanness. If these patterns have been fairly secured and rooted in care and a concern for oneself and others, they set the stage for genuine intimacy. They allow us to see the uniqueness of the other person and to develop a unique relationship with them. But even then, we all have our core issues, and these come up even in the best relationships.

The Importance of Transference to Psychodynamic Therapy

Transference is another important way, along with speech, that the other person's mind is revealed. As we noted earlier in this chapter, fostering transference from the first session is a core feature of psychodynamic psychotherapy. Via transference we can observe the patient's core issues active and in play, not as matters for speculation and theorizing, but alive in the room with us. Psychodynamic therapy does not create transference. Transference happens because we are human. But, psychodynamic therapy fosters and uses transference (in fact welcomes it), because transference brings much of what is unconscious to the surface, so that it can be observed. Transference allows us to see and feel how the patient is responding to us.

Some of the features of psychodynamic therapy are aimed at helping the transference come to the fore. The regularity of meetings, the relative anonymity of the therapist, the fact that the therapist keeps the majority of her personal needs in abeyance and strives primarily to understand—all these keep the therapist somewhat hidden, so the patient naturally creates an image of her that fits his pattern of relating.

Of note, transference tends to come with strong feelings—loving, contemptuousness, idealizing, and hating. As such, transference can make the therapist uncomfortable. Learning to understand, bear, and welcome transference is a key part of every therapist's development. Supervision is invaluable here.

Recognizing Transference and Enactments

How do we recognize transference? Typically, there are three features. The first feature is intensity of emotional reaction. Very strong reactions to us suggest the presence of transference. If you are a few minutes behind schedule and the patient erupts with anger over being left waiting, this suggests transference. The second feature is when the reactions do not really fit the situation. For example, if you are well rested, but the patient sees you as tired and overburdened, this suggests transference. The third feature is recurring, stereotypic patterns of relationship. If every boss is a tyrant, every teacher a dictator, and the patient begins to bristle at what he thinks you want him to do, this suggests transference.

7

Case Study—Applying Transference, Part 1

In an earlier section on obstacles to psychodynamic psychotherapy, we discussed how Mr. B reacted to me missing a session early in treatment. He assumed it was due to an emergency, and the suggestion that it might not have been was so threatening, he would not even think about it. This was an example of something so highly defended that we could not address it at the time. Over the next few years, we came to understand this reaction better. His father's career sometimes required him to unexpectedly be gone for days at a time to manage crises in his business. In contrast, his mother was experienced as fragile and unreliable, even though she was always home.

At a young age, Mr. B became acutely ill and was in quarantine. When he spoke of the hospitalization, he implied that his mother was to blame for leaving him at the hospital. His father was at the emergency room, but he had to leave for work. Why was he not angry at his father for leaving? "He had to go," he shrugged, explaining further, "His job was handling crises."

I remembered his reaction to my missing the session. The emotional intensity and lack of fit suggested transference at the time. But now, in the context of his childhood illness, it made more sense. I reminded him of the missed session, saying, "I understand better why you let me off the hook then, when I missed that session." He remembered, too, responding, "You couldn't be like my mother back then. You had to be like my dad. If you were gone, it was an emergency. If you were like my mom, I couldn't have stood it then. I couldn't have gone on working with you."

Here, the threat of me being like his mother was too much. He transferred to me instead the image of his strong father whose absence was forgivable. He was able to understand this more clearly now, and it gave him more insight into how persistent and pervasive the influences of early relationships could be.

Case Study—Applying Transference, Part 2

At another point in the treatment, Mr. B walked in with a large stack of books, stating, "I've been reading a lot about this other type of therapy. What do you know about it?"

"What got you interested in this therapy?" I asked.

He responded, "I don't know. I just heard about it somewhere. I thought it might be good for me."

I asked what about it appealed to him. He replied that he had been feeling more depressed lately, commenting, "Maybe what we are doing is making me worse. Maybe it isn't the right kind of treatment for me. Maybe talking about my feelings and my parents and my sister's death is just making me feel bad." He then asked abruptly, "So, what do you know about this other therapy?"

I told him what I knew, then asked him what he was feeling. He said he was anxious and then started talking about some software he had bought. It was not working, and the guy who sold it to him could not get it to work. He described him as an "idiot who didn't know what he was doing."

I replied, "Like maybe I don't know what I'm doing?"

He then talked about how much he feared being alone with his feelings, and his fears that I might lead him to some painful place and then leave him.

I suggested, "So, maybe it's better to try another kind of therapy?"

He nodded. "Yeah, but I think this is what I need to do, even if I don't like it."

Mr. B was afraid I did not know what I was doing. This fear led him to research other therapies and to consider stopping treatment. His coming in with a stack of books and questions about my knowledge on a different treatment, after a long period of treatment, was an intense reaction suggesting transference. I approached it by accepting that he felt this way, exploring why it had come up now, then pursuing the thoughts and feelings that followed. It became clear that I was like the software guy who could not make the program work. I would sell him something that led to a painful place where he needed help, then leave him.

We can speculate, based on what we know about his early life, that he feared I would react like his parents and send him off to deal with his feelings about his sister's death on his own. We can see how helping him talk about his reactions to me openly, without rejecting them or acting anxious myself, helped him have confidence in continuing treatment. Over time, we were able to make these connections more explicit, and thoughts about ending therapy were linked to his memories of being sent away after his sister's death.

Both of these examples illustrate that the way to address the transference is to explore the thoughts and feelings as presented, just as you would do with any other matter in therapy, through clarifying questions and gentle confrontations. It is also important to not be too quick to make the connection between past and present explicit. The main reason is that when we explicitly make these connections for patients, this tends to lessen the intensity of the current feelings and intellectualizes them, making it more a matter of speculation than experience for the patient. The best work comes from patients actively experiencing the feelings and evolving in their own insight.

However, *it is also important not to make everything be about transference.* Every comment about a caregiver is not necessarily about us. All complaints about us are not necessarily transference, either. Similarly, the patient's interest in changing to a different therapy may be rooted in present reality and not in transference. Mr. B might well have been right that we needed to switch tracks in therapy. It was only on exploration that we found his reactions were based on transference.

Therefore, it is important to understand that transference feelings are being felt about the therapist, not the person from the past. They may be related to past experience and learning and may involve important persons from the patient's past life, but they are currently *about* the therapist. To treat them otherwise too quickly diminishes them. Transference reactions tend to be in response to something that actually happened, like when the therapist forgot Mr. B's appointment. Sometimes we have actually made a mistake. It is usually best to deal with the patient's feelings first as realistic reactions, but this does not mean that there is not also transference involved. Our mistakes can become moments of fruitful exploration.

This brings us to the important concept of **enactments**. Enactments are complex interactional dramas where the therapist has been cast in a role by the patient and is then moved unconsciously to behave in a certain way.[5] Try as we might to be aware, we all have a tendency to fall into such patterns with others. It is our job as therapists to catch these enactments, after they have happened or while we are still in the midst of them, and make them an object of reflection, the main goal in all our psychodynamic work.

Enactments typically involve an interplay between transference and countertransference (the therapist's transference to the patient). Countertransference is a concept discussed in the next section. There I will describe an enactment in which Mr. B's wish to speak with me about philosophy touched upon wishes of my own, leading us to occasionally step outside the framework of therapy and resulting in an enactment.

Although enactments do happen, we should not be afraid of forming and maintaining the therapeutic relationship itself. Our main work as a dynamic therapist is to enter into a relationship with the patient, one motivated on our side by the desire to understand and to convey that understanding in a helpful way. To do this means to be involved with the patient so that their wishes, fears, desires, and sufferings come fully into play. Thought of in this way, enactments are likely to happen and then need to be both identified and turned into a vehicle of real insight and change.

7

These ideas about transference reactions and enactments are derived from psychoanalysis, where the patient is on the couch, not facing the analyst, four to five times weekly. In weekly, face-to-face therapy, such as the ones you will be doing in training, reactions are generally more muted. The reality of the therapist's face and her palpable social presence often mitigates transference reactions. In such cases, we can listen for what sounds like transference reactions to important people in the patient's life, knowing that this is where the most intense and significant feelings can be found.

Finally, it is important to remember that addressing transference once does not eliminate it. The nature of our attachments, the patterns we have learned, and the nature of our desires and fears, are all tenacious. Their rate of change is slow. It is not a matter of simply learning something once and being done with it. Transference reactions in various guises tend to recur throughout therapy. We will address this more fully in the section on working through below, but for now it is important to know that inertia and repetition are the norm, and dealing with various manifestations of transference is a key aspect of psychodynamic therapy.

What Is Countertransference?

Countertransference refers to the therapist's feelings in reaction to the patient.[15,16] Just as with transference, every reaction we have to a patient is not countertransference. The term is often used loosely in this way, but countertransference should be used to refer to stronger, less reasonable, more abiding reactions to patients, the source of which we tend not to be immediately aware.

Sometimes countertransference is a reaction to the patient's transference. For example, if you find yourself frequently irritated with the patient, this might be because the patient's hostile transference is leading them to be subtly aggressive.

However, therapists are not exempted from transference of their own. Transference, as we have emphasized, is an aspect of being human, of having learned to live in the social world that was already here before us. Countertransference can therefore also be the therapist's unconscious redirection of feelings about important people from their past onto the patient. Sometimes we will have reactions to patients that have nothing to do with them and everything to do with our past relationships. To make things even more complicated, both sources of countertransference can be involved at the same time. For example, I might be particularly irritated in response to my patient's passive aggressive behaviors because it brings up something of my own childhood.

Here are some common examples of countertransference manifestations:

- Having particularly strong feelings toward a patient, such as anger or attraction
- Being overly anxious with or about the patient
- Needing to "fix" the patient or get them to be a certain way
- Forgetting appointments or regularly running late
- Regularly letting sessions run past the scheduled stop time

- Focusing exclusively on one feeling or one important relationship while avoiding others

- Becoming overly chatty and personal

- Feeling recurrently bored or sleepy

Noticing countertransference is important. In extreme situations our feelings could lead us to violate boundaries and develop unprofessional relationships with our patients.[29] Or, we may be so angry or anxious that it is hard to think clearly or compassionately about our patient.[30] Fortunately, these extreme situations are not common.

Countertransference more often does not involve strong conscious feelings. Because many therapists are reserved and wary of being too aggressive, countertransference more often manifests itself by omission. We may avoid bringing things up or pointing things out or exploring certain areas because they make us anxious. We might not even notice we are doing this, and typically we will have very reasonable sounding rationalizations. But, it is countertransference that is leading us to avoid. For example, we do not talk about the patient's repeated lateness or cancellations. Or in other cases, we talk about their anger, but not their sadness. We might talk a lot about the father, but the mother never comes up. Or finally, we ignore clear references to us in their talk.

Countertransference feelings, though, can be an important source of information about the patient. Sometimes, we are reacting to things that we have not been consciously aware of. The more we understand our own issues and what typically triggers them, the better we can understand what the patient might be doing. Exploring our reactions can help us see things more clearly and better help the patient. We can then learn to welcome our countertransference feelings as a path to better understanding our patient, just as we learn to welcome transference as an important vehicle of change in therapy.

Sometimes, countertransference reactions can be subtle and move more into unconscious processing of undercurrents in the patient's talk. This is an important issue. You will notice as you listen, various things will run through your mind. They may be related to your personal situation and the preoccupations of the day, but they may also be associations to what the patient is saying. As you develop as a therapist, you will learn to assess these thoughts to see if these thoughts might be referring to the patient in some way. The answer may not appear during the session itself.

7

Case Study—Countertransference, Part 1

As mentioned above when discussing enactments, Mr. B was an intelligent, well-read man. He would sometimes want to discuss philosophical issues, some of which were very interesting to me. He would want to know my opinion about these things, and a few times I found myself discussing my views about some abstract matter. It was very pleasurable to talk this way with him, but I found myself recurrently stepping outside my role as his therapist.

My first job was to catch myself when I was tempted to talk with him in this way. Then I examined my own wish to step outside my role as a therapist and to be either an authority or his friend. I was then better able to explore with him what was going on with him when he would try to engage me in this way. Sometimes, we found he was simply trying to avoid some loaded emotional issue by intellectualizing. At others, he told me he felt lonely and wished that we could have a beer together and just talk. As he became more aware of these feelings, he became less embarrassed about his intellectual interests and was able to find some like-minded friends.

Case Study—Countertransference, Part 2

Another example of countertransference, albeit a more subtle form, involved my tending to forget about his sister. When thinking about him, I would regularly forget about how traumatic the event had been and how destructive the aftermath had been to his family. It was relatively deep into treatment before I actually asked him more details about the event. While it may have been wise not to charge into this defended and emotionally fraught topic early in therapy, I think I was mirroring his forgetfulness and avoiding the topic. Repeatedly noticing my own forgetfulness helped me eventually explore her death with him.

Therapists are human. We are going to feel anxious, angry, aroused, and confused at different times with different patients. Sometimes, this has to do more purely with us and the circumstances of our lives. But sometimes, we are reacting to something important in the patient.

Dynamic therapists should regularly monitor for countertransference because it is unavoidable, because it can interfere with the therapy, and because it offers potential insights into how the patient is relating to us. Countertransference can manifest itself by strong feelings, but it more often shows up quietly as omissions, avoidance, or changes in our manner, like when I talked about philosophy with Mr. B or when I forgot about his sister's death. When we are feeling strongly, it is best to be cautious, to stay relatively quiet, and focus on asking pertinent questions. This helps us avoid acting on what may be distortions coming from our own issues until we are better able to understand them.

FINALLY—THE TASK OF "WORKING THROUGH" IN PSYCHODYNAMIC PSYCHOTHERAPY

As we said before, the rate of psychological change tends to be slow. Our wishes, fears, and tendencies are deeply ingrained, and a single moment of self-recognition rarely leads to a lasting transformation. In therapy, this means that an insight into one's problematic behaviors rarely leads to their abolition. Say your spouse wants you to get less angry while driving. You make a vow and do better for a while. But then you are tired, you have had a long day, and that idiot in the other lane is on his phone, and… you make another vow and try again. Over time, if it matters to you, you get better. But, rarely is the change permanent the first time. **Working through** is the process of revisiting and reexamining the conflict so that gradually you are able to make a different set of mental connections that allow greater flexibility and autonomy in your choices.

Truly important issues often show up in a variety of situations that may not initially appear related. In therapy, we may come to understand a certain issue as it arises in a specific context. Later, we may be working on what seems to be a different issue when we suddenly realize it is, in fact, another version of something that we had seen before. This process of recognizing the same issues showing up in various guises and dealing with them repeatedly is part of working through.

Case Study—Working Through

Mr. B, the man who felt nothing about the sonogram, recognized quickly that having no reaction to something so significant was odd. However, this did not immediately lead him to recognize his feelings. Much of the ongoing work with him involved noticing situations where feelings would be expected, recognizing their absence as a sign of meaningfulness, asking questions about the situation, and helping him to wonder about his reactions. Gradually, his feelings came more and more into his awareness.

As our patient noted more and more lack of feelings, he talked more about the loss of his sister. By his account, the family acted as if nothing had happened. He could recall no emotional scenes, no anguished conversations, and no real mourning. It was as if his sibling was just gone and that was that. We could see in this a possible source of his tendency to blot out feelings. By his account, he had grown up in a family that did not value feelings, or was not comfortable with them, and certainly did not talk about them. He had learned to live that way. Over time, he began to feel things, and the work involved helping him clarify what he was feeling and better deal with this new range of experiences.

7

It is important for the therapist not to be discouraged by this necessary repetition. It is important to recognize repeated patterns as they show up in therapy. The patient will often be surprised to see these previously recognized issues showing up again in different guises, and they will have a greater appreciation both for the tenacity of important issues for us but also for how covert these issues can continue to be.

In reality, very primal issues for us often never go away completely. Under the right amount of stress, these issues may be reactivated. Therapy helps this to be less likely and helps us recognize and tame them when they are resurrected. Our reactions tend to become less intense and to certainly last a shorter time, with less destructive consequences.

As we got to the end of our work together, Mr. B told me, "We spent a lot of time getting me to recognize that I had feelings. Then, we worked on actually feeling them. Now I've come to realize, they're just feelings. I don't need to fear them, but they're not always the best guides to action." This sums up very nicely the course of psychodynamic therapy.

CONSULTATION, SUPERVISION, AND PERSONAL THERAPY IN PSYCHODYNAMIC PSYCHOTHERAPY

Consultation

De-identified case consultation with a good colleague not only helps with the burden of working with traumatized patients, but it helps with the burden of doing psychodynamic work in general. Working as a psychodynamic therapist can be difficult in general, not only with traumatized or grieving patients. The pain that is uncovered, the loss and conflict that many people live with, the intensity of feeling, and the often self-inflicted misery take their toll at times. Sharing this with an understanding colleague eases the isolation greatly and will enrich your work, not just during training but for your entire career. It will also help you address any countertransference and boundary issues that might be developing.

Supervision

Supervision is critically important in becoming a psychodynamic therapist.[31] To truly learn any skill you have to practice, and practicing is best done with the help of an experienced teacher. Every individual supervisor has their own way of approaching supervision, but what I have found most helpful is as follows. First, it is important to use some form of process notes, a term referring to the therapist's account of the session. I prefer not to take notes during the therapy session, as I feel this interferes with my concentration on what the patient is saying, as well as interferes with the free flow of my own reactions to what is going on. Going without notes also gives you a chance to use the listening techniques we talked about earlier. Other therapists feel differently about this—you may want to try both approaches to see what fits best for you. If you do not take notes, writing an account right after the session usually works well enough. Increasingly, training therapists have been recording sessions with informed consent and precautions with information security. I do not think recording sessions unduly distorts the flow of the session after both parties get used to it.

The reason detailed process notes are important for dynamic therapy is that they keep the supervision focused on the flow of thought and feeling in the session, as well as what was said and when. Without this, supervision can become too impressionistic. We might tend to leave out things we are not comfortable with or do not yet see the significance of. We might tend to present the case so that our interpretations of what is going on seem right but leave out information that suggests other ways of seeing things.

In addition, the best way to monitor for countertransference is through supervision, as well as your own personal therapy. In supervision, you should be able to talk freely about feelings and reactions to the patient. It is important to be receptive when your supervisor points out possible countertransference reactions. As you learn what to watch for through supervision, you will become increasingly adept at noticing when you are avoiding things and when you are interacting differently with your patients.

Personal Psychotherapy

Supervision should focus on what you are reacting to in the patient as a therapist, not on exploring your own personal feelings or history separately—that is the role of your personal therapy. Therapy can help you learn to think about your reactions to your patients and help you to wonder why you respond the way you do. The better you understand your own reactions, the more quickly and deftly you can use them as guides to noticing more about your patients.

All psychodynamic therapists should also enter into therapy themselves. Many helpful things come from this. The most obvious reason is that the better you understand yourself and your reactions to a variety of emotional issues, the better you will be able to help your patients. You will become more in touch with your own thoughts and feelings, be better able to think clearly in stressful situations, and be less likely to express your countertransference reactions. It will also help you learn to process your reactions to your patients more reflectively outside of the sessions because often we do not really appreciate what has been happening until we are able to think about it later.

Being in therapy also gives you invaluable lessons in technique. You will better appreciate the power of silence, of well-focused questions, and of gentle but clear confrontations. You will better appreciate the persistent ubiquity of resistance, despite your best efforts as a patient. You will also experience how healing it is to be listened to by someone who is being genuinely attentive without any other agenda. It is rare to ever be listened to in quite this way. Having experiences like these in your own therapy will give you much greater confidence in the efficacy of psychodynamic methods and will make them feel substantially less awkward for you.

7

Conclusion

Let us return now to the beginning. We started by way of a microcosm—the scene of Mr. B not having any feelings about a sonogram. We talked about this lack of feelings, and he began to wonder about himself and his reactions. We then offered a map of psychodynamic psychotherapy that begins with two people talking. We listen to the patient's stories, noting how they shape them, what they emphasize, and what they leave out. With our knowledge of developmental theory, relationship patterns, and defenses, we notice things that help us focus the patient's attention on recurrent themes, on how they manage their feelings, and what they try to avoid.

We saw Mr. B become increasingly aware of how much he shunned his feelings and feared he would be left to manage them alone, even by his therapist. This process of repeated and expanded noticing is the path of psychodynamic therapy. For Mr. B, this involved repeatedly seeing the ways in which he avoided his feelings in a variety of different situations. It involved seeing how he had been affected by the death of his sister and how his family had dealt with it. The more work he did, the more he would catch himself avoiding feelings. He then began to have more feelings and to feel closer to his family and friends.

As therapy progressed, Mr. B's attitude toward himself began to change. The goal of psychodynamic therapy is learning this new attitude toward one's own mental life. This attitude is characterized by a sense of questioning and wonder. The majority of this chapter has been devoted to showing you some of the concrete ways in which this attitude is manifested, at first by the therapist, and more and more by the patient. This growing curiosity about one's own mind is the key outcome of psychodynamic therapy. Learning and embodying this new way of questioning oneself led to greater patience, greater tolerance for unpleasant feelings, more compassion toward others, and a greater depth to relationships. These changes flow naturally from learning this new attitude.

We then offered a metaphor for psychodynamic therapy in the form of a person going up to her private room where all the figures of her imagination came out to play. The therapist joins the patient in their trip to their hidden room, bearing witness to the drama as it unfolds. This metaphor was meant to bring out the creative, open-ended, often mysterious aspects of psychodynamic therapy. We really cannot be sure where the therapy might lead us; we cannot be sure what new things may come to light. With Mr. B, this involved helping him find the stairway and the inner room. In that inner room, we explored the interactions of his memories and representations of his father and mother and his dead sister, as well as many other important people in his life.

Mr. B made great progress in his treatment. He gained the ability to wonder about himself. He began to experience more genuine feelings and was able to incorporate them into his sense of who he was. The story of his life changed. He had a greater appreciation for the impact of his sister's death, and he had more compassion for his parents. All of this helped him be more at ease with himself and with others. His relationship with his wife, his children, and his friends became richer.

As we were ending treatment, a major financial event hit him and his family, one that was outside their control. They were forced to make major adjustments in their lives. Mr. B talked openly about the stress and fears, but he did not become depressed, saying, "We'll do what we have to do to get through this. It's not going to be easy and I wish this hadn't happened, but we'll get through. We'll be alright. I think I can manage this."

Mr. B had worked hard in psychodynamic therapy and was, in many ways, a different man. With the new attitude he had learned to take toward himself, he was better equipped to deal with what life handed him.

That is the goal of psychodynamic therapy.

Self-Study Questions

1. After reading this chapter, how would you define the purpose and process of psychodynamic psychotherapy?

2. List and describe at least three strategies or tools commonly used in dynamic therapy.

3. Within psychodynamic therapy, what is the therapeutic impact of being listened to carefully? What results from this type of listening?

4. List at least two conditions for which psychodynamic therapy is indicated and two for which psychodynamic therapy is contraindicated.

5. Why are both transference and boundaries important to the process of psychodynamic psychotherapy? (Hint: review the concept of *relative anonymity*.)

6. List at least five defenses, and describe at least one patient behavior that could reflect each of these defenses.

7. Why is personal psychotherapy and supervision/consultation important to the psychodynamic psychotherapist? What are some potential barriers you might have in seeking either one of these suggestions?

7

RESOURCES FOR FURTHER LEARNING

Cabaniss DL, Cherry S, Douglas C, Schwartz A. *Psychodynamic Psychotherapy: A Clinical Manual.* 2nd ed. Chichester, England: Wiley-Blackwell; 2016.

Freud S. *The Interpretation of Dreams: The Complete and Definitive Text.* 1st ed. New York, NY: Basic Books; 2010.

Kohut H. *The Restoration of the Self.* Reprint ed. Chicago, IL: University of Chicago Press; 2012.

McWilliams N. *Psychoanalytic Psychotherapy: A Practitioner's Guide.* 1st ed. New York, NY: The Guilford Press; 2004.

Mitchell S, Black M. *Freud and Beyond: A History of Modern Psychoanalytic Thought.* Updated ed. New York, NY: Basic Books; 2016.

REFERENCES

1. Bhikku Bodhi. *The Noble Eightfold Path.* Kandy, Sri Lanka: Buddhist Publication Society; 1994.
2. Peake M. *Titus Groan.* 1st rev ed. New York, NY: Ballantine Books; 1968. *Gormenghast Trilogy,* vol. 1.
3. American Psychiatric Association. *Diagnostic and Statistical Manual of Mental Disorders.* 5th ed. Arlington, VA: American Psychiatric Association; 2013.
4. Leichsenring F, Klein S. Evidence for psychodynamic psychotherapy in specific mental disorders: a systematic review. *Psychoanal Psychother.* 2014;28(1):4-32.
5. Mitchell S, Black M. *Freud and Beyond: A History of Modern Psychoanalytic Thought.* Updated ed. New York, NY: Basic Books; 2016.
6. Erikson E. *Childhood and Society.* Reissue ed. New York, NY: W. W. Norton & Company; 1993.
7. Brenner C. *Elementary Textbook of Psychoanalysis.* Rev ed. New York, NY: Anchor; 1974.
8. Freud S. Inhibitions, symptoms, and anxiety. *Psychoanal Q.* 1936;5(1):1-28.
9. Kohut H. *The Analysis of the Self.* Chicago, IL: University of Chicago Press; 1971.
10. Kohut H. *The Restoration of the Self.* Reprint ed. Chicago, IL: University of Chicago Press; 2012.
11. Fink B. *A Clinical Introduction to Lacanian Psychoanalysis: Theory and Technique.* Cambridge, MA: Harvard University Press; 1999.
12. Epstein M. *Thoughts Without a Thinker: Psychotherapy From a Buddhist Perspective.* 12th printing ed. New York, NY: Basic Books; 1995.
13. Cabaniss DL, Cherry S, Douglas C, Graver R, Schwartz A. *Psychodynamic Formulation.* 1st ed. Chichester, England: Wiley-Blackwell; 2013.
14. Hall JS. *Deepening the Treatment.* Northvale, NJ: Jason Aronson, Inc; 1998.
15. McWilliams N. *Psychoanalytic Psychotherapy: A Practitioner's Guide.* 1st ed. New York, NY: The Guilford Press; 2004.
16. Cabaniss DL, Cherry S, Douglas C, Schwartz A. *Psychodynamic Psychotherapy: A Clinical Manual.* 2nd ed. Chichester, England: Wiley-Blackwell; 2016.
17. Meissner WW. The problem of self disclosure in psychoanalysis. *J Am Psychoanal Assoc.* 2002;50(3):827-867.
18. Brenner AM. Listening: an underlying competency in psychiatry education. *Acad Psychiatry.* 2017;41:385-390.
19. Greenson R. *The Technique and Practice of Psychoanalysis.* New York, NY: International Universities Press; 1967.
20. Lewis B. *Narrative Psychiatry: How Stories Shape Clinical Practice.* 1st ed. Baltimore, MD: Johns Hopkins University Press; 2011.
21. Bal M. *Narratology.* 3rd ed. Toronto, ON: University of Toronto Press; 2009.
22. Vaillant G. *The Wisdom of the Ego.* Reprint ed. Cambridge, MA: Harvard University Press; 1998.
23. Freud A. *The Ego and the Mechanisms of Defense.* Rev ed. New York, NY: International Universities Press; 1967.
24. Schafer R. *The Analytic Attitude.* New York, NY: Basic Books; 1983.
25. Freud S. *The Interpretation of Dreams: The Complete and Definitive Text.* 1st ed. New York, NY: Basic Books; 2010.
26. Shengold L. *Soul Murder: The Effects of Childhood Abuse and Deprivation.* New Haven, CT: Ballantine Books; 1991.
27. Herman J. *Trauma and Recovery: The Aftermath of Violence – From Domestic Abuse to Political Terror.* New York, NY: Basic Books; 1997.
28. Thornton W, Cain J, Litle M. Trauma, certainty, and exile. *Contemp Psychoanal.* 2010;46(3):355-379.
29. Gabbard GO. Countertransference: the emerging common ground. *Int J Psychoanal.* 1995;76(pt 3): 475-485.
30. Maltsberger JT, Buie DH. Countertransference hate in the treatment of suicidal patients. *Arch Gen Psychiatry.* 1974;30(5):625-633.
31. Jacobs D, David P, Meyer PJ. *The Supervisory Encounter: A Guide for Teachers of Psychodynamic Therapy and Psychoanalysis.* Reprint ed. New Haven, CT: Yale University Press; 1997.

AUTHOR ACKNOWLEDGMENT

I owe so much to the thought and spirit of my friend and mentor, Dr. Jeffry Andresen.

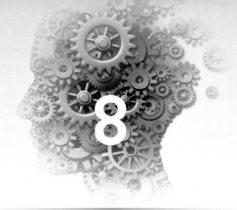

Beyond the Therapy Dyad: The Importance of Systems and Culture

MONA A. ROBBINS, PhD AND LAURA S. HOWE-MARTIN, PhD

Case Study

Mr. A is a 67-year-old new patient who comes to your office for a first-time evaluation and reports concerns about "fitting in" with his coworkers at a new job. He has a managerial position and has recently relocated to develop a task force focused on improving company production. When greeted in the reception area, he looks at you carefully, and then hesitantly follows you to the therapy room. Once seated, he expresses a reluctance to seek therapy "given all that is going on," and proceeds to take charge of the session, describing his preferences and opinions about therapy. After you interject to review limits of confidentiality and begin the initial evaluation, you ask about the reason for seeking therapy.

Mr. A goes on to share how important it is to make a good impression with colleagues, out of fear of not being considered for a potential promotion. He explains that fitting in has often been a problem for him, and he shares that his biracial identity has been "a blessing and a curse" in trying to connect with people. He appears solemn in demeanor and describes irritability, sleeping difficulties, and reduced appetite that all coincide with starting the new job. When asked about social support, he notes his spouse is his primary support person and who encouraged him to enter therapy. He also mentions having a distant cousin who lives nearby and a strong relationship with his former pastor, who lives in another state. He noted that taking this job opportunity meant moving away from family and everything familiar, which has left him feeling "empty." You ask about symptoms of sadness and anhedonia, to which he flashes a grin and replies, "You would say that, wouldn't

---

you?" Unsure of what is implied, you become uncomfortable and shift away from symptom assessment and move the conversation back toward Mr. A's interest in seeking therapy. He lets out a deep sigh and expresses fatigue at being rejected, overlooked, misunderstood, and states he wants to use therapy to cope and heal.

INTRODUCTION

How Do You Imagine Therapy?

When you think of therapy, what images come to mind from the case study? How did you envision the room or furniture? What was the focus of the session, and to what extent did prior expectations shape the treatment goals?

Prior to starting your first session or even learning how to "do therapy," you may have an *idea* of what therapy looks like. The image may include being seated in a chair across from your patient, looking intently as you occasionally nod and make associations between childhood, emotions, and present-day functioning. The office has comfortable furniture, is quiet, and is decorated with pictures. There is a clock nearby with a window for natural light to warm the room. The space is small enough to be cozy but large enough to include all the items (eg, furniture, desk lamp, bookshelf) needed to make the space feel welcoming.

Now, as you think about who attended the session, were there more people in the room besides the therapist and Mr. A? What ethnicity was the patient? And what gender was the spouse he mentioned?

All these questions and more are relevant to conducting therapy. Therapy is not just about the two-person relationship in the room (the "therapeutic dyad") but involves attention to the multiple—often invisible—layers of a person's identity and lived experiences. In addition, all patients exist and function within various systems—including their family of origin, community, workplace or school, geographic regions, and global society, to name a few.

In this chapter, we will focus on developing ways to incorporate systems and culture, using the case study ("Mr. A") to explore the layers of a patient's perspective and experience beyond the patient-therapist dyad. By the end of this chapter, you should be able to:

1. Consider the importance of systems in therapy, particularly family systems.

2. Acknowledge the role of cultural identity in understanding your patient's experiences based on their worldview.

3. Incorporate group-level identities and culturally relevant systems into the therapy process.

It is important to note here that the focus of this chapter is on individual therapy. There are a host of other therapeutic treatments, including marital and family therapy, group therapy, and community advocacy approaches that are excellent for specifically addressing issues within a system. We encourage you to use this chapter as a launch pad for exploring additional system approaches that could benefit your patient, over and above the individual therapy approach. For now, we will stick with the individual patient-therapist dyad to illustrate the importance of systems, context, and culture.

PART I: FAMILY SYSTEMS

Various professional organizations have highlighted the importance of considering broader systems.[1-3] Many guidelines for how to incorporate a systems approach in clinical care draw from the work of models that describe how systems interact across individuals, groups, settings, and over time. Adopting a systems lens helps us visually imagine the multiple systems that exist in your patient's life that involve the self, important others, and larger societal influences. We have included in the text box below one of the better-known systems models by Brofenbrenner[4,5] for a hint of the complex systems that involve an individual patient. In therapy, many patients may present with questions and concerns regarding their family, and it is on this family system that we will focus first.

Brofenbrenner's Ecological Model

We have chosen to use Brofenbrenner's ecological model[4,5] to illustrate the ways various systems exist and interact, including the small system of the therapeutic dyad and all the systems outside of it. This model may be fundamental for some of you, and perhaps new to others. Regardless, it can provide a useful way of remembering the large and small systems that influence the individual seated in front of you.

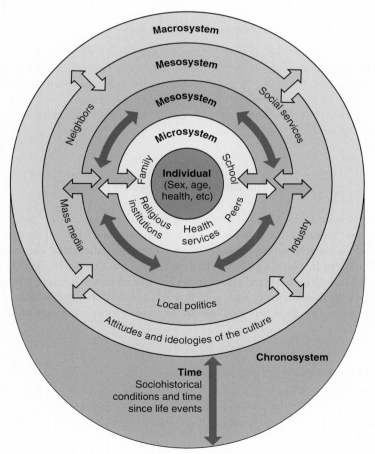

The immediate environment (**microsystem**) consists of your patient's close relationships. Early microsystems often involve parents, siblings, teachers, classmates, or peers, and current ones during adulthood can include close friends, intimate partners, spouses, children, and eventually even you as a therapist. These immediate environments represent the first place of learning that molds the basis of your patient's development.

Broader communities and immediate cultural environments (**mesosystem**) denote the interactions and connections formed across microsystems, such as the interaction between home and school, church and workplace, etc.

There are also interactions across systems, even when one of the systems does not include the patient (referred to as the **exosystem**). These interactions may not be well known to the patient, but still indirectly affect them. One example of this might be the relationship between the home and the parental workplace, in the form of a significant shift in a household through relocation or layoff.

Values, beliefs, and customs of society include broad cultural views of things like politics, institutional education, culture, and even fashion (referred to as the **macrosystem**). These play a significant role in an individual patient's thoughts, emotions, and behaviors. Your patient may mention something that happened on the current news, bring up a controversial topic trending on the news, or internalize images about beauty or acceptability portrayed in social media. Recognizing that this broader cultural or subcultural system affects your patient will help you learn what content is most important to how they see the world around them.

Finally, there are changes over time and history that impact your patient. The **chronosystem** involves the changes of the person over the course of their life, as well as the changes in their broader environment, situations, and settings across time. Knowledge of patterns and interactions with these systems over time, including the impact of important historical events, aids in conceptualization of the patient's problem.

The Role of Family Systems

When most people think about therapy, they have the image of one patient and one therapist seated together. You may also be aware of additional forms of therapeutic intervention, such as family, couples, group therapy, or consultation that can often include a room full of people who are involved in a patient's care. Of course, even in individual therapy, you know that there are always more people involved, because patients do not only interact with themselves or with you. But, if individual therapy is about the patient and their experiences, then how do these other people fit into the equation?

Nonindividual Therapy Approaches

This book does not focus on the numerous treatment options that involve groups, milieus, couples, families, communities, and treatment teams. However, it is important to recognize that these approaches can be preferred to individual therapy and take a different, systemic approach to identifying the source of the problem, challenge, and/or solution.

Group therapy—psychotherapy involving a patient in a group setting (eg, four or more persons) and a therapist where problems are addressed with the support of group peers. The group context allows validation and encouragement from others who may have similar concerns and provides opportunity for perspective taking and developing insight. Groups may be led by one or more therapists.

Couples/marital therapy—therapy aimed to help partners identify aspects of their relationship that can be strengthened for more rewarding interactions. Skills are provided to understand discrepancies the couple may perceive in the relationship with opportunity to problem-solve ways to address them.

Milieu therapy—a form of therapy that usually takes place in a residential facility where care is based on a group-support model to help patients develop skills for coping within their environment. Examples of facilities may include a day program, nursing home, or inpatient psychiatric hospital setting.

Family therapy—psychotherapy with a focus on addressing conflicts and improving the overall communication and interactions of the family. Various theoretical models exist that place emphasis on different dynamics of family composition and functioning (eg, Bowenian, Structural, Systemic, Strategic Family Therapy, to name a few).

8

Family Systems and Individual Psychotherapy. Some patients often make reference to their family of origin, whereas others focus on their currently defined family system. Understanding that family is an important aspect of your individual therapy patient's existence is vital. Family is one broader system that has a strong impact on your patient's presentation, even when you are not engaging in family therapy.

Family composition varies considerably from patient to patient and is best understood by asking the patient, "Who do you consider your family?" This highlights the fact that some patients consider family of origin and extended family as the only definition of "family" that counts, whereas others have been rejected or have walked away from their families of origin and have created a family with individuals not biologically related to them. Still others provide a combination of relatives and friends as their chosen definition of "family."

As noted in a prior text box, family therapy is a broad therapy approach that addresses conflict and discord within a couple or family by addressing the interactions of that system. Therapists who do a lot of this work develop additional expertise and training that allows them the title of family therapists. However, in the context of this specific chapter, we will consider how and why to incorporate family or other support members periodically into the *individual therapy* process in a manner that maintains integrity of your respective orientation and approach.

How and Why to Engage Family in an Individual Psychotherapy Session. The setting where you conduct therapy can greatly influence how you are able to engage with your patient. You may be seeing your patient in a private practice office where longer sessions and recurrent appointments are the norm. Or, you may be working within a medical setting where therapy sessions are briefer in duration and shorter in number of sessions (see Chapters 9-12 in this book). Either way, there are opportunities for engagement beyond the individual therapy dyad that include family and caregivers. Sometimes, having an additional set of eyes and ears can be helpful for obtaining collateral information, as well as a way to bolster potential resources for your patient. At other times, patients will specifically request that a family or support person be involved in treatment, either during the initial intake or at various points along the treatment trajectory. As a result, and with appropriate consent of the individual therapy patient, family members may be invited into a session as part of on-going care or a one-time point of check-in. You may also facilitate as a mediator to ensure that communication between the patient and their family remains as healthy as possible and to provide further psychoeducation around the proposed outcomes of therapy.

Bringing families into the therapy process may not resolve the broader family systems concern, but can begin to spark change. Below are three scenarios for how a therapist might include family in the individual therapy session:

1. *Include the family member(s) as a key part of the introductory sessions.* An example of this process might include welcoming the patient and family member(s) into the session to explain the therapy process, ensuring that everyone hears all information at the same time and are allowed to ask questions. You might discuss the option of having family members involved in some portions of therapy, with a collaborative understanding that the treatment focus is on the psychological care of the individual patient. As you conduct the initial evaluation, you may rely on collateral information from the loved one to supplement your findings while checking in with your patient along the way. However, be mindful that any paperwork or assessment forms are to be completed by the identified patient, unless additional assistance is needed (at which time you could volunteer, unless the familial culture indicates that a family member should be chosen to help).

   In this situation, it is also important to allow for one-on-one time between the patient and the therapist. This is for the purpose of developing rapport as well as a way to privately assess the patient (particularly for any concerns regarding domestic violence or coercion). One approach is to propose a plan to separate the therapy session into three parts—with both family and patient, patient alone, and time to debrief. You would then ask the family member to step outside of the room to wait in a separate area. The session may conclude with a collective debrief, or wrapping up with the patient alone. This sort of setup is commonplace when treating minors, but can also be used with patients who want family member involvement for a variety of personal and cultural reasons.

2. *Include family member(s) to address larger concerns that may require providing the family member a separate referral.* Bringing the family together to support the patient may reveal underlying emotional needs of other

family members that are best addressed in separate psychotherapy sessions. For settings where there are teams of therapists, it is optimal to provide a different therapist for the family member. In this case, concurrent sessions may be an option, with the patient receiving care from you in one room, and the family member engaged in their own session with another therapist in a separate room. This approach can be helpful particularly for families with limited time or transportation availability.

One note of caution—trying to treat two members of the same family unit, with you as the only therapist, in individual therapy is unwise. It can create boundary problems for you as the therapist. Keeping information truly "separated" in your head is a difficult task. It is likely that some thought or fact will slip through and cross over from one individual therapy session to another. Treating more than one member of a family in parallel individual therapy is *only* indicated in settings where there is a severe limitation on therapists with the necessary expertise and should certainly be discussed with your supervisor first.

3. *Include family members on an ad-hoc basis* (eg, *emerging concerns about safety, a need to obtain additional information*). For example, if a patient appears delirious or intoxicated, family support is imperative to assist with safe disposition home. In addition, if it becomes clear that a patient is at an increased risk for suicide, but is not imminently at risk (ie, does not require involuntary hospitalization), family member(s) can be involved in the individual therapy session as part of transparent safety planning discussion. Involvement of family in these situations is best done with the consent of the patient, but sometimes, safety and imminent risk of harm override confidentiality. Remember that while family members (in this instance) help to supplement the therapy, the focus of the therapy process is on the individual patient and their needs.

Family may also be included at the request of a patient. Sometimes, family is involved to provide additional support and comfort during a difficult time. For cultural reasons, it may be preferred to have several members of a family present when receiving information or clarifying details about treatment. At other times, family may demand to be involved, even at the objection of the patient. In these circumstances, it is important to revisit the treatment preference(s) of the patient and potentially even advocate for the patient's right to confidentiality.

Regardless of the scenario, when adding family members, you will still want to check in with your patient about their preferences and perceptions of how effective including an additional person has been in moving toward their goals. You will also want to keep in mind cultural considerations that could influence care such as hierarchy (eg, patient feeling the need to defer to requests of an older relative), language barriers (eg, family wanting to interpret for the patient), or transportation limitations (eg, patient's sole reliance on family for transportation in order to attend a session). These factors can affect the patient's interactions with you as well as the information you receive. As a result, you will want to be thoughtful about how and when to include family members. Ultimately, the focus of the treatment should

8

be on meeting the overall goals of your patient. If at any time you believe the scope of treatment has exceeded the bounds of your expertise, you will need to consider additional supervision and/or referrals to maximize best practices.

Finally, we would like to make a brief note here on the temptation to use family members or friends acting as interpreters. With the exception of rare and unique circumstances, it is never appropriate to rely on family members or close friends to provide interpretation for psychotherapy. This clearly creates issues with confidentiality, relationships, and boundaries in treatment. Instead, if an interpreter is required for therapy, we recommend you rely on trained interpreters who also have experience as cultural brokers. For additional recommendations surrounding interpreters in therapy, please see Refs. 6-9.

Case Study: Family Therapy Referral

Mr. A presents at his second therapy session with his spouse, and asks if they can be seen together to discuss further what the plans were for treatment, and also so that his spouse could provide some collateral information. As you have appropriate consent on file, you welcome Mr. A and the spouse into session, clarifying with both the purpose and scope of the session as a continuation of individual therapy for Mr. A. During the approximately 30 minutes or so that both Mr. A and his spouse are in the therapy room, you notice that there is notable marital tension and many of the concerns brought forward during that time centered on communication stressors and relationship issues. You are not a marriage therapist, but recognize this systemic issue could be better addressed by a marriage and family therapist. Involving the spouse during the intake session resulted in referring both Mr. A and his spouse to marital therapy as a best recommended treatment, to resolve issues specific to the relationship itself, while Mr. A continues individual therapy to address his own personal struggles. In this example, bringing the family into individual therapy allowed present opportunities for further therapeutic work that might not have otherwise happened.

PART II: MULTICULTURAL THERAPY

The Diversity of Our Patients

The lives of the patients you serve are as diverse and varied as the shades of a color. Whether royal, navy, sapphire, sky, or turquoise, all represent variations of blue, but differ based on how much or little other colors are added. A hint of purple can darken a blue to indigo, while a splash of green can create a vibrant teal. In its true form, the base color of blue remains, but it is enriched by the subtle nuances of variety.

Similarly, patients come to therapy with their own backgrounds, fears, possibilities, and goals, which have been dulled or brightened by variations in their lived experiences. They bring a history that, when effectively considered, can begin a conversation about how to provide optimal care. As discussed in Chapter 4, it is important to know "where to begin." It is vital to be aware of context, patient and therapist diversity, as well as the impact of broader systems on a patient's world-view, to help improve rapport with patients, establish a working alliance, and set appropriate boundaries. But where do you begin with such a seemingly broad topic as "culture"?

Cultural Identities and Worldview

What Do We Mean by "Culture"? It is helpful for you to think about culture in a comprehensive way that begins with how a patient sees themselves and the world around them. Culture consists of everything we do, how we do it, and factors that influence why we choose certain behaviors over others. In short, culture is how we live life. Formally, we are defining **culture** as global beliefs, values, habits, and practices that influence our thoughts, behaviors, and interactions. Culture forms our social and behavioral norms of engagement and is not only related to race, ethnicity, or gender, but can also include language, religion, food, clothing, and communication styles.

Every patient brings many intersecting cultural identities to a therapy session that can be expressed in numerous ways. Some aspects of cultural group membership may be more visible than others, such as the phenotypic traits of hair texture, facial features, or skin complexion. Other expressions may include accents, clothing choices, body language, or even subtle preferences such as the timing or tempo of therapy. Even more subtle are characteristics we cannot see but are revealed with trust, exploration, and a positive therapeutic alliance between patient and therapist, such as spiritual beliefs or political affiliation.

The point is, we all have multiple cultural identities that become more or less relevant based on the context. When our patients come to us in therapy, they carry a variety of cultural identities. As a therapist, we can learn about these identities by acknowledging the importance of culture and worldview, listening for ways our patients can educate us about their perspectives and the importance of their cultural identities in their lives. What may seem to be a significant cultural group identity on the surface may be less important to our patient.

This necessarily requires embracing the concept of cultural humility instead of viewing yourself as needing to develop cultural competence. **Cultural humility** is broadly understood as taking the stance as a therapist to "know what you don't know" in terms of your patient's cultural identity. Originally identified by Tervalon and Murray-Garcia,[10] this concept has been elaborated on more fully in recent writings by Hook and colleagues.[11,12] This stance allows a therapist to openly acknowledge areas of potential cultural similarities and differences, areas of cultural misunderstanding or ignorance, and further education by the patient to the therapist about their cultural background. This, in conjunction with ongoing cultural competency training and independent learning by the therapist, helps create a lifelong approach to multicultural care, instead of assuming this is a "one and done" set of information or skills. Some examples of exhibiting cultural humility include the following:

> *I know you are originally from the upper Midwest and grew up on a rural farm. Tell me what it was like to grow up on a farm.*

8

You recently immigrated to the US. What was the immigration process like for you? Can you help me understand what impact that has had on your life?

You were born right at the end of the Great Depression and grew up during World War II. How did being part of that generation affect you? What do you think about generations before and after yours since that time?

Note that although there is a certain amount of knowledge that comes from the patient, this approach goes hand in hand with you doing your own homework and increasing your own cultural knowledge. This includes being familiar with the treatment literature, maintaining knowledge of multicultural treatment guidelines, and learning more about areas of cultural identity important to your patient, in between sessions, so that you can draw upon an applicable treatment knowledge base.

Know Thyself and Know Thy Biases. As a beginning therapist, it benefits you to be honest with yourself and to notice your own biases. Therapists are often the last to admit they experience or specifically express bias. However, like all human beings, bias is a real and honest part of our existence. **Bias** can be defined as the personal preference you hold toward or against a person, situation, or idea and is usually thought to be unfair.[13] Often this preference happens without you even noticing, because it is a part of how you have learned to see the world. Biases are formed from experiences and are related to our individual perceptions of truth. Unfortunately, the term "bias" is frequently used interchangeably with prejudice or discrimination and sometimes becomes an ugly word that sparks discomfort.

Because the term "bias" is viewed as a negative and uncomfortable characteristic, this is a topic that can be difficult for therapists to explore and is often given limited attention in discussions about challenges in therapy. Although we all have personal biases, you have to decide what you want to do with this information and to what extent a particular bias can help or hinder your ability to connect with others. And ultimately, you can use your awareness of this process to help grow as a therapist.

Other words that tend to be used alongside bias include prejudice and discrimination. **Prejudice** is defined as a preconceived judgment or opinion that is based on limited information, and oftentimes directed toward one's group membership.[14] It is not uncommon for therapists to hold prejudicial beliefs or more systemic biases about specific groups and also carry these beliefs into therapy with them. This is why honest self-evaluation is necessary for improving your work in multicultural care. **Discrimination**, on the other hand, is defined as an actual behavior that treats a person belonging to a specific group or groups differently, and typically negatively. Discrimination, as a behavior, emerges from either implicit or explicit bias or prejudice.[14] Sometimes, therapists are unaware they are engaging in discriminatory behaviors. One example includes a therapist not returning initial therapy requests as quickly from patients who "sound less educated" in a voicemail.[15,16]

So, let us reiterate this point—*you will have your own biases about patients.* You may have developed biases about certain groups, populations, or disorders that make you less comfortable with initial engagement or ongoing treatment of specific patients. Even therapists who consciously hold very accepting or progressive views are not immune to implicit racism, sexism, homophobia, or even discrimination against individuals. Too often, therapists try to hide these biases from themselves, with the hopes the biases might resolve on their own or simply vanish. We believe that would be like asking you to unlearn the lyrics to your favorite song, just because someone tells you not to sing when you hear the music play. Try as you might, there is likely a murmuring background rendition playing in your head. The same principle applies to biases. We can try to ignore our biases, but it ends up taking far more energy and effort to dance around them than had we dealt with them head on.

Our recommendation for you is to constantly assess your own worldview, which includes acknowledging and exploring your own biases, stereotypes, prejudices, and even subtle actions of discrimination. How you handle every patient will partly depend on your comfort with acknowledging that biases can and do exist, and with the recognition that biases do not have to be the determining factor of success in therapy.

The Value of Cultural Immersion

One approach to increasing cultural awareness that is common in undergraduate and graduate level courses on multicultural therapy is to purposefully engage in an extended **cultural immersion** experience. These experiences are meant to increase understanding of another's perspective, reduce bias, and increase empathy via prolonged interpersonal cross-cultural interactions.[17] Participation in these sorts of experiences not only assists with learning valuable cultural knowledge, but also helps an individual highlight their own biases and therefore "know thyself" more deeply.[18,19]

Immersion experiences typically involve choosing a cultural group with which you are relatively unfamiliar or have a significant known bias, and engaging in activities with members of the group, preferably repeatedly and over an extended period of time. In addition, it is important for immersion exercises to allow you to engage as a true group member or immersed observer, instead of as a volunteer or treatment provider, as the latter roles create separation and a power differential. It is not uncommon to experience anxiety during the planning stages of an immersion experience, and to even procrastinate or intellectualize the experience itself, despite feeling overtly "excited" to begin. In addition, it is vital to not only complete the immersion experience, but to allow for a subsequent period of reflection and self-evaluation, either alone or with a trusted confidante. However, it is our experience that the immersion assignment is repeatedly highlighted as a very useful educational tool in learning environments involving multicultural topics (eg, in a graduate multicultural therapy course).

Dealing with Bias in Therapy. As much as you encourage your patients to "do the work," the effectiveness of therapy rests in the common factors that form the therapeutic relationship. The basics of these have been discussed already in Chapter 4 and consist of building rapport, establishing a therapeutic alliance, and maintaining boundaries.

Patients bring their own biases into sessions about expectations of therapy. At a basic level, a patient may have a bias about the quality of care provided based on a therapist's gender (eg, feeling more comfortable speaking with a female therapist based on perceptions of emotional capacity). Some patients may strongly advocate for seeing a therapist that holds the same faith-based or religious views (eg, Christian counseling). Other patients will hold biases that are more overtly negative, such as expressing racist, homophobic, or xenophobic views. Working with patients that hold and openly express prejudiced views can present a real challenge.[20]

So, how do you handle bias when it shows up in therapy? It depends. Keep in mind that the skills presented in this chapter are not expected to be utilized all at once nor all within the initial therapy session. These skills represent a holistic approach to working with patients beyond an initial question and answer intake interview. Learning these skills can arm you with tools to help you think about what transpired in one session and how you might take the next step.

Awareness and discussion of bias can open up opportunities for growth and deepening of therapy. Once you are aware of the biases at play, you are in a position to expand the growth of your patient (and yourself). You can choose the easier (and often more comfortable) route of ignoring the signs of bias, or you can use the signs as directions to guide your work. As you recall, bias in isolation is not the problem—it is how we use our biases to create discrimination and prejudice that becomes the problem.

In therapy, you will often teach patients how to develop more effective strategies to deal with a problem or how to enhance or restructure previous strategies to realign with what is now more feasible or effective. However, it is hard to change something you do not first understand. Acknowledging and understanding a patient's bias is the first step toward understanding the function bias may play in their lives, and whether or not this way of thinking has moved them closer to or further away from their goal.

You might be asking yourself at this point—is it my responsibility to point out *all* of the cultural biases or prejudices of my patients? The short answer is no. You cannot expect yourself to redirect the therapy session each and every time this occurs, or else you will not be able to effectively address the patient's presenting concern or need. The bigger question is: *what is the value in addressing this bias and how might addressing it help or hinder the patient's goals and therapy process?* Some patients may raise the issue themselves, as people are sometimes aware of their own biases and wish to address them. But other times, the patient will be unaware of the bias. For cases when your patient is unknowingly demonstrating a bias that seems to be impeding *their own therapy goals*, the decision to spend time unpacking and exploring the thoughts related to this issue becomes more clear.

For example, a patient may present with an initial concern of angry outbursts toward strangers. While describing the most recent incident that escalated into anger, she shares about experiencing road rage while driving behind someone from an ethnic minority group, using derogatory language about the driving incompetence of the group as a whole. Option A: This *could* be a springboard for discussing how their biased belief system affects (and possibly contributes to) their problems in functioning within a broader, shifting cultural environment. Option B: This incident *could* also be an example of poor impulse control with an opportunity to address stress management and de-escalation. Either response (and a host of other options not mentioned) could be therapeutic and patient-centered. However, the decision to pursue option A or B will depend on the overall goals of treatment and the extent to which the bias is impeding the patient's ability to function in a psychologically healthy way.

Bias and prejudicial comments can also arise and be directed toward you as the therapist. These comments can be in the form of fleeting remarks made about others who share an identity similar to you. In addition, it may be clear that your patient knows you are a member of that cultural group (eg, biological sex, racial identity, age), or may be completely unaware (eg, religion, sexual orientation). Regardless, this can put you into a bind and cause significant discomfort. Our recommendation is to be proactive in understanding and growing in your own self-knowledge (including self-reflection of the incident), consult heavily with trusted supervisors and advanced peers, and weigh the impact of addressing these comments in therapy against the likely consequences (both positive and negative). For further guidance on the ethical dilemma brought forth by these situations, see Ref. 20.

Case Study: Exploring Bias in Therapy

Let us return to the case study of Mr. A following his unclear remark to you. On additional probing he says, "Every doctor always assumes I'm depressed or thinks I'm going to go off and kill myself. But I'm just pissed off and sad. Why can't you people just let people like me feel angry and sad sometimes about the world?" A first pass would be to seek more clarity to understand the nature of who "you people" versus "people like me" might be. Mr. A may be referring to differences in your gender, race, sexual orientation, socioeconomic status, professional roles, or something else entirely.

During the session, Mr. A later explains his challenge in identifying as a biracial Dominican American man with a fair skin complexion. He states feeling like he lives in two different worlds, without being accepted in either one. Mr. A reports pride about being promoted to the new position which he attributes to his lighter skin. However, he expresses worry that he may not be given respect in his new role should his colleagues learn of his biracial identity.

This creates an opportunity for you to understand more about what "you people" means in his view of your ability to connect with and help him. You might want to gradually explore his thoughts about what it means to him for you to be (for example) a White female therapist in training, providing therapy to an older Dominican American male patient, and learn how perceptions of each identity affect the therapeutic relationship. In our experience, it sometimes helps to simply acknowledge the elephant in the room, instead of trying to act like cultural and worldview differences may not exist. If you do not, you could be building a higher barrier or modeling the belief that difficult discussions do not have a place in therapy. However, you will want to be thoughtful about your approach, as direct questioning or confrontation about these differences can result in defensiveness and an injury to the therapeutic alliance. This would also be a great time to do a self-reflective check of your own feelings about approaching the topic of cultural differences with your patient. Chances are if you are feeling unsure and nervous, then so is your patient. In this case, you might say to Mr. A, "I know there are a lot of similarities and differences between us. You made a comment about 'you people' during our first session and you brought up the same phrase again today—are you willing to talk with me more about that, so I can better help you?"

The Influence of Societal Systems on Therapy

As we mentioned earlier, patients develop and exist in a multitude of systems, with family being an important one. They may engage in one way within the therapeutic dyad, but have been raised or exist within a specific family structure, neighborhood, religious community, or broader context that affects how they understand the world. Therefore, it is important for therapists not to be naive about the larger social, national, and historical systems and events that impact our patients, as many will bring these experiences into the individual therapy session.

Identifying Cultural Trauma. **Cultural trauma** (sometimes referred to as historical trauma or racial trauma) is defined as experiences of atrocious events that have resulted in varied long-lasting effects for a group or generation of people.[21-24] Examples of events that provoke this sense of cultural trauma include slavery, the Holocaust, and 9/11. These national and international events evoke intergenerational feelings of hypervigilance, grief, and anger.

For example, indigenous groups in various countries, including the United States, have specifically been targeted for geographical relocation, often through genocide and later, through complete cultural assimilation. As a result, entire generations lost their cultural home and became marginalized. Cultural trauma can increase a sense of mistrust and anxiety of the dominant group, and plays a clear role in the rates of psychopathology observed among historically traumatized and marginalized indigenous populations.[25,26] These cultural traumas can be associated with an increased risk for suicide and substance use disorders, as populations avoid seeking treatment from "majority group" (usually White) providers or government organizations and instead resort to less effective coping mechanisms.[27,28]

Exploring a patient's membership in a historically traumatized group is something that may come up during a carefully completed cultural assessment (discussed later in the chapter). However, it may not be a concept or issue that would readily arise otherwise, or even something many culturally traumatized patients recognize as potentially explanatory for deep feelings of distress and marginalization. Therefore, the therapist is in a useful position to not only recognize the *individual* psychology of the patient, but also the broader *historical* and *systemic* context in which the patient operates.

Case Study: Cultural Trauma

Mr. A mentions during his third session that he was denied time off by his new boss for a religious holiday that is specific to his family's home country. He starts by commenting, "I shouldn't be mad. It's just a holiday." He further notes that his boss explained to him, "It isn't really a company or recognized religious holiday here, you know? And you're still new. I don't want to show preference." Mr. A then feels disappointed, because he gathers for this holiday annually to celebrate with his extended family and community. However, he has been careful not to mention his religious affiliation at work because of the history of persecution associated with his faith community. This denial of time off may evoke not only individual feelings of anger, but also feelings of grief that have roots in broader cultural group tradition and remembrance. Helping Mr. A understand the relationship between the here-and-now experience of irritation about a day off with the historical importance of the cultural celebration may be one way Mr. A can better understand what he initially described in therapy as an "overreaction to a holiday."

The Impact of the Ever-Changing National Landscape. One trend that has been commented upon by therapists in recent years is the impact of ongoing political dialogues and national demographic trends on the current American culture, and therefore the behavior of our patients in therapy. Some patients have reacted to this trend by making increasingly politicized commentary in the therapy session. Others have expressed increased feelings of confusion or anger at the changes in America. Regardless of the opinions and beliefs of the patient or therapist, these national trends and events can and do find their way into the therapy dialogue. A therapist who is aware of the impact of these broader systems can remain sensitized to and aware of national events that may promote feelings of malcontent or reaffirm beliefs.

For example, what if a patient voices frustration about the political climate and asks for your thoughts about the matter? How might you respond, particularly if you find yourself internally agreeing or strongly disagreeing? You could acknowledge this frustration with a reminder that your role in the therapy process is to focus on and support our patient's mental health care, irrespective of any of your personal beliefs, needs, or background. Often, this is a very difficult topic to discuss given a need to maintain professional boundaries with your patient (eg, see Ref. 29, on therapist political self-disclosure). However, there is a way to validate their personal concerns, hold your own beliefs privately, and address the presented content without feeling obligated to side with one argument or another. You might respond by saying, "It is hard not to notice the political climate of the country right now. If you are willing, I would like to understand how these changes have affected you in your life."

Multicultural Applications in Therapy

Cultural Views of Psychotherapy. The Cultural Formulation Interview (CFI) was published as part of the Diagnostic and Statistical Manual of Mental Disorders (DSM-5)[30] and provides one way to explore a patient's view of treatment through the use of a brief interview (see also CFI mention in Chapter 2 on conceptualization and assessment). This interview is quite similar to the explanatory models of distress work of Kleinman[31] and uses several open-ended questions to understand a patient's view of mental health and mental illness, mental health treatment, and the idea of their family and cultural community about mental health issues.

While it might be thought that interviews such as the CFI would only be applicable with patients who appear "different from" the therapist, we recommend routinely implementing this approach in your clinical care. What emerges from using interview approaches such as the CFI is often a reevaluation of assumptions about patients and a clearer understanding of how psychotherapy fits into *the patient's* preferences about mental health treatment.

Also, as we noted in the beginning of this chapter, it is important for you to understand your own perspective and experience, so as to better understand how it may be similar or different from the view of your patients. You might consider completing the CFI on yourself prior to completing one with a patient, to increase your own self-awareness.

Case Study: Using a CFI-Informed Approach

It is assumed that Mr. A has had prior experiences with psychotherapy before, but perhaps he has only viewed psychotherapy stereotypes in the media or has heard about psychotherapy from friends or family. Due to time limitations, you opt to not complete an entire CFI at the initial session. Below is an example dialogue that might emerge when using an explanatory model of distress to assess Mr. A's perceptions of mental health treatment and, importantly, the perspective of those in his immediate environment.

Therapist: What do you see as the problem or challenge at this time?

[This question seeks to understand how the patient defines the problem or challenge in their own terms, instead of yours.]

Mr. A: I don't really have a problem—they do. I mean, the people at work do. But you probably think I'm crazy for coming to see you.

Therapist: Sounds like you think therapy is only for people who are crazy. What would your family and friends say about you seeing a therapist?

[This response helps elaborate on how Mr. A views therapy and provides a prompt to learn more about what others in his life might say.]

Mr. A: Well, that's just it (laughs). In our family we don't go to therapy. It's just for crazy people. My grandmother would say I should pray about my problems. Either way, I'm here and talking to you. So, isn't it up to you to tell me what you think is wrong?

Therapist: Not exactly. But it's a good time for me to ask you what you expect your treatment providers to do for you in general.

[This opens the door to learning (1) what kind of therapist-patient relationship Mr. A expects and/or desires, and (2) how his cultural identity has shaped expectations (benefits or barriers) of this experience.]

Mr. A: I don't know. No one has ever asked me that before, and I'm new to this therapy thing. I sort of assumed doctors just tell you what's wrong, give you a prescription, and then you do it. And if you don't get better, it's your fault. But I would rather that I have a say, you know?

This interchange, however brief, gives us a lot of information we may not know about Mr. A's view of mental health care and the perspectives of others important to him. It also tells us a bit about his fears about the process and the desire to have a collaborative relationship in treatment, despite perceptions that this level of collaboration is not allowed. This is the purpose of initially using the CFI with any patient, or at least an approach informed by the CFI.

Ways to Assess Cultural Identities. Our cultural group identities are one important way we define ourselves or how we make sense of who we are. Beyond the therapy dyad, our patients are members of a larger world where they are faced with decisions and tasks that will highlight or hide various parts of their identity. Even just noting cultural similarities and differences that may exist within the therapeutic dyad communicates that identity matters to your work together.[32] This approach can be very powerful in establishing rapport. When we are allowed to present in a manner consistent with how we view ourselves, we experience more comfort and security. However, when our cultural group identity is unknown, questioned, or even negatively received, we can develop feelings of insecurity and distress which can present in the form of depressive or anxious symptoms or other behaviors.

So, how do we begin to assess something as vast and broad as cultural identity? We find Pamela Hays'[33] ADDRESSING framework to be one very useful model for assessing the complexities of an individual and the cultural group identities they represent. This mnemonic is as follows: **A**ge/generational influences, **D**evelopmental or other **D**isability, **R**eligion and spiritual orientation, **E**thnic and racial identity, **S**ocioeconomic status, **S**exual orientation, **I**ndigenous heritage, **N**ational origin, and **G**ender.[33] The ADDRESSING mnemonic highlights potentially important areas of a patient's cultural group identity membership that can prompt further exploration. These cultural identities may be expressed in the context of psychotherapy in specific ways that are similar or different from day-to-day interactions. Understanding how these identities are expressed may also provide information about strengths and insecurities in other contexts.

When we use this model in practice, we incorporate this concept into the routine therapy intake and also in subsequent therapy sessions. This serves two purposes. First, it allows us to listen for important clues to a patient's cultural identities that they perceive as important. In addition, asking more about cultural identity and worldview opens the door to acknowledging to the patient that you believe culture has an important space in therapy.

We usually start off by saying something like, "Understanding my patient's cultural identities is important because it tells me more about you, and also helps tailor your treatment, so I might ask you more about your history and background throughout therapy." Below are further examples of how to incorporate a few parts of the ADDRESSING model using additional information you learn from Mr. A. If you are further interested in this model or approach, we refer you to several texts written by Hays[33] and other colleagues in the field of multicultural psychotherapy.

Age and generational influences: Age and generational cohort impact life experiences, technology exposure, and perceptions by others of their role within broader society. For example, stereotypes and expectations may exist about Baby Boomers and Millennials with age-dependent expectations regarding age.

Case Study: Age and Generation

Mr. A tells you he identifies as an "older" member of the work team, with extensive experience but less technology expertise. This causes him to struggle to connect with a younger employee more accustomed with the current media interface. He further elaborates that the misunderstanding in communication with colleagues has resulted in failed assignments or missed deadlines. This information regarding generational cohort can allow you to recognize the impact of age and generation on Mr. A's identity and the presenting complaint of "fitting in."

Religion and spiritual orientation: Religious identity and/or spiritual beliefs have an extraordinary impact on a patient's viewpoint and their explanations for the environment, their purpose, morality, and coping strategies. Even patients who deny any religious beliefs, per se, may have views on broader spiritual questions such as why we exist. Sometimes, we ask fairly directly, "Do you have any specific religious or spiritual beliefs that will help me better tailor your therapy?" However, depending on your own comfort in discussions of religion or spiritual orientation, questions about religious affiliation can be received with defensiveness (especially if the religion or spiritual belief is not well known or often misunderstood).

Case Study: Religion and Spirituality

Mr. A mentions the importance of prayer and faith in his family to deal with life's stressors. Later, he notes feeling distanced from church because of the relocation and being without a "church home." You begin to explore with him whether or not finding a new church home or problem-solving ways to reconnect with his church in other ways may be helpful for his overall feelings of loneliness and isolation.

Religion, Therapy, and Boundaries of Competence

Some therapists are uncomfortable discussing religious or spiritual issues as part of therapy. However, to truly understand your patient's outlook, it is necessary to also consider religious and/or spiritual beliefs patients use to understand the world around them, the purpose of life, and views on life after death.

It is important to also recognize there are limitations to how much you can address about specific religious or theological questions that may arise. Some licensed therapists also have a background in pastoral counseling, theology, and other religious education that qualifies them to fully discuss specific questions about religion in the context of psychotherapy. Most do not. In our experience, it is usually best to defer pointed questions about theology or religion to the experts (eg, a hospital chaplain or the patient's spiritual leader). If you work in a setting with a chaplain, this is a wonderful relationship to cultivate as much of the time you will both be addressing similar questions patients bring to the table. It is helpful to understand where the mutual boundaries of competence arise between the two of you.

There are many wonderful resources available that address ethical and practical questions regarding spirituality, religion, and therapy. We would direct you to your professions' ethics code and this useful framework by Plante[34] as springboards for reviewing more recent writings in the literature on this issue.

Ethnic and racial identity: Race and ethnicity tend to be at the forefront of conversations about cultural group identity. Usually, these are the first (and sometimes only) identities considered when thinking about culture with less focus on ethnic identity across all groups. For example, ethnic identity may be less commonly discussed among White Western cultural populations.[35] Instead, patients may identify by their **race** (biological and phenotypical characteristics of a group) or **nationality** (ancestry based on country of origin) with less awareness of their **ethnicity** (shared cultural norms of a group). The reasoning behind this could be variable. Someone's specific ethnicity could be unknown, or ethnicity is not a prominent identity for that person.

8

Case Study: Ethnic Identity, Racial Identity, and National Origin

At first read of the medical chart, Mr. A is described as a Black male. On the therapy clinic intake paperwork, he checks "other" and writes in "biracial" in the race/ethnicity category. This provides you very few clues as to his specific racial or ethnic identity. In reality, you might make immediate conclusions about his race and/or ethnicity upon meeting for the first time.

However, through learning more about Mr. A's family and personal history over the first two sessions, you find out he identifies as "Dominican American" and has a strong cultural group pride. You then learn that he was the first and only Latinx employee to hold a managerial position in the current company, but is often perceived as "African American." This knowledge shifts your conceptualization of Mr. A's concerns about "fitting in," difficulties with feeling marginalized, and begins a dialogue about his experiences as a Dominican American at work and elsewhere in his life.

Gender identity: **Gender** refers to culturally ascribed definitions of what it means to be a man or a woman. Most intake forms ask a patient to identify as either male or female, although it is important to offer a broader array of gender identity options than male and female, such as "prefer not to say" and "prefer to self-describe." Therapists must be mindful of the various ways a patient may gender identify and to not assume that outward presentations match internal gender identity.

Case Study: Gender Identity and Perceived Role

During your first few sessions with Mr. A, he makes a comment or two about being the "breadwinner" within his family, and how his job is vital to his idea of what it means to be a man. However, because of the recent relocation and job stressors, he is wondering if he is even in the correct vocation or job position and is doubting his abilities. Although Mr. A mentions he and his spouse have discussed the possibility of downsizing and relying solely on her income, he refuses to entertain that idea. Understanding Mr. A's gender identity, the strong gender roles he ascribes to, and perhaps how these intersect with his Dominican American identity certainly help you understand his perspective and experiences, and therefore shape your potential interventions. For example, you would not simply explore or challenge Mr. A's perspective about these issues in therapy without considering the ongoing impact of masculine identity and traditional gender roles on his thoughts, feelings, and behaviors.

Patient Names and Preferred Pronouns

What do you call your patient? We tend to err on the side of formality when meeting adult patients for the first time, as this generally confers a sense of respect. Patients will sometimes correct you or spontaneously provide a preferred name or title, but you can also directly ask how your patient prefers to be addressed by you.

However, what if you are unclear as to your patient's gender identity? As most formal titles (eg, Mr. or Ms.) are clearly gendered, there is a decision point to be made upon meeting a patient for the first time, or even when continuing to work with a patient who identifies as transgender and/or is undergoing gender-confirming interventions.

Our solution is relatively simple—use both the first initial and last name listed in the patient record when meeting any patient for the first time (eg, when retrieving a patient from the waiting room). Then, when in private, always ask what the patient's preferred address or title is. This is good practice in general. In some cases, particularly in the aforementioned case of patients who identify as transgender, preferred titles, names, and pronouns may shift over time or procedure. Asking can feel interpersonally awkward, but remember—you are not required to know everything in order to be a good multicultural provider. In fact, knowing what you don't know is a wonderful approach to take and can provide your patient a sense of comfort in exploring issues that they may feel are taboo in other relationships.

The Importance of Acknowledging Multiple Identities. The aforementioned examples are not exclusive nor are these the only ways patients can express their group identities. In fact, many cultural identities do not exist in a vacuum and can overlap or take turns in how much or little is expressed, given the context. **Intersectionality** refers to the way our cultural identities are related and intertwined with one another.[36-39] Think of intersectionality as the weaving of these threads together, sometimes creating very different fabric patterns for different people. Intersectionality provides a context for understanding patient interactions, relationships, and perceptions of dynamics in their environment. Depending on a situation, it can be challenging for a patient to disentangle themselves from the complex overlap of identities that may appear to be unified (eg, Black and female).

Take a moment to think about yourself and how you might describe your identities using the ADDRESSING model. Now, imagine you were told you could only pick one cultural identity to assume for the day and that this was the way you must present at all times with little to no connection or reference to the other parts of yourself. How would you decide which identity to prioritize? Are you curious about who you would be interacting with that day or what roles you would be assigned?

The exercise to select one cultural identity is a life challenge we face each and every day, more so for those with multiple minority cultural group statuses. While not always explicitly stated, patients may feel obligated or strongly encouraged to select specific cultural identities they will "own" for the day, setting, or purpose. Beneath this presentation, there may be an inclination to hide, conceal, or ignore the other identities for a variety of reasons. Some may do so out of anxiety and a need to assimilate in order to gain acceptance among groups. Others may do so out of fear that recognition of an identity may lead to negative consequences or reactions, leading to distress or isolation. Still others may not even be aware of the multidimensional nature of identity and see themselves as one identity or another. This may lead to unconscious rejection of important parts of themselves, which may later surface in therapy as an opportunity for identity exploration. Regardless of why a patient chooses to embrace or suppress a form of their cultural identity, what matters is whether the decision brings them joy or pain.

As a culturally informed therapist, you will not know everything and will make mistakes or say something you felt jeopardized the therapeutic alliance between you and your client. The point is to be *aware* of your influence and notice when additional understanding may be needed for healing the alliance, as you both adjust to working together. For example, a client may describe adjustment (or "present differently") from setting to setting (eg, changes in their language, dialect, or dress) as they seek comfort and "feel out" their identity within that space. It does not necessarily mean a person is being less genuine. They may just need to establish comfort and safety to feel open in sharing various aspects of their identity with you. Still other patients may prefer to speak in a style most comfortable for them based on that particular setting (ie, "code switching," which is the practice of alternating between different languages or language styles) and may only start shifting their speech style when they become more comfortable with you.

8

Case Study: Intersectionality

Let us return to the case study of Mr. A. You may already have a working agenda or idea of how this session is supposed to go. From the information you obtained via chart review and the intake paperwork, you formed a hypothesis about the presenting concern. However, after meeting with Mr. A for a few sessions, and using a culturally humble approach, you have learned that central to his identity is that of an older married man, with a strong religious faith and strong ties to his Dominican American heritage.

None of these identities are singularly impactful or more important than another, and they clearly influence his learned views of himself and the world around him. For example, he has a strong view that he needs to be the primary financial provider within his household, as well as spiritually strong for his family. However, his age (and perceptions of others about his age) has caused him to feel somewhat obsolete at work, which increases anxiety about his ability to fulfill his role. You as the therapist have only learned this by acknowledging the importance of these additional cultural group identities and creating the space for your patient to collaboratively understand how these roles and identities intersect to affect the patient in the here and now.

Lifelong Learning and Multicultural Considerations in Psychotherapy

As you can see from this chapter, we are describing an overarching approach to therapy, by viewing your patients as part of a broader context and with a host of cultural identities. Infusing this approach into therapy on a routine basis takes quite a bit of practice and a level of conscientiousness. However, it also requires a commitment to lifelong learning as a therapist who practices cultural humility.

What we did not cover in any great detail in this chapter was the literature on evidence-based therapies for various cultural groups. Most research completed on psychotherapy has historically used convenience samples of relatively educated White patients. As such, there remains a large gap in what we know about the cross-cultural validity of assessment and treatment approaches that are based on research. There is quite a bit of developing interest in the application and cross-cultural utility of commonly used psychotherapy techniques (eg, CBT[40]) and adaptations of therapies to better fit a specific group's needs (eg, dialectical behavior therapy for adolescents[41]). However, it is insufficient to assume that *all* therapies by *all* therapists are appropriate for *all* patients. Therefore, it is important to be aware of the emerging research literature and studies that *have* been done with various groups that are traditionally not involved in clinical trials and to use treatments created and adapted for specific groups when applicable.

It is unusual to find that a randomized controlled trial on any given therapy approach has been completed on a group of people with Mr. A's specific cultural identities. So, what do you do then? Sue[42] coined a term **dynamic sizing** to describe the careful and thoughtful application of broad, population-based research unique to the individual and patient sitting in front of you. For example, you might read a study that indicates the incorporation of *dichos* (or *sayings*) may be helpful when working with patients who have emigrated from Central America and whose primary language is Spanish. Yet, the patient in front of you may dislike this approach or struggle with metaphors. Therefore, while knowing the larger population-based literature on various cultural groups is extremely important, you still need to know when and how to apply it. We encourage you to keep an eye on the multicultural therapy literature as it grows and develops, and a similarly keen eye on the individual in front of you.

At the end of this chapter, there are a list of helpful resources to further your learning, as well as a list of the references used throughout this chapter. We hope this content sparks an interest in continuing to learn more about systems and cultural humility. Literature, films, consultation, supervision, and cultural immersion experiences can all work together to make cultural humility a lifelong learning practice.

Conclusion

This chapter has set the groundwork for understanding that your patients are involved in systems and cultures that exist beyond the individual psychotherapy dyad. So often, we become engrossed in the therapeutic relationship to the point of ignoring important developmental and family influences on the here-and-now behaviors of our patients. We fall into the same trap when we fail to incorporate the influence of broader cultural and systemic factors into understanding how our patient approaches the world. In addition, as a culturally informed therapist it is necessary to continue to "know thyself," know one's own worldview, and continue to broaden a sense of cultural humility so as to better serve our patients.

A word of comfort—we cannot be all things to all patients at all times. Simply opening up the door for your patient to realize that their way of life and cultural experiences do have a place in your therapeutic relationship is a strong starting point. The tools we introduced in this chapter should help you on that journey.

8

Self-Study Questions

1. What systems exist in a patient's life that are external to the individual therapy relationship? Why are these important?

2. Complete a self-assessment of your own cultural identities, using the Hays' ADDRESSING model mnemonic. Then, complete this for a patient you have recently seen or observed. What do you notice?

3. Make a written plan for a brief cultural immersion activity (perhaps 1 or 2 hours) that you could realistically complete in the next month. This could include a festival, a cooking or meal opportunity, a performance or play, an interview, or simply an observation experience in a new cultural environment.

4. Have you ever heard a patient make a prejudicial remark about you or another person? How did you respond in the moment? How might you discuss this with your supervisor or another trusted mentor?

5. When might you involve a family member in an individual psychotherapy session? When might you choose to not involve them?

RESOURCES FOR FURTHER LEARNING

Comas-Diaz L. *Multicultural care: a clinician's guide to cultural competence. Center for Excellence for Cultural Competence.* Washington, DC: American Psychological Association; 2012. Available at https://nyculturalcompetence.org/cfionlinemodule/

Hays P. *Addressing Cultural Complexities in Practice.* 3rd ed. Washington, DC: American Psychological Association; 2016.

Lewis-Fernández R, Aggarwal NK, Hinton L, Hinton DE, Kirmayer LK, eds. *The DSM-5 Handbook on the Cultural Formulation Interview.* Washington, DC: American Psychiatric Publishing; 2016.

Sue DW, Sue D, Neville HA, Smith L. *Counseling the Culturally Diverse: Theory and Practice.* 8th ed. Hoboken, NJ: Wiley; 2019.

REFERENCES

1. American Psychiatric Association. *Practice Guidelines for the Psychiatric Evaluation of Adults.* 3rd ed. Arlington, VA: American Psychiatric Association; 2016.
2. American Psychological Association. *Multicultural Guidelines: An Ecological Approach to Context, Identity, and Intersectionality.* 2017. Available at http://www.apa.org/about/policy/multicultural-guidelines.pdf.
3. National Association of Social Workers. *Standard and Indicators for Cultural Competence in Social Work Practice.* Washington, DC: National Association of Social Workers; 2015. Available at https://www.socialworkers.org/LinkClick.aspx?fileticket=PonPTDEBrn4%3D&portalid=0.
4. Bronfenbrenner U. Toward an experimental ecology of human development. *Am Psychol.* 1977;32(7):513-531.
5. Bronfenbrenner U. Ecological models of human development. *Readings on the Development of Children.* 1994;2(1):37-43.
6. Martin WB, Benedetto NN, Elledge DK, Najjab A, Howe-Martin L. Beyond the language barrier: Recommendations for working with interpreters in individual psychotherapy. *Prof Psychol Res Pr.* 2020. doi:10.1037/pro0000350.
7. Bauer AM, Alegría M. Impact of patient language proficiency and interpreter service use on the quality of psychiatric care: A systematic review. *Psychiat Serv.* 2010;61(8):765-773. doi:10.1176/appi.ps.61.8.765.
8. Becher EH, Wieling E. The intersections of culture and power in clinician and interpreter relationships: A qualitative study. *Cult Divers Ethn Minor Psychol.* 2015;21(3):450-457. doi:10.1037/a0037535.
9. Miller AB, Hahn E, Norona CR, et al. *A Socio-Culturally, Linguistically-Responsive, and Trauma-Informed Approach to Mental Health Interpretation.* Los Angeles, CA: National Center for Child Traumatic Stress; 2019.
10. Tervalon M, Murray-Garcia J. Cultural humility versus cultural competence: A. critical distinction in defining physician training outcomes in multicultural education. *J Health Care Poor Underserved.* 1998;9:117-125.
11. Hook JN, Davis DE, Owen J, Worthington EL, Utsey SO. Cultural humility: measuring openness to culturally diverse clients. *J Couns Psychol.* 2013;60:353-366.
12. Hook JN, Davis D, Owen J, DeBlaere C. *Cultural Humility: Engaging Diverse Identities in Therapy.* Washington, DC: American Psychological Association; 2017.
13. Major B, Townsend SM. Coping with bias. In: Dovidio JF, Hewstone M, Glick P, Esses VM, eds. *Prejudice, Stereotyping and Discrimination.* London: SAGE Publications; 2010:410-425.
14. Dovidio JF, Hewstone M, Glick P, Esses VM. Prejudice, stereotyping and discrimination: theoretical and empirical overview. In: Dovidio JF, Hewstone M, Glick P, Esses VM, eds. *Prejudice, Stereotyping and Discrimination.* Thousand Oaks, CA: SAGE Publications; 2010:3-28.
15. Kugelmass H. "Sorry, I'm not accepting new patients": an audit study of access to mental health care. *J Health Soc Behav.* 2016;57(2):168-183.
16. Shin RQ, Smith LC, Welch JC, Ezeofor I. Is Allison more likely than lakisha to receive a callback from counseling professionals? A racism audit study. *Counsel Psychol.* 2016;44(8):1187-1211.
17. Tomlinson-Clarke SM, Clarke D. Culturally focused community-centered service learning: an international cultural immersion experience. *J Multicult Couns Dev.* 2010;38(3):166-175. doi:10.1002/j.2161-1912.2010.tb00124.x.
18. Barden SM, Cashwell CS. Critical factors in cultural immersion: a synthesis of relevant literature. *Int J Adv Counsell.* 2013;35(4):286-297.
19. Canfield BS, Low L, Hovestadt A. Cultural immersion as a learning method for expanding intercultural competencies. *Fam J.* 2009;17(4):318-322.
20. Mbroh H, Najjab A, Knapp S, Gottlieb MC. Prejudiced patients: ethical considerations for addressing patients' prejudicial comments in psychotherapy. *Prof Psychol Res Pr.* 2019;51(3):284-290. doi:10.1037/pro0000280.
21. French B, Lewis J, Mosley D, et al. Toward a psychological framework of radical healing in communities of color. *Counsel Psychol.* 2019;48(1):14-46. doi:10.1177/0011000019843506.
22. Mohatt NV, Thompson AB, Thai ND, Tebes JK. Historical trauma as public narrative: a conceptual review of how history impacts present-day health. *Soc Sci Med.* 2014;106, 128-136.
23. Nagata DK, Kim JH, Nguyen TU. Processing cultural trauma: intergenerational effects of the Japanese American incarceration. *J Soc Issues.* 2015;71(2):356-370.
24. Wilkins EJ, Whiting JB, Watson MF, Russon JM, Moncrief AM. Residual effects of slavery: what clinicians need to know. *Contemp Fam Ther.* 2013;35(1):14-28.

8

25. Brave Heart MYH, Chase J, Elkins J, Altschul DB. Historical trauma among indigenous peoples of the Americas: concepts, research, and clinical considerations. *J Psychoactive Drugs*. 2011;43(4):282-290.

26. Gone JP. Redressing First Nations historical trauma: theorizing mechanisms for indigenous culture as mental health treatment. *Transcult Psychiatry*. 2013;50(5):683-706.

27. Ehlers CL, Gizer IR, Gilder DA, Ellingson JM, Yehuda R. Measuring historical trauma in an American Indian community sample: contributions of substance dependence, affective disorder, conduct disorder and PTSD. *Drug Alcohol Depend*. 2013;133(1):180-187.

28. Morgan R, Freeman L. The healing of our people: substance abuse and historical trauma. *Subst Use Misuse*. 2009;44(1):84-98.

29. Solomonov N, Barber JP. Patients' perspectives on political self-disclosure, the therapeutic alliance, and the infiltration of politics into the therapy room in the Trump era. *J Clin Psychol*. 2018;74(5):779-787. doi:10.1002/jclp.22609.

30. American Psychiatric Association. *Diagnostic and Statistical Manual of Mental Disorders*. 5th ed. Washington, DC: Author; 2013.

31. Kleinman A. *Patients and Healers in the Context of Culture: An Exploration of the Borderland Between Anthropology, Medicine, and Psychiatry*. Vol 3. Berkeley, CA: Univ of California Press; 1980.

32. Comas-Diaz. *Multicultural Care: A Clinician's Guide to Cultural Competence*. Washington, DC: American Psychological Association; 2012.

33. Hays PA. *Addressing Cultural Complexities in Practice: Assessment, Diagnosis, and Therapy*. 3rd ed. Washington, DC: American Psychological Association; 2016.

34. Plante TG. Integrating spirituality and psychotherapy: ethical issues and principles to consider. *J Clin Psychol*. 2007;63(9):891-902.

35. McIntosh P. White privilege: unpacking the invisible knapsack. In: Plous S, ed. *Understanding Prejudice and Discrimination*. New York, NY: McGraw-Hill; 2003:191-196.

36. Crenshaw K. *Demarginalizing the Intersection of Race and Sex: A Black Feminist Critique of Antidiscrimination Doctrine, Feminist Theory and Antiracist Politics*. Vol 1989, Article 8. University of Chicago Legal Forum; 1989.

37. Cole ER. Intersectionality and research in psychology. *Am Psychol*. 2009;64(3):170-180. doi:10.1037/a0014564.

38. Gutierrez D. The role of intersectionality in marriage and family therapy multicultural supervision. *Am J Fam Ther*. 2018;46(1):14-26. doi:10.1080/01926187.2018.1437573.

39. Grzanka PR, Santos CE, Moradi B. Intersectionality research in counseling psychology. *J Couns Psychol*. 2017;64(5):453-457. doi:10.1037/cou0000237.

40. Iwamasa GY, Hays PA. *Culturally Responsive Cognitive Behavior Therapy: Practice and Supervision*. Washington, DC: American Psychological Association; 2019.

41. Rathus JH, Miller AL. Dialectical behavior therapy adapted for suicidal adolescents. *Suicide Life Threat Behav*. 2002;32(2):146-157.

42. Sue S. Cultural competency: from philosophy to research and practice. *J Community Psychol*. 2006;34(2):237-245.

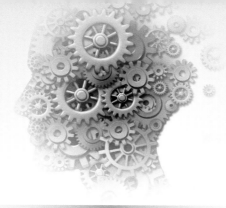

Section 3

PSYCHOTHERAPY IN NONTRADITIONAL SETTINGS

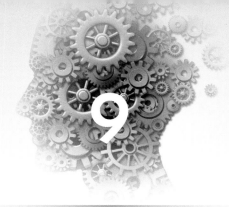

Psychotherapy in the Community Mental Health Setting

AMY S. BRENNER, MSW, LCSW

Case Study

Mr. N is a 40-year-old Latinx man living in a large Northeastern city. He is the oldest of nine children from a Roman Catholic family. He was a quiet, studious kid, and did well in school. His parents described him as "a bit odd, but he had friends and did normal kid and teenage things." During his freshman year at a large university, he started to have difficulties with his temper. He often yelled uncontrollably at his roommate, and also his girlfriend, but would then settle down for a while. He started sleeping and eating less, and threw himself into rugby, eventually making the varsity team. While good for the team, his teammates found Mr. N "intense and vicious," especially when the team was not doing well. His parents noted these changes at the time but attributed them to the normal stresses of college and sports. Although his behavior became more remarked upon by family and professors, his grades did not suffer, and he ended up graduating with honors.

He moved home to live with his parents while he made his next life decision—job or graduate school. His yelling and fighting with others intensified, especially with his parents and the younger siblings still at home. He began to think his parents were plotting to have him killed and that his siblings were spying on him. He also experienced periods of catatonia, where he would stare into space for hours on end, often hearing voices that were not there. He was unable to work, and his ability to maintain activities of daily living (ADLs) became quite poor.

One day, he hit his father without provocation, and the police were called. He then struck a police officer while he was being arrested, simultaneously screaming about his civil rights and government plots against him. At that point, it was just luck and good judgment by the police that he was taken to a psychiatric ER to be evaluated, instead of the city jail.

He was diagnosed with bipolar disorder at that point. His mania had a very strong psychotic piece to it. This was the start of numerous hospitalizations, followed by discharges back to the family home. Tensions at home continued to rise, as Mr. N's mother tried to prod him to take his medications, and to bathe and change clothes regularly. Some hospitalizations were short, with a focus on getting Mr. N stabilized on medications. Others were longer term at the state hospital as he awaited a substituted judgment, usually to require him to take a depot Risperdal shot (a long-acting injectable antipsychotic medication). Of note, a "substituted judgment" is when the inpatient psychiatrist declares to a court of law that a patient is not competent to make medical and medication decisions. At this point, a guardian is appointed by the judge, usually a family member or a lawyer. The guardian can then decide if psychotropic medications can be administered against the will of the patient.

Mr. N experienced significant symptoms of tardive dyskinesia, which were bothersome to him and led him to often discontinue his medications. He had slowed speech and walking, and extrapyramidal symptoms that impacted his mouth and arms. He often reported that his head was "filled with cotton" and that he was "moving through honey." His joy of reading diminished and his self-esteem, previously based on intelligence and personal appearance, had hit rock bottom. He often believed he was not actually sick, and the medications were just "the government's way of controlling [him]." Numerous substituted judgments only served to reinforce paranoia about the government as a whole.

Often, even in a psychotic state, Mr. N had the means to fight these judgments. He hired a lawyer who secured his release from the hospital unit with just a promise to take his medications or would assist him with getting the substituted judgment dismissed after discharge, when he would appear competent in court. After a few days, he would quit taking the medications and the entire process would start again. After 4 years of this, and over 12 hospitalizations, the family no longer felt like they could let him return to their home. The hospital applied for Mr. N to be placed in state services, which were granted.

INTRODUCTION

This chapter will introduce you to the role of psychotherapy in community mental health (CMH) treatment. You will learn about some of the common experiences and stressors of people with serious mental illness (SMI) who are often treated in these settings. While it is common to see comorbid depression, addiction, and personality disorders in CMH settings, I will primarily focus on patients with psychotic illnesses such as schizophrenia, schizoaffective disorder, and bipolar disorder in the chapter. You will also learn about the continuum of care that your patient may move through. (Of note, the use of the term "patient" has some controversy attached to it; see further details under section Importance of the Recovery Movement and Trauma-Informed Care) In order to do this, you will need to understand some basic facts about the ideas that drive CMH care, and about how this care is structured. I will focus throughout on how to work in alignment with these systems, and how to adapt psychotherapy to be effective and useful to your patients in these settings. Throughout this chapter, I will use the case of Mr. N to illustrate not just movement through the CMH system, but how one might engage in therapeutic interactions with him as he is served at each step.

You may arrive at reading this book having had very different prior exposure to people with SMI. Perhaps you have finished a rotation on an inpatient unit, a psychiatric emergency department (or ED), or in an outpatient clinic, and you may wonder how your patients with SMI get support in the community once they leave your care. Perhaps you have been assigned to a homeless outreach rotation or a PACT (Program for Assertive Community Treatment) team, or to provide medication management in one of these settings. It is going to be important to understand both the unique culture of the SMI patient and the unique stressors they go through in order to help them therapeutically.

If you are familiar with CMH settings, you will recognize that traditional outpatient psychotherapy is not always the treatment norm. Often, you will see patients as part of a multidisciplinary team and will be involved in many aspects of overall care that may include case management, advocacy, and engagement with others in the system. You will also see patients perhaps more or less frequently than in a traditional outpatient private practice, and sometimes in very unstructured environments (eg, in an ACT team office or a patient's supported housing apartment). Without having a designated "therapy session," you may wonder how your patient interactions may be of help.

In this chapter, I will show that every patient interaction you have is therapeutic on some level, and that many of these interactions can be profoundly beneficial. You can help your patients with SMI maintain their integration in the community and increase their independence. Compared with the experience in a hospital or general outpatient clinic, a patient moving into CMH care will receive therapeutic interventions in a variety of settings, throughout their care. As with every site, there are new acronyms to learn and new ways to think about how patients/clients/consumers get treated in the community. Some of these ideas dovetail with current ideas of inpatient care, and some are specific to the community. You will need to achieve a basic cultural competence in understanding the world of the seriously mental ill patient. I will first discuss what you need to know about the CMH culture so you can maximize your helpfulness and understanding.

9

PART I: THE CULTURE OF COMMUNITY MENTAL HEALTH CARE

Continuum of Care

Before you understand your role, you need to understand what is referred to as the *continuum of care*. This phrase is used in both the SMI/CMH communities and the homeless care communities to indicate the pathway a patient may travel toward both housing and independence. These services vary greatly depending on the extent of state funding. Depending on the state in which you are training, this continuum may be a fully fleshed out set of programs through which patients move fairly seamlessly. Other states have not allocated nearly as much for appropriate care of the mentally ill and homeless populations, and therefore services are fractured and cobbled together as best as they can be.

Due to the transitioning of the mentally ill from long-term hospitals in the 1960s and 1970s to community settings (known as *deinstitutionalization*), many more persons with SMI began to live outside of institutional care.[1] Ideas began to promulgate about how best to care for these clients in the community, and these ideas continue to be refined, challenged, and revolutionized today. Many in the first wave of deinstitutionalized patients, who were used to the structured environment of a state hospital, found adjustment to community settings fairly easy, as it basically recreated similar types of caretaking in a different community setting.[1] Patients were warehoused in clusters of segregated, supported apartments and group homes without treatment goals and without the idea of graduating to more independence. As more progressive thinking came into play, movement through the continuum became more the norm. Ideas about independent living, real community integration, and vocational rehabilitation started to thrive in CMH agencies that saw the potential for patients to not just leave the hospital, but to gain back pieces of lives lost to mental illness.

Although deinstitutionalization was mostly a positive idea, the reality is that over time, cities and towns became overwhelmed in trying to fund and support all the persons who were unable to cope with living alone in an independent housing situation and to take care of themselves entirely. As newer generations of the SMI population came of age in a world of short-term hospital stays, cities found themselves with jails and homeless shelters full of persons with SMI who had different needs and were struggling to succeed in the community. These later waves of patients were also not as accepting of limited community resources and many became effective advocates for newer models of care.[1]

Navigating the Care Continuum: Finances, Medical Care, and Housing Stressors

Let us take a look at what stressors and challenges a patient might face in this transition into the community. Funded through the Social Security Administration, many in the SMI population qualify for what is known as *Supplemental Social Security Income* (SSI). This provides a monthly income for disabled persons of $771, as of 2019.[2] Some patients, who have a previous work history and work credits, receive *Social Security Disability Income* (SSDI) instead, which can range in amount.[2] Additionally, through a city or state program, patients can be eligible for transportation vouchers and discounts on electricity, gas, oil, and food (via food stamps).

Patients who qualify for SSI may also be eligible for a state government's *Medicaid* healthcare insurance plan due to unemployment or lack of financial resources. Some patients who qualify for SSDI or are aged 65 years and older may also qualify for *Medicare* healthcare insurance through the Federal government. Both of these provide medical care and prescription coverage, and often, these benefits are filed for during an inpatient hospitalization. Already you can see one stressor emerging—this population tends to exist at the very lowest levels of poverty. As a result, making treatment recommendations that cost additional money (yoga classes, vacationing, massages) is not helpful to a person who cannot afford them, nor do some patients have stable access to phone, internet, or other technology that would make teletherapy a universal access point.

Another major stressor for SMI patients is their health. Many are not in good physical health, in addition to their struggles with mental health. Much of this population smokes cigarettes, and although there are many theories why this is so, there is often little in the way of assistance to effectively quit.[3] Illnesses of the heart and lungs are prevalent, exacerbated by a lack of exercise and poor diets (brought on through a tangle of diminished finances, lack of education, medication side effects, and mental illness symptoms). Many patients therefore become obese, with diabetes and other metabolic syndromes becoming their norm. Some of the medication side effects contribute to these health issues, with weight gain and diabetes among them.

Housing is another major stressor for patients with SMI. A patient who has exhibited SMI and has met the criteria to be engaged in a state's mental health services will often need a step-down service as they are discharged from a psychiatric hospital stay. While a patient may be discharged to their own home, or back to live with family, many are in need of supported housing. One early step-down service after discharge from a psychiatric hospital stay might be a *respite facility*, staffed 24/7 to make sure a patient remains stable while a more permanent housing option is sought. A *group home* (where patients live in a communal setting with staff support) may next be in place for patients registered with a state's mental health services, usually run by nonprofit CMH agencies. These group homes can include 24/7 residential staff who dispense medications, help clients with ADLs, and work on treatment planning with them. A patient might "graduate" to a less restrictive group home, perhaps only staffed at night, or with staff just checking in during the evening hours. The next step might be a *supported apartment*. Some of these might be owned and operated by an agency that creates a cluster of supported apartments.

Other patients might receive their Section 8 voucher and move into any *independent apartment* in the city that will take these vouchers. *Section 8 vouchers* are provided by the state as a housing subsidy to people without economic means, usually requiring the recipient to pay 30% of their income toward rent. Not surprisingly, these are highly sought-after vouchers for which there are years' long waitlists and many bureaucratic hoops through which to jump. Sometimes, a CMH agency will own some of these vouchers, which they can use for patients. Some drawbacks to Section 8 subsidies include the fact that many property owners will not take them, due to bias against low-income tenants. Although cities often require new buildings to "set aside" a specific percentage of the property as low-income housing, this percentage is generally inadequate to meet the needs of all the people who qualify for them. Therefore, a patient might get their voucher and have to relinquish it due to not being able to locate an apartment that will work with them.

Even the most capable person would have extreme difficulties navigating this complex world of regulatory, bureaucratic, and economic obstacles. Imagine how this must be for a person with SMI, who may have cognitive or executive functioning impairments. Think about how stressful it is every time you have to look for an apartment. Now multiply that by lack of transportation, possible lack of organizational capabilities, lack of financial resources, and a diminished stock of affordable housing!

9

Let us say you are working in one of the states that does not fund a comprehensive and integrated continuum of care. A patient is then likely to be discharged from the hospital to a homeless shelter, where they will enter a different continuum of care, transitioning from a regular general population shelter, to perhaps a transitional living arrangement where they are learning skills for self-management and taking care of their own place to live. After this, they may enter a similar path of supported to independent apartments.

Homelessness adds additional stressors to those mentioned previously. Shelters are generally closed during the day, forcing an SMI patient to pass the hours outside. In addition, homeless people with mental illness are highly vulnerable to physical and sexual assault.[4] As many shelter beds are at a premium, lining up for a bed may start several hours before the shelter opens in the evening. If one arrives late, they may not get a bed. Again, patients in the throes of a mental illness may not have the wherewithal to successfully run this gauntlet.

Another option is that your patient may be discharged from the hospital to a *boarding house*, some of which are set up to handle the needs of a person exiting the hospital, some of which are not. Regulation of boarding homes for people with SMI varies widely from region to region. Another housing option is called a *single-room occupancy* (SRO). This is often a room in a building set up for this type of living, with communal bathrooms and as often as not, no kitchen facilities. Both types of housing are at least "housing" and can decrease the risk of assault associated with homelessness. But, lack of support services for the patient, as well as an advocate to the landlord, can make tenancy for those with SMI difficult in these environments as well.

Case Study: Navigating Housing

Mr. N had qualified for Medicaid during his last hospitalization. At the end of the most recent hospitalization, his SSI benefit had been approved. He was eligible for the state continuum of care. Due to his level of functioning, it was determined that he might be able to manage a supported apartment with an ACT team providing support and medication management. A group home was not determined to be a good fit, because he was higher functioning than most of the residents but could also be quite difficult to get along with in many group situations. Although he had a current substituted judgment at the hospital, he was already working with a lawyer to have this dismissed upon discharge. This would mean he would not be required to receive a depot injection of Risperdal once discharged.

He received a Section 8 voucher that was held by the CMH agency that provided his services. He had previously applied for his own Section 8 voucher and was told the waitlist was 5 to 7 years. He was crushed by this and felt he would be beholden to the CMH agency for longer than he felt comfortable with. He was concerned how the agency's control over his housing situation would impact him. However, he knew he didn't have enough money to get an apartment on his own. In addition, his parents had been clear that he could not come back to the family home.

> On discharge, he was sent to a respite facility while he waited for the supported apartment paperwork to be finalized. He hated the respite program—it was loud, three patients shared a room, and some residents seemed like they should be in the hospital. He also believed the other men in the room were talking about him, touching his belongings, and generally plotting to murder him in his sleep. He called his case manager frequently, asking when the apartment would be ready and how soon could he get out of here.

Meeting the Patient Where They Are: Outreach Teams

A very important principle of CMH care is the need for meeting a patient where they are at, both psychologically and geographically. Outreach teams can help bridge the gap between hospital and clinic and housing, while adding valuable resources.

In a CMH setting, your training will often involve placement with a multidisciplinary outreach team of some sort. It is important to remember you are part of a team. You each have a role to play and each contribution is valuable in the recovery process for the patient. Try to leave your preconceptions about other mental health disciplines at the door. Let the team help you learn and help you move from the symptom-focused treatment view, which may have been emphasized in your education, toward seeing patients as whole people, just as you see others in your own life.

Homeless outreach teams often start to engage with clients on the streets or at homeless shelters. Often clients who are too paranoid to attend treatment at a CMH clinic can be engaged on the streets and gently brought toward more stability as an alliance is made, and trust is established. These encounters can be part of the homeless continuum of care or can be contracted out through a mental health agency to identify and engage clients with SMI. As mentioned previously, the SMI population has specific obstacles to overcome with regard to obtaining housing and treatment. Outreach teams can help patients sort through the litany of paperwork in order to get housing and benefits, help with transportation to appointments, coordinate with the shelter to make sure medication is obtained and taken, and provide medication management through a team psychiatrist or psychiatry resident.

Likewise, outreach teams are set up to continue to engage patients "where they are" once housed. These teams can go by many names: ACT (Assertive Community Treatment), PACT (Program for Assertive Community Treatment), ASH (Assertive Supported Housing), or Supported Housing Outreach. ACT teams tend to take the form of a replicable, evidence-based program that follows certain guidelines for service provision.[5,6] Therefore, I will use the term "ACT" as I discuss outreach. However, be aware the team you work on might be called something different yet have very similar goals.

ACT teams are multidisciplinary treatment teams, comprised of mental health professionals and paraprofessionals that are available to a client 24/7. The team works together to support every aspect of a patient's community needs. Evidence shows that these types of teams can lead to decreased hospitalization frequency for most types of patients with SMI (patients with certain personality disorders do not seem to benefit as much).[7] Quality of life is also improved, as is the ability to maintain housing.[7] Members of the 10- to 12-person team include a psychiatrist or psychiatry resident or psychiatric nurse practitioner to provide medication management, social workers, psychologists, vocational rehabilitation specialist, substance abuse counselors, and outreach staff.[7] Typically, each member of the team carries a small caseload of patients, which they case manage, meaning they are responsible for engaging with the patient, creating treatment plans, and completing documentation. However, each member of the team is familiar with every patient, so any staff member can engage and be useful to every patient. This is called *cross-training*.

As you might expect, ACT teams provide a great deal of supportive psychotherapy. The therapy is generally not administered in 50-minute sessions (although some well-funded teams can do so) but rather is distributed through and integrated into all of the team's meetings with the patient. The teams can be deployed more directly to assist a patient, as opposed to a therapist waiting to engage at a clinic.[8] This also creates a more patient-centered approach, as opposed to many other settings where a patient will find themselves that are more clinician driven.

Many ACT teams employ the *Housing First* model of intervention, which was started by Pathways to Housing.[9] It is the idea that a person should be in stable housing first (regardless of their willingness to take medication, give up alcohol or substance abuse, or participate in treatment or treatment planning goals). The stability of a home often gives patients a reason to mitigate risks and cooperate with treatment as much as possible. This is the idea of harm reduction—increasing client choice while at the same time decreasing the detrimental effects of mental illness and substance abuse.

Some continuum of care housing models are more demanding. A patient must be treatment compliant, sober, and on medications prior to entering any kind of housing (even some transitional housing). Only then are they considered ready to move through the continuum. Unfortunately, these requirements often convey a stance that patients make poor choices and therefore require more oversight.[10] This idea remains controversial, but evidence shows a direct relationship between the Housing First approach and decreased homelessness.[10] This philosophy dovetails into the greater ideas of the recovery movement, which I will discuss shortly.

In order to help patients become more independent, many programs require extensive treatment planning, which focuses on providing the least restrictive care possible. These treatment plans are usually state mandated, both for the agency to show that they are actually working with patients, but also to justify movement of the patient toward more independence. These treatment plans can range from the everyday (taking care of ADLs, taking medication, being on time to appointments, managing money, social skills) to larger goals (obtaining a supported job, taking a college class, volunteering, working on relationships). Treatment planning is based on the patient's current needs, meeting them where they are, and creating plans that help with forward movement, no matter how small. Treatment plans are important because they provide the goals that all of your therapeutic interventions will work toward.

Case Study: Treatment Planning

Mr. N was very eager to get a job. He was very good at math and accounting and felt like he could handle a job in this area. The long-term treatment plan goal for Mr. N was to get a job in accounting by working with the vocational rehabilitation counselor. However, this long-term goal was broken up into many smaller short-term goals that addressed the steps he needed to complete to be ready for a job. For example, he needed to address his ability to shower and dress in clean clothes consistently, so as to be appropriate for a work environment. Next, he needed to address inconsistencies with taking his psychotropic medications. Keeping his symptoms managed was viewed as contributing to his larger goal of maintaining a job and dealing with the daily stressors of working.

Importance of the Recovery Movement and Trauma-Informed Care

In understanding treatment planning and interventions, there are two additional perspectives and skill sets that are necessary for work in the CMH field. The first is a strong understanding of the recovery movement perspective. The second is the recognition of trauma in the lives of many of your patients in this setting, which necessitates the ongoing practice of trauma-informed care.

In the past, treatment plans were often dictated to a patient by the staff, based on their perceptions and priorities. Sometimes, these could be coercive in tone and effect, such as tying a patient's access to their money to good behavior or taking medications. In addition, the treatment plan was often focused on improvement in discrete symptoms, as this is what providers had been taught to focus on. Over time, this created a tension with patients and their advocates, who felt that clinicians were missing what was most important—the patient's ability to live a satisfying and fulfilling life. Out of these ideas was born the recovery movement.

The *recovery movement* is a way of thinking about SMI that emphasizes social empowerment and getting people back to work. It is an approach that rejects the images of incapacity and worthlessness that can foster adoption of a disabled role.[9] This approach is central to our work as therapists for patients with SMI, as recovery focuses on generating optimism and empowerment through both peer and professional support.

I will pause here to note many in the recovery movement have rejected the term "patient" and prefer to use "client," "consumer," or other terms because they feel "patient" has diminishing or dependent connotations. Instead of the unequal power dynamic of patient versus doctor/agency provider, people are "consumers" of a provider's services.[11] The idea is for patients to be partners in their care, to be involved in all aspects and to help make decisions about treatment, treatment planning priorities, to even have the option not to accept treatment if they wish. (Although appreciative of this perspective, I have used "patient" throughout the chapter both for consistency and because the word best captures the sacred professional responsibility of the clinician.)

The recovery movement is meant to convey *hope*, that people can recover from SMI, and that they can regain a functional place in society. Studies show that community integration—really being a part of where one lives and works—increases self-esteem, self-determination, and hopefulness.[12] Hope is an important message to maintain as you work with patients with SMI in the community. Hope is not a strategy; it cannot be a substitute for a careful treatment plan, and there is a lot of hard work that goes into recovery. However, hope is an emotion that should be fostered throughout the process of recovery.

There are limits to what the recovery model can encompass, as consumer choice, involuntary commitments, and court-ordered treatments inherently do not go together. At times, the tension between recovery movement ideas that advocate for increased consumer choice and the need for involuntary interventions can become stark. In the community, however, you have a chance to make the biggest impact on increased consumer choice, and as a trainee you should always keep this principle in mind. Studies have shown that consumer choice increases well-being and decreases psychiatric symptoms over time.[9]

However, there will always be patients who need involuntary interventions. For example, the Social Security Administration can decide that a person is not competent to handle their own money. A *representative payee* (aka rep payee) may be put into place to pay a person's bills and manage their money received from the government. This representative can be a family member or friend, or an agency where a person is receiving treatment. Of course, this relationship will have its own tensions, and the patient may end up feeling coerced and angry (and unfortunately, there is little oversight from the SSA as to when the need for this monitoring should cease). On the other hand, many a disorganized or impulsive patient has made choices in the moment that left them destitute, and this financial oversight arrangement can prevent these outcomes.

A more extreme example of involuntary intervention is court-ordered outpatient treatment, also known as a *substituted judgment*. As you saw in the case of Mr. N, a court can declare a patient incompetent to make medical decisions and appoint a guardian to do so for them. Generally, this is in order to have medications forcibly given to the patient, usually by injection of a *depot* (ie, long-acting) psychiatric medication. The idea is that once a patient is less symptomatic, they would realize that they would have agreed to take the medication in order to return to baseline. While substituted judgments can be relatively straightforward in a hospital setting, implementation in the community is more fraught. Often, a patient may be decompensated but able to manage ADLs and home life on a relatively stable basis for some time before an intervention is deemed necessary. Recovery movement advocates might argue that this patient should have the right to refuse medications and continue as they are, whereas a medical model perspective might argue for more intervention.

As noted, trauma plays a specific role within CMH settings. In each setting you work in, it is important to always be practicing *trauma-informed care*, defined as an awareness of how patients have been impacted by violence and abuse, and how this trauma has made them more vulnerable.[13] Patients with SMI may have had experiences of childhood abuse or bullying that increased their risk for illness. In addition, having SMI greatly increases the patient's vulnerability to assault as an adult.[13] Research indicates that upward of 50% of psychiatric patients have a history of trauma, so using a framework of trauma-informed care is crucial.[13] Recognizing and accommodating these vulnerabilities to trauma can help the patient engage in and participate more fully in treatment.[13]

This does not mean you are necessarily treating these traumas directly, unless that is specifically your role in the patient's treatment. Rather, your priority is to make sure the patient is not further traumatized by interventions, situations, and settings while they are receiving your services. Homelessness and unstable housing environments, mental illness, and poverty are already traumatic stressors. Trauma-informed care has been shown to both decrease the need for crisis interventions and increase stability in housing,[14] so integrating these ideas into your every interaction with a patient with SMI can be beneficial. In addition, further approaches to integrating trauma-informed care with patients with SMI are elaborated upon in Chapter 12 on psychotherapy in inpatient psychiatric settings. For more information on trauma-informed care, see the National Center for Trauma Informed Care at https://www.nasddds.org.[14]

PART II: EVIDENCE-BASED PSYCHOTHERAPEUTIC INTERVENTIONS IN COMMUNITY MENTAL HEALTH

Now that you are familiar with the context and unique stressors facing your patient with SMI in the community, and you have looked at some of the tensions in that system, let us look at some of the psychotherapeutic treatment you may offer in community settings. Remember, a patient may not receive all of these treatments or may receive them at different points as they move through the continuum of care. Certain interventions are specific to the setting in which they occur, while others can be used across the myriad settings in which you may find yourself working. Yet wherever you meet a patient along their journey, you can have a positive impact on their recovery. I will illustrate this by returning to the case of Mr. N and discussing several evidence-based psychosocial interventions that often integrate supportive therapy techniques (case management, family psychoeducation, social skills training, vocational rehabilitation/supported employment), as well as how to use individual psychotherapy itself.

The Importance of Therapeutic Alliance

First, let us focus our attention on something that will be crucial to every intervention: the therapeutic alliance (also reviewed in Chapter 4 of this book). You may not be versed or trained in all of the interventions described in this section. Most of these modalities take time to work and create change, and you are not going to fully treat a patient during your short rotation through their lives. Many of your interactions will be aimed at short-term change or support. Where should you begin?

Forming an alliance is the best place to start. Research shows that the alliance is the most "robust predictor of outcomes,"[15] and patients who formed good alliances tended to continue to be engaged in treatment and compliant with medications after 2 years.[16] However, patients with SMI tend to have the most difficult time establishing these alliances, which may be different from patients you may have seen in a clinic or in short-term treatments who do not suffer from SMI.[15] Your time with the patient may be relatively short term, and this alliance may always be fragile, as SMI patients do not always come to treatment ready to engage and may in fact have been court remanded or otherwise forced to participate.

This alliance is about providing support and setting goals. This will start with asking questions in a nonjudgmental way and listening to the patient's answers without assumptions. It is often best to ask questions that simply let a patient tell you more about the situation. The goals you and the patient set together should focus on their continued recovery, past the idea of you, the trainee after you, etc. Have a plan that advances their broad, long-term recovery goals, not your goals for them. These goals could include help with medication adherence, perhaps challenging a delusion, or helping create program compliance. Also, learn what you can from your team so that you can be a contributor to the patient's long-term recovery, instead of just a custodian.

Case Study: Building a Therapeutic Alliance

Mr. N was meeting with the new psychiatric resident, Dr. W, on the ACT team for an intake. During their discussion, Mr. N mentioned that he often plugged the bottom of his bedroom door with towels at night to go to sleep. Dr. W said, "Tell me more about this, so I can understand." Mr. N proceeded to tell him that the towels blocked out the voices. Dr. W replied, "Which voices?" Mr. N answered, "The voices in the hall, the walls of my apartment are very thin." Although Dr. W was primed to hear a psychotic patient who mentions "voices" as dealing with something in his head, it turned out to be Mr. N's way of dealing with external problems.

Mr. N still had a difficult time connecting with Dr. W, although he appreciated his willingness to listen and learn about him. He was acutely aware that this particular doctor would be here 6 months, then another would come, and then another. It became tiresome telling his story over and over and being asked the same questions in each introductory assessment. Did this guy not read the chart? Does he actually think he is going to have a fabulous new insight into the problem that forever cures Mr. N and restores all he has lost? Additionally, Mr. N's tendency toward paranoia always made him question these experiences—was he being tested? Were these successive doctors trying to catch him out or trip him up?

However, Dr. W, in anticipating reactions such as these, knew not to take Mr. N's reluctance to connect personally. He was, in fact, only on the ACT team for 6 months as part of a succession of doctors who had been and would be helping on this team. As a result, he was honest with Mr. N about these realities. He did not promise to be there in the future, to handle Mr. N's care outside of his current commitment, and did not deny the feelings Mr. N had about the situation. He acknowledged the anger and disdain Mr. N felt, the feeling that he deserved better or different care, and that he was just a poor person for the new trainees to "experiment on." Dr. W allowed Mr. N to voice all of his concerns.

Dr. W made sure to read the chart, to familiarize himself with Mr. N so that he was not always asking basic questions Mr. N had answered several times before. This helped Mr. N not feel that he was being used for "practice" or that Dr. W was making each interaction about his own training. Instead, focusing on how to help Mr. N in their short period of time together, Dr. W found it helpful to highlight Mr. N's goal of getting a job. At each session, he tried to explore different facets of Mr. N's experience as these related to finding and keeping work. This brought out many painful feelings for Mr. N—of loss, of incompetence, of fear, of humiliation—that made for rich therapy sessions as they worked through these together.

At the end of their work together, Mr. N was able to see and be proud of a discreet piece of work they had done together. Dr. W was able to feel like his short time with Mr. N had been valuable and contributed to the longer-term goal of greater independence.

Case Management

Case management is generally thought of as a person or group that helps a patient navigate the service continuum, to connect with and continue with services that fit the patient's particular needs. There is evidence for the helpfulness of case management in improving housing and decreasing time spent in the hospital, especially with intensive case management.[17]

In some locations, a case manager is assigned by the state or the local CMH provider to see a patient once or twice a month. They are responsible for coordinating the care of the various treatment and service providers, linking the patient with resources and programs, and generally keeping the patient moving smoothly through the continuum. These case managers tend to have larger caseloads, and patients often come to them at their office or facility. Other programs provide for a more intensive case management, with smaller caseloads so that patients can be seen weekly. Often, these case managers will see patients in the patient's home settings or in the community. Sometimes, they will act in roles similar to ACT teams, providing transportation assistance, money management assistance, help looking for housing, etc. but differ from ACT in that they are not usually a part of a multidisciplinary team.

As mentioned before, some states do not provide a lot of services, so case management may be the only contact other than a medical provider that a patient has. Case managers are often burdened by unmanageable caseloads and hampered by bureaucratic rules in terms of the care they can or cannot provide. As a trainee, case management in this specific format will probably not be your primary role, but you will have contact with a patient's designated case manager throughout your time caring for the patient. It is important to see them as an ally in the patient's therapy.

Case management is about building an alliance with the patient, engaging them in services, and connecting them to those services. As a result, there are important elements to supportive therapy happening in any effective case management, such as enhancing coping strategies and developing collaborative problem-solving.

Case Study: Case Management

Mr. N was assigned a case manager, Mr. D, when he was accepted for services in the local office of the state's department of mental health. Mr. D set up interviews for him with various service providers and attended these appointments with him. When Mr. N decided he was interested in the supported housing program, Mr. D met with the providers to help Mr. N complete the paperwork. Once Mr. N moved into his apartment, which was managed by a local mental health agency, Mr. D saw him once a month to check on his progress. Mr. D was in contact with Mr. N's outreach team several times a month by phone to make sure Mr. N was meeting with the outreach worker and adherent to medications.

Family System Interventions: Expressed Emotion and Psychoeducation

There is much empirical evidence for family interventions. Family interventions also incorporate some of the core aspects of supportive therapy, such as an emphasis on psychoeducation. Psychoeducation involves helping the family and patient understand the illness, explore the unique stressors of mental illness, recognize strengths, and create coping mechanisms. It also helps family members decrease their expressions of criticism, anger, and guilt, the importance of which is discussed below.

Whether living in the home with family, or in a continuum of care situation, SMI patients and their families often have a long history of tension. The concept of *expressed emotion* (EE) refers to hostility and criticism within a family system that may have always been present or has evolved as the patient's illness has stressed the family unit. In addition, overinvolvement in a patient's life can lead to higher EE.[17] This concept of EE forms the basis for family therapy interventions that aim at helping SMI patients and their families decrease EE. Previous studies showed that high EE situations in the home were predictive of relapse in schizophrenic patients, regardless of adequate medication treatment.[18,19] Family interventions focused on decreasing EE have been shown to subsequently decrease frequent rehospitalization, without increasing the family's burden of caring for the patient, and to decrease their overinvolvement.[4]

It may be your role to intervene with the family, perhaps on an ACT team or in a clinic situation. Therapy in any setting with more than one patient is a delicate balance of alliances (see Chapter 8 for more on the topic of integrating family/support persons into treatment). Your primary alliance should be with the SMI patient, but that does not mean you take the patient's side in any disagreements. It can be helpful to gently point out to the patient the ways in which their behavior is impacting the family. However, it may also be your role to prevent the family members from "ganging up" on the patient.

It is important to maintain good boundaries in family therapy, as in all therapies (see Chapter 4 for a more in-depth explanation of boundaries). Everyone in the therapy is considered your patient. As a result, it is not appropriate to have outside relationships with any of the family members even though they are not the primary SMI patient. It is also important to not ally with the other family members against the patient. Some patients have difficult personalities or ways of relating, even aside from their illness, and you may not particularly feel aligned with or fond of them. You may feel sympathy for what the family has had to endure. However, the goal of family therapy is to help the entire family decrease their EE. Tending to the well-being of the family unit is a first start in enlisting them to assist with an SMI patient's recovery goals.

Case Study: Family Interventions

When Mr. N returned home after college, continuing conflicts with his parents led to high EE in the home. His parents often yelled at him about his perceived "laziness," criticizing the way he smelled due to failing ADLs. His brothers commented that Mr. N's teeth were rotting out, and it was "his own damn fault" or that "he was disgusting."

Through bringing the family and Mr. N into therapy, the therapist was able to educate the family as to the symptoms of Mr. N's illness. The therapist explained how the medications dried out his mouth, and often caused tooth decay, as well as how his illness impacted his motivation to care for himself—something he was working on in his treatment goals. They discussed ways in which the family could be supportive of cumulative successes and reinforce positive steps, instead of focusing on the negative. Mr. N's therapist also pointed out to Mr. N that his lack of showering was unpleasant for family members when he would visit home. Together they discussed ways in which he could present with clean clothes and freshly showered and make each visit less unpleasant for his other family members.

It was also noted that Mr. N's parents and brothers would often yell at him as a group, which both frightened and enraged him. He often felt cornered and would lash out verbally, then physically, until they stopped. The therapist was able to explain this dynamic to the family, and to suggest new ways of interacting that avoided the appearance of "ganging up" on Mr. N. His mother, for instance, needed to be very concretely told that criticizing Mr. N for wearing a dirty shirt, then calling in his brothers to support her statements, felt both belittling and bullying to Mr. N. She was educated that her approach was unlikely to change his behavior and would likely lead to an outburst. Mr. N's mother had said she was trying to avoid the outbursts, as the situations frightened her. Yet, she could not see her own role in them until the therapist walked her through it. At the end of the session, Mr. N's mother was able to see her role in exacerbating the hostility in the house, and pledged to work harder to be less critical of Mr. N.

9

Social Skills Training

Social skills training is a broad area, addressing not just how people interact in relationships, but how they manage work, leisure, and activities of daily living. It also includes how one manages their time, attends appointments or work regularly, and in general plans their life. Social skills training can be an important step toward higher functioning in the community for an SMI patient and is a crucial component of supportive psychotherapy (see Chapter 5). Social skills become impacted for various reasons in SMI patients, but deficits can encompass basic self-care (such as cleanliness and hygiene), conversational skills and social cue recognition, and the ability to manage one's time.[17] Many patients will have treatment goals that fall under this heading, such as taking care of personal hygiene, taking medication as prescribed, balancing personal interactions with alone time (for some increasing the amount of time they socialize, for others learning to self-manage times of anxiety or need), or meeting with their treatment providers as scheduled.

Sometimes, social skills training seems like it should be intuitive, or that people will naturally pick it up through social cues and interactions. Gaining and improving social skills requires instruction and conscious intention throughout a healthy life. It is important to keep in mind the destructiveness of SMI and the absolute necessity to help patients rebuild, sometimes from scratch, their ability to function in society.

As a trainee you can begin by asking yourself—how do I help this patient improve their skills in this area? Some social skills training involves structured modules with prescribed interventions. However, if you do not have access to these, you can still make an impact on functioning through role-playing and modeling, corrective feedback, and eventually extrapolating and rehearsing these skills to a more natural setting. This teaching may take place in an individual therapy session, in a group session (such as at a day program or intensive outpatient program), or in more informal ways, such as during a meeting with another ACT team member. The goal is to help the patient address problems in a range of skills needed to live independently, with the idea that improvements in all of these areas support recovery and community integration, and hopefully are protective against relapse.

Case Study: Social Skills Training

When Mr. N started with the ACT team, he began to go to a vocational program to work on his goal of eventually becoming employed again. However, due to auditory hallucinations, he often ignored people when they were speaking to him or laughed at times when it was inappropriate to the conversation. Others found this behavior off-putting and avoided him, and the program counselors felt they could not proceed with moving him into a supported employment situation. His ACT case manager helped him break down exactly where these interactions were going awry and gave him specific language for responding when he became distracted.

For example, if he did not hear someone, instead of yelling "What?" he learned to ask them nicely to repeat themselves. His case manager also taught him to explain what he was responding to when he was laughing and to reassure others he was not laughing at them. At first Mr. N found this rather belittling; after all he saw himself as an educated person who had navigated the world well until this point. But, as he and his ACT case manager started to role-play these scenarios, he saw how much of a positive impact these small shifts in behavior were having with the other patients and staff at the program. He was also able to see how these behaviors were going to positively impact getting and keeping a job, which he was eager to do.

Vocational Rehabilitation With Supported Employment

As patients recover and become more a part of their communities, the goal of employment becomes more prominent. In the past, it was more common for people with SMI to work in contained workshops that made certain allowances for social issues and time management concerns. Some of the criticisms of these models were the ways in which patients were kept in protected settings, instead of being integrated into community settings and held to real-world expectations.[12] As the recovery movement took hold, so did the idea of patients with SMI gaining competitive employment.

One of the ways to achieve this is known as *vocational rehabilitation with supported employment*. These programs aim to help a patient gain a competitive job, help them learn the necessary skills and responsibilities, and continue to support them through employment. These are jobs in the general community, not work groups or sheltered teams overseen by an agency. Outcome measures have found that supported employment of competitive jobs tends to have more positive results for patients with SMI than traditional sheltered work programs.[17] This is due to many factors, with patient choice and individually tailored job support being among them. The more their work experience feels "normal" and the more they feel they are contributing and giving back to the world at large, the more positively their integration in that community will progress. If you are working on an ACT team or homeless support team, you may have a vocational counselor on the team. Mr. N, for example, worked with the ACT team vocational counselor to obtain a job working as a seasonal tax preparer with a national company.

Individual Psychotherapy

You might provide individual therapy sessions as part of an ACT team, an outpatient clinic situation, or in an intensive outpatient day program. Individual therapy has often been experienced as a highly valued service for SMI patients. Although patients are not always initially eager to participate, families often feel that the additional support and professional expertise can be of value to both the patient and the supporting members of the family. Often, a therapist's role is to support what other providers are trying to help the patient gain and stabilize the environment for the patient, beyond the exploration common to individual psychotherapy. For example, a patient struggling with housing may have a case manager or outreach worker assisting them with the specific tasks involved in finding or keeping housing. The therapist needs to both be in contact with these team members and be supporting those goals in treatment.

Individual therapy for patients with psychotic illnesses has undergone a transformation in the wake of the recovery movement. Traditionally, patients with SMI were not seen as able to tolerate intense psychotherapy. Instead, only supportive therapy was considered an option, and the therapist was thought of as an attachment figure who might be able to link the patient to reality over time. This idea has changed over time, with benefits to illness management and recovery seen in different types of therapies. Several specific therapies have good data for their effectiveness. I will discuss some here, but be aware that currently no particular therapy is proven more effective than another. You may be trained in supportive psychotherapy (see

Chapter 5), cognitive behavioral therapy (see Chapter 6), and/or psychodynamic therapy (see Chapter 7). Other evidence-based treatments include reality adaptive therapy and personal psychotherapy,[20] which are not covered in this book.

There have been a number of CBT therapies implemented and studied for psychosis. These methods continue to have challenges in fidelity to chosen strategies and a consensus of methodology.[21] Central to CBT for psychosis is the idea that the way an SMI patient interprets their psychotic symptoms is what causes distress, not the actual symptoms themselves.[21] As you saw in Chapter 6 on CBT, challenging these symptoms, such as distortions of reality and modifying core beliefs, comprises the basis of this therapy. (Note: please review this concept of "challenging" in Chapter 6 and what this entails in a CBT framework, before negatively confronting a patient who expresses delusional beliefs.)

On a practical level, however, many clinicians in CMH settings use an eclectic approach, or what has been described as "flexible psychotherapy."[20] The idea is to use specific interventions that are based on the research evidence for various forms of therapy, but to also use general ideas in psychotherapy that have been experienced historically as beneficial to patients with SMI. It does not really matter whether you call it "flexible" or "eclectic" or something else, as long as you stick to principles and techniques that are found throughout the scope of psychotherapy, because many different therapies actually have common factors (see Chapter 4).

So, what is crucial for a productive and useful psychotherapy in CMH settings? Remember that a patient-centered approach is critical. This means respecting your patient's preferences about the therapy approach. Some patients will want a more unstructured, conversational style, while others will prefer to have a schedule of tasks to work on together. Of course, being listened to is often the most important factor in successful psychotherapy, regardless of how symptomatic or disorganized the patient may seem. Additionally, bringing respect, warmth, and ability to admit when you are wrong will greatly enhance the therapeutic alliance, which is always a key to success. Your patient with SMI does not need you to have all the answers or to always be right, but they do need you to be an authentic and honest person that they can depend on. With SMI patients, ideas of transference and countertransference are not generally explored in early therapies, especially with trainees who may be on rotation with the treatment team for only brief periods of time. It is, however, important to talk to your supervisor about your feelings of countertransference (see Chapters 7 and 14).

In terms of goal planning, your priority should be to restore any immediate deterioration to pre-acuity levels of functioning. Long-term goals would certainly be to return to premorbid or near premorbid levels of functioning. To do this, you and your patient should identify and build on existing coping strategies. If those are few, you will want to help your patient establish new strategies, using current strengths as a base.

You can also help your patients who are having trouble recognizing or are in denial of their illness identify "symptoms" (in quotes here, as your patient may not call them this) or patterns of behavior that are causing trouble in their lives. This is often called *reality testing* and it consists of gently questioning and exploring how

real a distorted thought may be and offering other more realistic ways of thinking about a situation. Helping SMI patients reality test and correct distortions of
thinking can lessen acute episodes and crises. As your patient learns to self-identify
symptoms, you will then be able to help them learn how to self-manage symptoms
(eg, through specific CBT techniques).

Allowing and helping a patient to bear the sadness and loss of having a chronic
illness and to grieve the life expectations that were lost is also important.
Ultimately, you are helping a patient accept the loss of one version of life, and
plan a different, but hopeful, new life. Along with losses, some patients will have
experienced significant trauma in their past. However, as noted previously, working through trauma requires that the patient is in a psychiatrically stable place,
with the ability to have insight into the process and be motivated for this kind of
challenging work.

Case Study: Individual Therapy

Mr. N felt that in acknowledging his mental illness, he had to also acknowledge
all he had lost (a rugby career, a wife and children, financial stability). This felt too
painful, so initially it was easier to deny these feelings of loss. In working through
these issues in therapy, he was able to reach a place of not only acceptance, but
the ability to see a different, but still good, future waiting for him.

However, Mr. N's paranoid feelings remained a significant obstacle in therapy.
Mr. N often felt that his family, the government, the psychiatric resident, and other
ACT team members were in some way out to get him. He felt persecuted but was
unable to articulate why or to what end. Discussions with Dr. W, which initially
focused on getting a job, started to bring out these feelings of paranoia. Mr. N was
a high-functioning individual brought low by his illness. Certainly, this had to be a
conspiracy or an alternate universe?

Dr. W very gently asked Mr. N to explain these ideas, without judging or laughing or telling Mr. N he was silly. The simple fact that someone was listening without
immediately trying to put him off felt good to Mr. N. He was able to then talk more
deeply to Dr. W, about the unfairness of this affliction and why did it have to happen to him when he had everything ahead of him. Through their talks, Dr. W very
gently challenged Mr. N to think about why the government would want specifically to punish him, why the ACT team would want to keep him sick, and what gain
there would be for his parents to have their eldest child be frequently hospitalized.
Through a combination of a strong therapeutic alliance, nonjudgmental stance,
and gentle confrontation, Dr. W was able to get Mr. N to acknowledge and look at
some of the distortions in his thinking.

9

This kind of therapeutic work is not magical, and it does not cure psychosis.
However, over time a patient can become able to see ways in which their mind is
distorting things. Often, they are then able to do this work on their own as they
become progressively better, but a therapist can help them progress in a more clear
and supported manner.

Conclusion

In this chapter, you have examined some issues related to persons with serious mental illness, and how psychotherapeutic interventions are managed throughout the continuum of care. The continuum of care provides for housing and psychosocial support services that help patients with SMI integrate into their communities and live more fulfilling lives. You have looked at some of the specific stressors that challenge the SMI patient population. These stressors include poverty, unstable housing, and comorbid health issues that make living with SMI even more difficult. Lastly, you have looked at the evidence-based interventions a trainee can use during their treatment of patients in this population. These include case management, family systems interventions, social skills training, vocational rehabilitation, and individual psychotherapy. These interventions, coupled with the empowerment of patients in their treatment, lead us to reasons to be hopeful and why we should continue to work with patients toward recovery and independence.

Self-Assessment Questions

1. What is the "continuum of care"?

2. What stressors do patients face as they move through this continuum?

3. What additional difficulties does a poorly funded continuum create for a patient? How does your state fund and support SMI patients?

4. How might the therapeutic alliance be impacted by having a multidisciplinary treatment team in which individual providers may cycle through every few months?

5. Describe at least two ways in which a family systems intervention would be helpful to patients with SMI.

6. What is the "recovery movement"? How does this look similar to and different from other perspectives on mental health care?

RESOURCES FOR FURTHER LEARNING

National Alliance on Mental Illness. Available at https://www.nami.org
National Center for Trauma Informed Care. Available at https://www.nasddds.org
Mental Health America. Available at https://www.mhanational.org

9

REFERENCES

1. Lamb HR, Bachrach LL. Some perspectives on deinstitutionalization. *Psychiatr Serv.* 2001;52(8):1039-1045.
2. *Supplemental Security Income (SSI) Benefits.* Social Security Administration; 2019. Available at www.ssa. gov/benefits/ssi/
3. Banham L, Gilbody S. Smoking cessation in severe mental illness: what works? *Addiction.* 2010;105(7):1176-1189.
4. Tsemberis S, Eisenberg RF. Pathways to housing: supported housing for street dwelling homeless individuals with psychiatric disabilities. *Psychiatr Serv.* 2000;51(4):487-493.
5. Nelson G, Aubry T, Lafrance A. A review of the literature on the effectiveness of housing and support, assertive community treatment, and intensive case management interventions for persons with mental illness who have been homeless. *Am J Orthopsychiatry.* 2007;77(3):350-361.
6. Salyers MP, Tsemberis S. ACT and recovery: integrating evidence-based practice and recovery orientation on assertive community treatment teams. *Community Ment Health J.* 2007;43(6):619-641.
7. Phillips SD, Burns BJ, Edgar ER, et al. Moving assertive community treatment into standard practice. *Psychiatr Serv.* 2001;52(6):771-779.
8. Thornicroft G, Susser E. Evidence-based psychotherapeutic interventions in the community care of schizophrenia. *Br J Psychiatry.* 2001;178:2-4.
9. Tsemberis S, Gulcur L, Nakae M. Housing first, consumer choice, and harm reduction for homeless individuals with a dual diagnosis. *Am J Public Health.* 2004;94(4):651-656.
10. Greenwood RM, Schaefer-McDaniel NJ, Winkel G, Tsemberis SJ. Decreasing psychiatric symptoms by increasing choice in services for adults with histories of homelessness. *Am J Community Psychol.* 2005;36(3-4):223-238.
11. Tomes N. The patient as a policy factor: a historical case study of the consumer/survivor movement in mental health. *Health Aff (Millwood).* 2006;25(3):720-729.
12. Bond GR, Salyers MP, Rollins AL, Rapp CA, Zipple AM. How evidence-based practices contribute to community integration. *Community Ment Health J.* 2004;40(6):569-588.
13. Butler LD, Critelli FM, Rinfrette ES. Trauma-informed care and mental health. *Dir Psychiatr.* 2011;31:197-210.
14. Hopper EK, Bassuk EL, Olivet J. Shelter from the storm: trauma-informed care in homelessness services settings. *Open Health Serv Pol J.* 2010;3:80-100.
15. Howgego IM, Yellowlees P, Owen C, Meldrum L, Dark F. The therapeutic alliance: the key to effective patient outcome? A descriptive review of the evidence in community mental health case management. *Aust NZ J Psychiatry.* 2003;37:169-183.
16. Frank AF, Gunderson JG. The role of the therapeutic alliance in the treatment of schizophrenia: relationship to course and outcome. *Arch Gen Psychiatry.* 1990;47:228-236.
17. Bustillo JR, Lauriello J, Horan WP, Keith SJ. The psychosocial treatment of schizophrenia: an update. *Am J Psychiatry.* 2001;158(2):163-175.
18. Brown GW, Birley JLT, Wing JK. Influence of family life on the course of schizophrenic disorders: a replication. *Br J Psychiatry.* 1972;121(562):241-258.
19. Butzlaff RL, Hooley JM. Expressed emotion and psychiatric relapse: a meta-analysis. *Arch Gen Psychiatry.* 1998;55(6):547-552.
20. Fenton WS. Evolving perspectives on individual psychotherapy for schizophrenia. *Schizophr Bull.* 2000;26(1):47-72.
21. Morrison AP, Barratt S. What are the components of CBT for psychosis? A Delphi study. *Schizophr Bull.* 2010;36(1):136-142.

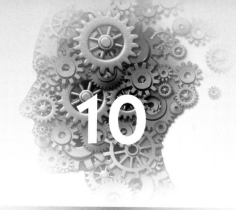

Psychotherapy Within Consultation-Liaison Settings

LINDSEY PERSHERN, MD AND BEN LIPPE, PhD

Case Study

Mr. R is a 73-year-old Hispanic male who was referred for a psychotherapy consultation during his medical hospitalization, due to concerns regarding depression and anxiety after new cancer diagnosis. He prefers to communicate in Spanish though is able to speak English conversationally. He has no known psychiatric history, but was recently prescribed an antidepressant medication to help manage mood and anxiety symptoms. However, he is still complaining of low mood and high anxiety, which he finds difficult to manage. He also described a recent development of problems with concentration and memory, to the point that he often forgets relevant information from his medical team about his medical treatment plan. Additionally, one of the patient's nurses overheard the patient making a statement to a friend over the phone that he was having thoughts of suicide to "just end this pain," but he subsequently denied having said this and became irritable with the nurse for "eavesdropping." You are asked by the medical team to see this patient to begin psychotherapy during his current hospital stay. He informed the team that he would be open to speaking with you, but wondered aloud how talking with a therapist could help him feel any better.

INTRODUCTION

This chapter provides a framework for effective psychotherapy in consultation-liaison settings, with a primary focus on hospital settings. There are a range of factors that make this work both challenging and gratifying. Therapists in these settings share the important role, along with the patients themselves, of promoting wellness through recognition and treatment of psychological factors impacting medical outcomes and overall quality of life. The initial portion of this chapter will focus on ways to conceptualize medically ill patients, including common responses to illness, stressors inherent in hospital environments, and distinguishing between preexisting versus developing mental health concerns. This chapter will then define the role of therapists and finally outline the basics of conducting psychotherapy in consultation-liaison settings.

Privilege and Possibilities

As mental health providers, the privilege and opportunity to work in the consultation-liaison setting is rewarding and important work. This work offers the opportunity to intervene and make significant differences, as improvements in a hospitalized patient's distress have a much larger scale impact on their physical health and quality of life. The potential emotional needs of patients who are experiencing medical illness are many and varied. As a result, the provision of psychotherapy in the hospital requires understanding of the stress of illness and the hospital setting, as well as consideration of the many factors contributing to the patient's subjective experience.

Not all hospital environments provide psychological treatment or consultation-liaison psychiatric services. For those that do, the therapist's role is to optimize the ability of the patient to successfully traverse the course of the hospital stay and to also create a springboard for seeking services post-hospitalization, if needed. The judgment of therapeutic success is made by the patient and their families, the primary treatment providers and staff, and the hospital system as a whole. This reality places the therapist in a unique position to consider the roles and functions of broader systems outside of the individual therapy relationship, and integrate them into the therapeutic treatment plan.

The primary role of mental health providers in consultation-liaison settings is direct patient care. This means that in addition to patient evaluation and recommendations to the referring medical team, therapists in consultation-liaison settings have the opportunity to provide individual, family, or group therapy to help alleviate emotional distress for patients in the context of acute or chronic health problems. Sometimes your initial role will include working collaboratively with other medical services, such as combined sessions with a physical therapist to help assist a patient dealing with emotional distress related to fear of falling. Additional roles include activities such as screening for psychological distress, educating the patients on how psychological factors can influence medical outcomes, conducting presurgical psychological assessment, and teaching or training medical staff on basic identification of mental health needs.

Preexisting or Developing Psychiatric Comorbidities

In addition to the impact of psychological responses to illness and hospitalization, patients may also require treatment due to preexisting psychiatric symptoms. Mental illness is prevalent in the hospital setting, but often underrecognized. However, the inherent stresses of the hospital can be magnified in those with underlying psychiatric diagnoses. As therapists in the hospital, we serve to provide support and intervention for those with active psychiatric symptoms.

Frequent diagnoses made in the hospital setting include anxiety disorders, mood disorders, somatic symptoms disorders, delirium, and substance use disorders.[1-3] Patients with comorbid psychiatric symptoms often have longer hospital stays, slower recovery, and greater risk of poor outcomes after discharge.[4] Patients with depressive disorders might present needing admission for management of medical consequences of their depressive symptoms (eg, low appetite/weight loss, poor self-care including management of medical problems). In addition, patients who pose acute safety concerns in the hospital due to acute suicidal ideation require mental health evaluation and management of risk. Patients with anxiety disorders or posttraumatic stress disorder (PTSD) are often challenged by the stressors of the hospital environment related to control, privacy, and trust.

Effectiveness Research

What does the research literature say about the effectiveness of psychotherapy in consultation-liaison settings? As noted previously, psychological and psychosocial factors play a key role in the etiology, diagnosis, and treatment of medical illness.[5] Research on psychotherapeutic services for medically ill patients indicates therapy can provide a range of clinical improvements in health outcomes across a variety of medical conditions, including cancer, diabetes, heart failure, obesity, and solid organ transplantation.[6,7] From an economic standpoint, therapist involvement in medical settings has demonstrated utility including reduced medical costs, decreased length of hospital stays, faster return to employment, and reduced functional disability.[8] An interdisciplinary approach to patient care, including the involvement of a mental health treatment provider, has been shown to improve health outcomes, improve the relationships between patients and providers,[9] improve adherence to medical recommendations, and result in improved quality of life.[10] As a result, the number of therapists serving on consultation-liaison services has increased over the past decade, as evidence in support of the utility of having mental health providers in hospital settings continues to expand and proliferate.[11]

CONCEPTUALIZING MEDICALLY ILL PATIENTS

Mind-Body Connection

The exploration of the mind-body connection has a long history. Even ancient civilizations considered the significance of the processes within the body and brain on an individual's mental state. Put simply, the mind affects the body and the body affects the mind.

Illness has psychologic consequences, resulting from both the direct impact of disease processes and the experience of being ill. Disease processes, as well as their treatments, can have a direct impact on the patient's mental health. For example, patients who have experienced a stroke have an increased risk of developing depression. Another example is the increased incidence of anxiety in patients with pulmonary disease due to physiological effects of hypoxia, as well as the stimulating side effects of broncho-dilating medications. Patients also invariably respond emotionally to the experience of being ill. Thoughts and feelings about themselves emerge as do efforts to cope with a multitude of potential stressors. These thoughts and feelings can be painful and may conflict with how they usually see themselves. Their coping efforts can sometimes be maladaptive and that makes the experience even worse.

Biopsychosocial-Cultural Framework

Patients respond in unique ways to being ill and in the hospital. Evaluation and intervention require exploration of the individual experience, which can be organized around biologic, psychologic, social, and cultural factors. The patient's response can manifest as a direct expression of what they are feeling or as changes in behavior, which then need to be understood and interpreted by others. It is helpful to consider a patient's level of distress as well as the impact on their hospitalization. If a patient is anxious, for example, exploration of their symptoms will include how their anxiety affects their interactions with staff and their ability to tolerate the needed medical treatments. As mental health providers, our work is predicated on the reality that human beings are unique. Application of the biopsychosocial-cultural framework in these cases often reveals a complicated web of factors influencing personal adjustment to the medical illness and management.

Let us revisit Mr. R to illustrate the contribution of biological, psychological, social, and cultural factors in his case, as exploration of these elements is helpful to the development of an effective treatment strategy.

Biological factors. Psychiatric symptoms in cancer may represent a normal reaction, a psychiatric disorder, *or* the somatic consequence of the cancer itself or related treatments. Faced with a serious diagnosis, patients often respond with a variety of emotions that are considered a normal or expected consequence. When symptoms exceed a certain threshold of severity and cause dysfunction, patients will exhibit symptoms that meet criteria for a psychiatric diagnosis.

If we apply this specifically to Mr. R, we know patients with cancer have increased rates of depression and anxiety, with variability noted in prevalence based on gender, age, stage of cancer illness, and type of cancer.[12] Differentiating a primary mood or anxiety disorder from one caused by the cancer itself can be challenging, but is important when considering treatment and prognostic expectations. Certain cancers are known to cause mood and anxiety symptoms, as are chemotherapy treatments. If primary or metastatic lesions are present in the brain, this risk increases. For Mr. R, his reported symptoms reflect potential consequences of his cancer and chemotherapy treatment, especially his neurocognitive symptoms. Discussion with his primary team about head imaging, as well as the plan for continued chemo treatment, will inform the therapist's role in managing these symptoms.

Psychological factors. We know that cancer is a new diagnosis for Mr. R, which infers a period of great uncertainty and stress. In addition to subjective distress, his low mood and high levels of anxiety and cognitive symptoms influence his experience of the hospital, which is a completely new environment. Depression and anxiety can also result in disengagement and avoidance, which can impact the staff-patient relationship dynamic.

Mr. R's response to this challenging cycle depends on many factors, including personal resilience. For the therapist, there are opportunities to validate Mr. R's experience, support effective coping strategies, and align priorities for safety and wellness. Exploration of these psychological factors will include questions about his response to being ill in the past, current experience of the hospital, and his emotional responses.

Social and cultural factors. Social and cultural factors impact Mr. R's experience of being ill, as well as his acceptance of support and psychiatric interventions. His ambivalence about the benefits of psychotherapy reflects a more generalized rejection of mental health interventions stemming from the stigma of mental illness within his community. Factors that will influence his response include family support, health literacy, spiritual beliefs, and communication with the medical team. The involvement of supportive family members provides stability and comfort both in the hospital and when discharged.

On the other hand, Mr. R's limited understanding of the medical system and lack of medical knowledge create additional stress, which becomes more significant when his cultural norms encourage acquiescence to the authority of medical professionals. Any past experiences involving racism and marginalization may become reiterated in the hierarchical system of the hospital. In addition, communication challenges between patients and staff in the acute medical environment are heightened by language barriers and provider time pressures. For Mr. R, the experience of having the nurse react to his voicing desire to end his pain further deepens the staff-patient divide.

COMMON PSYCHOLOGICAL RESPONSES TO MEDICAL ILLNESS AND HOSPITALIZATION

The subjective experience of the hospitalized patient is variable and influenced by multiple factors. Each patient is different, as is each hospital stay. Some patients facing very significant medical issues and complicated hospital courses respond with highly effective coping skills and sail through seamlessly. Others with minor conditions requiring relatively simple interventions can decompensate significantly during their stay and require much support to tolerate medical treatment. We will focus on two key factors that contribute to a patient's response, (1) the stress of medical illness and (2) the stress of the hospital environment.

Patient Understanding of Illness

A patient's response to illness starts with their understanding of the diagnosis and treatment. Within the dynamic hospital environment, there are many barriers to communication of facts regarding diagnosis, workup, and treatment planning. Patients often have a relative knowledge deficit regarding their medical illness and prognosis, which can cause unnecessary anxiety and/or miscommunication. It is important for mental health providers to have a factual understanding of the patient's medical conditions, prognosis, and treatment plan, prior to meeting with

10

the patient for the first time, to avoid further miscommunications. Then, as in other psychotherapeutic contexts, the therapist assumes a position of curiosity about the individual, first exploring their basic understanding of their condition and what is happening in the hospital, prior to providing any sort of psychoeducation.

Patient Perspective on Illness and Treatment

In addition to a patient's factual understanding of their illness, we need to consider their personal perspective on the illness and hospitalization. What does being sick enough to need to be in the hospital mean to them?

When we consider the inherent challenges of being ill, it is helpful to think about the time course of disease. Patients are hospitalized when the needed management of their medical problems exceeds what is considered safe or deliverable in the out-patient setting. This threshold can be met when a patient experiences a transient medical problem, or when a chronic medical problem acutely worsens. Admission to the hospital may result in a new diagnosis or signal the progression of a known illness.

Sometimes, patients who have struggled to maintain their functioning outside of the hospital see the hospital admission as a relief, saying to themselves, "Thank goodness I am finally going to get the care I need." Others have had limited awareness of their medical issues and may see admission as an inconvenience. For others, the medical diagnosis can be challenging to their self-concept and sense of mortality. The meaning of medical illness can stimulate a variety of reactions, depending on factors such as age, level of education, presence of comorbid medical problems, and extent of social support. We describe many of these reactions below.

Common Reactions to Illness

Patients confronted with the reality of their own vulnerability and mortality may respond with denial, fear/anxiety, grief/sadness, guilt/shame, or anger.[13] The individual patient's experience of and response to illness provides an opportunity for the therapist to dramatically influence the course of illness, both during and after the hospitalization. Emotional reactions to illness serve as opportunities for the therapist to provide support and promote acceptance and meaning-making adaptation to medical illness.

Denial. Patients may fail to achieve acceptance and demonstrate varying degrees of denial of their illness. Denial in the medical setting can be fundamentally troublesome to primary providers, staff, and even family members. The patient may minimize their symptoms, lack emotional reaction, overtly reject a diagnosis, or refuse necessary medical treatments.

For example, during your initial assessment with Mr. R, you discover he does not believe that he really has cancer, but instead is primarily focused on alleviating his pain. He specifically states, "I don't know why they keep going on and on about cancer. They thought my uncle had it and it wasn't until after surgery that almost killed him that they realized he was fine. I just hurt like crazy when I eat, that's all, doc."

As a result, his frustration may stem from his disagreement with providers about the recommended treatment, which can result in him feeling anxious, frustrated, and hopeless about getting relief from the pain.

Fear/anxiety. Anxiety is often the prevailing emotion when patients are in the hospital. Anxiety can manifest and impact the medical treatment in a variety of ways. Initially, this anxiety is usually centered on the experience of being ill (pain and discomfort), rather than longer term fears around prognosis or mortality. Anxiety can interfere with the development of the provider-patient relationship and lead to miscommunication regarding symptoms and treatments. The fearful patient may avoid certain discussions or procedures and even question the benevolent intentions of providers and staff.

For example, anxiety will be an important area of exploration with Mr. R, as anxiety can be disabling and may need to be a large area of focus in his care. If Mr. R is not able to adequately describe his pain to his providers due to feeling anxious or overwhelmed during their sometimes too brief interactions, it will impact the efficacy of medical pain interventions.

Grief/sadness. A medical diagnosis represents a loss in many ways resulting in grief and sadness. The potential losses include loss of future goals or dreams, loss of control, loss of love or approval, and loss of life. There are actual physical losses to many patients, as well, such as loss of health or function, or loss of a limb or organ. All of these are sources of grief and sadness that can be overlooked within a fast-paced medical system. When sadness is accompanied by hopelessness, a patient may consider death as a desired outcome. Even when patients do not report symptoms of a major mood disorder, they may still experience thoughts of suicide that place them at risk.[14] For Mr. R, the therapeutic interview would ideally explore actual and anticipated losses, his emotional reactions, and his statements of wanting to die, recognizing grief may play a significant role in his emotional and behavioral reactions while hospitalized.

Guilt and shame. Guilt and shame are emotions that are confronted often in psychotherapy situations and are commonly seen in reaction to medical illness. Some patients may perceive illness as a form of punishment or retribution for past wrongs. Others may focus on their position of dependency and feel overwhelmed by a sense of burdensomeness on their family members, caregivers, and/or hospital staff. In some circumstances, guilt and shame can be related to factors contributing to the development of worsening of their medical problems.

Anger. Expression of anger by patients is met with intolerance by some medical providers, although this is a very common response to illness. In an acute medical environment, patients are often (unreasonably) expected to behave in a specific, predictable way, such as demonstrating immediate acceptance of an acute medical problem and its associated treatments.

For example, Mr. R's nurse describes him as angry and paints the picture of a "difficult" patient whose room she finds herself tip-toeing past or even circumventing to avoid getting yelled at. At the same time, Mr. R describes an environment where he feels ignored, not able to get what he needs when he needs it, and a general sense that providers do not care about him. Continuation of this cycle can lead to Mr. R's disengagement, refusal of recommended treatments, and ultimately his request for a discharge against medical advice, or AMA. Without effective intervention, the consequence of anger may be failure of medical care for Mr. R.

10

The Stress of Hospitalization

Many aspects of being in hospital are stressful, including loss of independence, control, predictability, and privacy. Patients in a hospital setting lose much of what is considered central to independent adult life. They rely on others for most of their needs and are expected to relinquish control of even basic decisions. Patients are expected to shift into a position of unequivocal trust of those who they do not know and accept a variety of uncertainties. Those who need assistance with activities of daily living (ADLs) depend on staff who are caring for other patients and may not be available when needed. Patients have little control of daily activities. Food is delivered when it is available, medications are administered at provider-specified times, and procedures are performed on an unpredictable schedule. Patients come to expect interruptions that disrupt sleep and interfere with visits from family and friends. The hospital environment invariably limits personal privacy.

In reaction to these stresses, you will see patients respond in a wide variety of ways. Some patients react to the demands of hospitalization with confusion and frustration. In an effort to cope, these patients may refuse care, request discharge against medical advice, or demonstrate overt hostility toward medical caregivers. These can all be ways to regain some sense of control, even if it comes at a cost to the patient. On the other extreme, some patients become overly dependent and regressed in response to hospitalization. These patients seem to cope with the loss of control and independence in the hospital by embracing it, as it may feel like a relief to surrender completely to another's care.

We see many of these factors affecting Mr. R's hospitalization. He reacts to the loss of privacy during his phone conversation, as well as the confusing sequence of the early stages of workup and treatment of newly diagnosed cancer. Mr. R's depressive symptoms center around a sense of burdensomeness due to physical and functional limitations. He cries as he describes the humiliation he feels every time he presses the button to call a nurse or aid to assist with toileting. His anxiety also stems from a sense that he will not get what he needs from his care team and a practical worry that his autonomy in making medical decisions will be taken away.

Broader Hospital System Pressures

We cannot forget that patients within a hospital are interacting with individual providers, who are themselves influenced by pressures from the hospital system. Medical providers must balance efficiency and productivity pressures with comprehensiveness of patient care. This impacts the ability of individual providers to develop therapeutic relationships with their patients, by limiting the number of providers to patients, time available to spend per patient, and availability to address urgent issues. Patients whose care challenges the limits of time and available resources in a stressed system may not get what they need emotionally. As a result, patients with unrealistic expectations of the system may believe that they are being dismissed or ignored by their care team. Mental health providers can assist by providing psycho-education, suggesting communication strategies for both parties, and normalizing the experience for the patient.

Impact of Health Disparities

Disparities in how healthcare is provided also influence the individual patient's experience. The factors that lead to uneven care include mental health stigma, race, ethnicity, cultural background, and socioeconomic status. These factors influence the referral of patients for psychiatric assessment as well as the success of therapy. Consideration of these factors by the consulting therapist will assist in management of patient and provider expectations as well as facilitate communication of recommended interventions.

Mental illness stigma. The stigma of mental illness impacts the care of psychiatric patients in the hospital. Patients are stigmatized based on cues that infer mental illness[15]: psychiatric symptoms, social skills deficits, physical appearance, and labels. The hospital environment contributes to these cues, making patients even more vulnerable than in other settings. Patients with psychiatric symptoms in the hospital are often perceived as difficult or too time-consuming. Medical illness can impair communication, social engagement, and limit self-care. In the acute setting, patients are often reduced to labels of their diagnosis or the level of their care needs.

Returning to Mr. R, we find that the nurses, in response to his comment of "end(ing) the pain," reflexively removed all potential harmful objects in his room and ensured close staff supervision for safety by placing a staff person in his room at all times. Mr. R was then labeled "the suicidal patient in room 304." The potential consequences of public stigma, even among healthcare providers, include stereotyping, prejudice, and discrimination. In addition, stigmatized patients are referred less often for psychotherapy in the hospital.[16] The role of the therapist in these situations extends to include liaising with staff, to provide support and education for providers, as well as providing support and education for the patient regarding the reasoning for these reflexive measures.

Racial/ethnic factors. Race and ethnicity influence access to healthcare, medical workup and management, psychiatric diagnosis, and referral patterns for psychotherapy. Racial/ethnic minority groups consistently have fewer physician visits, less healthcare expenditures, and lower rates of overall healthcare use compared with whites.[17] When patients are hospitalized, these disparities are evidenced by differences in medical care and treatment outcomes. Beyond the role of implicit bias, research has shown that white providers apply a racial framework to medical decisions for nonwhite patients,[18] contributing to this disparity and systemic racism. Racial minority patients with psychiatric symptoms are less likely to be referred to a psychiatrist and receive a psychiatric diagnosis.[19]

If we apply knowledge of these disparities to Mr. R, we can assume that potentially limited access to care outside the hospital likely contributes to progression of his disease and impacts future treatment plans and prognosis. While in the hospital, his care could also be influenced by cultural incongruence with providers, language barriers, and possibly overt discrimination. These factors would clearly increase the stress of his hospital stay and contribute to his anxiety and would require further assessment with Mr. R to clarify if these broad problems have been his experiences on an individual level.

10

Sexual minority disparities. Significant healthcare disparities exist for sexual and gender minorities both in and outside of the hospital. This designation includes many different terms of identification, which we will consider under the umbrella of lesbian, gay, bisexual, and transgender (LGBT). LGBT patients have increased health risks, increased prevalence of smoking and substance use, delays in healthcare seeking when ill, and chronic stress due to overall marginalization.[20] When these risks culminate in a medical admission, disparities perpetuate due to overt discrimination, health insurance disparity, and lack of adequate training in LGBT health.[20,21] Implicit preferences for heterosexual patients in healthcare workers influence communication and patient-provider interactions. Culturally competent care of the LGBT population in the hospital is improved by educational programs. Considering the personal experience of patients who identify as LGBT will aid in overcoming some of these challenges and supporting health and recovery.

WHAT IS YOUR ROLE?

Definitions and Overview

Mental health providers offer a range of services and roles within inpatient medical and surgical settings. Services provided may include psychotherapy, which may be done by clinicians assigned this role (eg, graduate psychology or clinical social work trainees) or by clinicians as part of their broader general management of the case (eg, psychiatry residents). Psychotherapists typically assess, diagnose, and treat mental disorders that may be impacting physical health status.[22] Services rendered may include patient assessment, provision of psychotherapy, working with the patient's family or caregivers, and recommendations for therapeutic changes to the environment (eg, recommending limited interruptions by staff at night, as medically feasible, in support of addressing the patient's concerns regarding sleep disruptions). In addition to providing individual or family psychotherapy interventions, another primary role for therapists in these settings is that of consultant to the doctors, nurses, and other hospital staff about any patient issues that are considered behavioral or psychological in nature.

Furthermore, therapists serve as a liaison and sometimes an advocate for the patient and can help to bridge the gap between the patient and medical team, as well as the gap between hospital and outpatient care. One way this is accomplished is through dialogue with the patient regarding expression of needs and improving communication with their medical providers. Another is the provision of outpatient resource information prior to leaving the hospital, to help facilitate initiation of outpatient mental healthcare. Accordingly, the range of roles for psychotherapists in these settings reflects the diverse nature of presenting problems and needs of the patient, medical team, and healthcare systems.

Limitations to the Scope of Practice

In addition to knowing what therapists in consultation-liaison settings do, it is also important to understand what they do *not* do. For example, despite well-intentioned personal requests for professional emotional support or therapy from medical staff with whom therapists work, it is considered inappropriate and unethical to provide formal psychotherapy to medical staff colleagues, as it would represent a dual relationship (ie, work colleague/friend and therapist). The recommended approach here is to acknowledge the colleague's distress, while remaining careful not to present yourself as offering professional therapeutic services. Instead you can be very helpful by making referrals to other mental health professionals that might be appropriate to help support the colleague.

As mentioned previously, it is important for therapists to have a factual understanding of the patient's medical diagnosis, prognosis, and medical treatment plan. However, it is not the role of the therapist to provide medical diagnosis on behalf of the medical team, to educate patients about their medical condition, or to make medical recommendations regarding their medical problems. It is also not the role of the therapist to explain details of surgeries or to consent patients for medical procedures. You can help clarify information from the medical team in terms that are more understandable to the patient or help facilitate additional communication strategies between the patient and medical team.

Also, psychologists and other nonpsychiatrist therapists may be asked to provide pharmacologic recommendations. It is not uncommon for another treatment team member to say, "Hey, I know you're not a psychiatrist but I'm sure you know about these medications. Please tell me what medication you recommend for this patient to start taking." It may be tempting to provide specific medication recommendations, as you may indeed have a strong education in psychopharmacology, but nonpsychiatric psychotherapists generally do not make medication recommendations or prescribe medications. Exceptions include psychiatric advanced care providers (eg, nurse practitioners, physician assistants) and psychologists with additional training and certification in certain states in which psychologists currently have prescription privileges. Alternative ways to be helpful in this case include recommending a medication consultation, consulting with the prescribing provider, and/or addressing behavioral or cognitive issues impacting medication adherence. Check with your state licensing board if you have any questions regarding prescription privileges or other questions about staying within your scope of professional practice.

10

REASONS FOR CONSULTATION

There are many potential reasons for referral in consultation-liaison settings. Consultation referrals are most often generated by the primary team, not the patient themselves. Many factors contribute to the perspective that a patient may need or benefit from psychological support/psychotherapy in the hospital.

Assessment of these factors starts with clarifying the consult question—*what prompted the concern of the referring provider*? This requires the synthesis of information from multiple sources. Requests for mental health assessment in the hospital can be notoriously vague and often require a search for more information. This is best done by speaking directly to the referring provider and reviewing the medical chart. In this discussion, it is helpful to orient the conversation toward symptoms (patient-reported or perceived by others), behaviors, and the impact of these on the current hospitalization.

One way to evaluate the concern is to categorize consultation referrals into four broad categories: (1) patient emotional distress, (2) provider emotional distress, (3) problematic behaviors, and (4) medically unexplained symptoms.

Referral Reason #1: Patient Emotional Distress

Patients are often stressed by illness and hospitalization, and their emotional response impacts their treatment. Providers who interact with a distressed patient can identify their emotions as sad, worried, or angry and request support. They may also seek assistance when these emotions negatively impact medical care, for example, a sad patient not wanting to eat or take medications. Patients themselves may directly communicate distress leading to referral for therapy.

For example, in our patient case, we learn that Mr. R made the team aware of his low mood and high anxiety, which were troubling and affecting him. A distressed patient may request the involvement of a mental health provider during the hospitalization. Sometimes a patient's distress is related to communication or care issues. In these cases, the initial interview serves as an effective intervention of support and validation, as the therapist assumes the role of listener and ally. Although less common than a provider-generated request, a patient-identified need can be fertile ground for the development of the therapeutic relationship.

Referral Reason #2: Provider Emotional Distress

It is often more difficult to elicit information related to provider distress. When a consult is requested, there is something troubling that the primary team needs assistance with. Providers may perceive a patient as withdrawn and depressed if, for example, the patient is less engaged or not improving as anticipated. For example, we know that Mr. R has experienced depressive symptoms since his diagnosis and can expect these symptoms to impact the medical team's experience of him. Some depressed patients activate an increased sense of compassion and empathy in providers, while others experience frustration and detachment. Both often result in a request for mental health services, but require different approaches.

In acute treatment environments like intensive care units, providers may struggle to identify or verbalize their own reactions to patients. Most physicians receive some education on the concept of countertransference, often focused on the example of the patient with a personality disorder engendering anger and frustration. Unfortunately, this singular emphasis on personality disorders may lead us to miss the many other kinds of patients that can trigger similarly strong feelings.

Let us return to our case. Mr. R is under the care of a family medicine team with consultation by the oncology service. On admission, the primary physician discovers that Mr. R had signs of early skin cancer starting 10 years ago, but did not seek care due to his lack of concern and limited access to medical services. Since his admission, this same physician has spent very little time with Mr. R. She sees her role as secondary to the oncology team. She also finds using an interpreter and attempting to communicate with Mr. R challenging, as he often answers with brief, one-word answers and appears to not realize the significance of his medical diagnosis. She placed a consult for a mental health assessment after a nurse reported concerns that Mr. R may be at risk of harming himself. When you talk with the physician, she communicates that she is not concerned about Mr. R's mental health. She rapidly describes Mr. R's medical case, stating that his prognosis is poor due to his late stage of cancer and his "noncompliance." When you inquire if she perceives Mr. R as depressed or anxious, as he is currently taking medications for both of these conditions, the provider responds "No, he's not depressed, he just doesn't take care of himself." She is seemingly unaware of Mr. R's symptoms and instead appears both detached and frustrated by his perceived lack of self-care.

We can hypothesize many potential reasons for this physician's feelings toward Mr. R. First, patients with cancer can challenge any physician's sense of mortality. Second, patients whose path to medical care is delayed, regardless of the reason, can activate a sense of frustration that leads to patient-blaming and low expectations for their future behavior. These emotions can lead to provider avoidance and disengagement, and a resulting cycle of poor doctor-patient interactions. Third, providers who do not know their patients well will have difficulty accurately assessing the patient's emotional states. In this case, it seems that the provider's feelings have resulted in having little interest in exploring mental health needs with the patient.

Our role in liaising with providers includes asking questions to elicit information, as well as model more mental health-centered methods of patient assessment. In addition, we can ask this physician about patient behaviors that demonstrate his interest in and expectations of treatment. Is the patient refusing medications or procedures? Has he communicated wishes through an advanced directive? Is the sense of Mr. R not caring about himself driven by Mr. R's symptoms of depression? Providing tactful, appropriate feedback and treatment recommendations to his physician after interviewing Mr. R can be very helpful ways to appropriately challenge the provider's assumptions.

Referral Reason #3: Problematic Behaviors

In the busy hospital setting, potential problematic behaviors by patients are varied and typically include the following: (1) apathy or disengagement, (2) inability to tolerate treatments or procedures, (3) refusal of care or disagreement with treatment plans, (4) demonstration of anger through aggressive or agitated behavior, (5) acts of self-harm, (6) odd/bizarre behaviors, or (7) impulsive behaviors. Any of these can interfere with adequate medical treatment and raise concerns for the staff. The withdrawn/apathetic patient may not engage to answer questions accurately or may stop eating or participating in medical care. The anxious patient may prematurely terminate a breathing treatment due to feeling overwhelmed and short of breath.

Loss of control and uncertainty often drive behaviors that are in opposition to a medical plan of care. Patients who feel ignored or misunderstood may react with refusal of medications, blood tests, or other procedures. These refusals of care are often troubling for staff and providers but are less commonly explored. On the other hand, patients sometimes request treatment that the medical team does not feel is appropriate. A challenging example is the patient reporting uncontrolled pain despite the recommended intervention. When a patient demonstrates overtly dangerous behavior, such as physical aggression, staff and systems struggle to manage safety while maintaining empathy and compassion for the distressed patient.

10

Sometimes the referring provider is unclear about what is behind the problematic behavior and may make comments such as, "There is just something off." In these cases, the provider is typically correct in that there is something unusual happening. Patients who are disengaged or respond oddly can be delirious or have a chronic underlying neurocognitive problem that is undetected. Patients who behave and communicate in unexpected ways may be psychotic or manic. The request for mental health consultation for vague concerns does not mean the consultation request is inappropriate, but it may be a signal that optimal patient care is compromised. This makes the work of the mental health consultant particularly important. In the initial assessment, the therapist will ask questions that may reveal underlying neurocognitive deficits, acute psychosis or mania, or suicidality. In these cases, involvement of a psychiatric provider is appropriate, as well as rapid feedback to the primary consulting team that further medical workup may be indicated.

Referral Reason #4: Medically Unexplained Symptoms

Consults are commonly generated when the process of medical evaluation does not yield a clear explanation of the patient's complaints. In some of these cases, the referring team may have appropriate knowledge and consideration of somatic symptom disorder diagnoses. In others, the referral to a mental healthcare provider may represent a last resort effort to "do something" for the patient. These types of consults can be accompanied by team and patient frustration, and sometimes even feelings of failure by the referring provider. However, patients with functional somatic symptoms are also more likely to be depressed or anxious, compared with patients with alternative diagnoses,[23] and require intervention.

In contrast with symptoms that are medically unexplained, somatic symptoms that are judged to be in excess of what is expected by providers are often minimized or ignored. This is particularly common with pain, which leads to an unfortunate perception or blatant labeling of a patient as "drug-seeking." Goals in these cases include collaboration with primary teams to optimize education about diagnosis and treatment and to provide support and guidance regarding patient-centered care.

WHAT TREATMENT CHOICES ARE AVAILABLE?

Research on Specific Therapies

The most widely utilized and most commonly studied approach within health psychology in terms of psychotherapeutic interventions is cognitive behavioral therapy (CBT). CBT has demonstrated effectiveness in treating related symptoms across a wide range of medical conditions including chronic pain, rheumatic diseases, smoking cessation, cancer, and eating disorders,[24] as well as diabetes management[25] and even solid-organ transplantation.[26] The structure of CBT, with primary focus on identification of thoughts, emotions, and behaviors, as well as skills development to help cope with associated emotional distress, lends itself well to medical environments (eg, typically time-limited in nature) and patients with a need for more immediate symptom relief.

Motivational interviewing[27] is an approach that has demonstrated utility across a range of behavioral health presenting issues[28] (see Chapter 3 for more on this approach). Acceptance and commitment therapy (ACT) is another empirically supported approach for a variety of behavioral health concerns (see Chapter 12 for reference to ACT).[29]

Similarly, psychodynamic psychotherapy has demonstrated effectiveness with a diverse range of medically ill patients.[30] There is also a historical lineage of effective psychodynamic practice with medically ill individuals by consult-liaison psychiatrists, although psychodynamic therapy is not exclusive to psychiatrists. The time-limited nature of therapy in medical settings may lend itself more favorably to brief psychodynamic approaches, however, rather than long-term psychoanalytic psychotherapy.

Supportive psychotherapy, primarily geared toward helping patients cope and manage emotional distress, is another important empirically supported treatment approach when dealing with medically ill populations.[31] Much of your therapeutic work in a hospital context may reside in this category given the focus on coping skills development and emotional support. Although typically brief and broadly supportive in nature (eg, provision of psychoeducation and practical problem-solving over a few sessions), a common misconception is that great depth of assessment and therapeutic work do not occur in supportive psychotherapy. In reality, it takes a tremendous amount of clinical skill and knowledge to choose this type of therapy with a hospitalized patient, as supportive therapy is not always indicated. However, for patients in the hospital experiencing emotional distress, supportive psychotherapy can be of great benefit.

Another form of psychotherapy in medical contexts is group psychotherapy. Often, groups are formulated based on themes of presenting mental health concerns (eg, a "depression group") or by medical issue (eg, a "cystic fibrosis support group"). In group psychotherapy, it is important to address goals and themes relevant to all group members rather than the typically more narrow goals as in individual psychotherapy.[32]

As you can see, therapeutic approaches are not a "one size fits all" when working with patients in medical settings. Lean on your educational and training background, as well as your supervisor and careful case conceptualization, to make sure you are cognizant of the benefits and limits to your selected approach with an individual patient. Also, for additional information regarding the basic tenets and practice of these therapy orientations, see the corresponding chapters in this textbook.

10

Modifications to Psychotherapy in Medical Settings

There may be times when elements of psychotherapy need to be modified. For example, sometimes the patient's medical issues can contribute to challenges in psychotherapy and accurate diagnostic conceptualization. Consider, for example, when patients have certain medical problems that may be contraindicated for certain types of coping skills (eg, difficult for patients to do diaphragmatic breathing exercises when they have significant pulmonary problems), or when medical devices impact the patient's ability to effectively communicate (eg, tracheostomies with or without speaking valves). These are cases in which psychotherapy can still be effective and valuable, although consideration of the impact of the medical condition must be taken into account and the intervention selected accordingly. For example, the patient with impaired ability to communicate due to intubation may need creative problem-solving such as using written expression or simplified hand signals to bolster the patient's ability to communicate with you.

Also, certain disorders in the *Diagnostic and Statistical Manual of Mental Disorders*, Fifth Edition (DSM-5) specify that the cause of the psychiatric symptoms is due to an underlying medical condition.[34] For example, depressive disorder due to another medical condition clarifies that the depressive symptoms are due to direct effects of underlying medical issues (eg, hypothyroidism), in contrast to a depression caused by a nonmedical cause such as negative interpretation of stressors. Accordingly, psychotherapy may be less effective in those cases, as the etiology of the psychiatric symptoms is physiological. With that said, etiology is not the sole predictor of therapeutic outcomes. Recognition and understanding of medical etiology of any psychiatric symptoms is important, but does not mean that supportive therapy cannot be helpful. For example, development of the therapeutic alliance and providing empathic validation of emotional distress (examples of common factors in psychotherapy) and encouraging engagement with helpful social support (example of optimization of environmental/social factors) can help relieve severity of depression regardless of underlying medical etiology.

SPECIFIC CONSIDERATIONS FOR PSYCHOTHERAPY IN CONSULTATION-LIAISON SETTINGS

Practical Barriers

Psychiatric assessments in the hospital require a few important adaptations. The aspects of the hospital environment which challenge a patient's functioning and communication will invariably impact the first visit. The physical space of a hospital room is determined by the design of the hospital. Typical inpatient hospital spaces are busy, loud, and provide limited privacy. The scheduling and need for medical treatments may also impact the patient's ability to participate in therapy. Patients may require continuous oxygen that interferes with communication or experience distressing medication side effects that are distracting.

Mental health assessment in the hospital setting requires creative strategies when communication is impaired due to speech or motor problems. Patients with hearing impairment may benefit from closer proximity than typical in the clinical interview or require use of written communication. Patients with impairments in their speech ability may utilize pen and paper. Those who are unable to hold or manipulate a writing instrument can be assisted with a communication assistance board that has letters or symbols and can be used through pointing (either by the patient or the provider). Intubated patients who are not sedated, although difficult to interview, often can communicate using hand gestures, mouthing words, or other assisted communication device. Finally, gathering additional collateral information from treatment providers and other available sources can be invaluable in these situations.

Self-Stigma, Shame, and Refusal

In addition to practical barriers, individual factors may prevent patients from accepting mental health support or services in the hospital. For many patients who are distressed in the hospital, the involvement of any mental health provider may spark feelings that they are crazy, weak, or incompetent. These self-perceptions often result in feelings of shame, which can contribute to refusal or avoidance of psychotherapy treatment. This response is magnified when a patient is afraid of the judgment of involved family members.

However, as a mental health consulting service in the hospital, it is possible to help patients create a new frame for viewing mental healthcare. Validation and normalization go a long way with reluctant patients and families, when their reluctance is rooted in shame. We can inform patients of some of the facts presented in this chapter, such as the fact that being sick and in the hospital is stressful and that attending to patients' emotional needs, in addition to their physical/medical needs, leads to better outcomes. We can also play a role in increasing a patient's likelihood of continuing mental healthcare after being discharged, if it is indicated.

Cultural Humility

Incongruence of culture, ethnicity, and primary language may challenge the therapeutic relationship. Hospitalized patients come from all walks of life and cultural backgrounds. Patients often experience the medical culture of a particular inpatient setting as very scary and foreign. Lack of adequate communication and support can perpetuate this defensive position and contribute to overall distrust of the healthcare team. For example, we can think of Mr. R's interpretation of the nurse as "eavesdropping" expanding into a sense of mistrust that extends to other providers and the system at large. These concepts were covered in Chapter 8 in this book, but are reiterated briefly here as applied to therapy in hospital settings.

Cultural factors also influence the experience of illness, hospitalization, and treatment. Assessing the impact of cultural factors on the individual patient requires exploration of their personal narrative in order to avoid presumptions and stereotyping. Beyond encouraging patients to explore and explain their subjective experience in respect to their culture, discussion with family and the use of translators as cultural brokers can be very helpful. Chaplain services play the same role when exploring the role of spiritual and religious constructs of illness and health. These aspects of culture can be particularly important in management of distress in patients with terminal illness and at the end of life.

Self-awareness. For the therapist, self-awareness of cultural attitudes, beliefs, and potential biases is critical in developing a culturally sensitive therapeutic approach. Ethics workshops, supervision, coursework, and other similar training environments are wonderful places to increase your knowledge base regarding cultural influences in therapeutic outcomes as well as support your ongoing quest to develop cultural competence. You should also be mindful of opportunities to consult with professional colleagues regarding any current or foreseeable cultural conflicts that may arise during the course of therapy.

10

Use of interpreters/cultural brokers. Recognition of how cultural factors interact with medical systems and providers is important in the therapeutic framework. For example, when a patient prefers to speak in a language that the therapist is not fluent in, this may present inherent challenges in psychotherapy, as subtleties in meaning can become lost in translation. In a medical context, the need for accurate interpretation of medically complex jargon, in addition to the psychotherapy terms you may be using, becomes all the more pronounced. Thus, it is ethically important to utilize trained interpreters whenever feasible. Although family members may willingly offer to assist with interpretation, this is not recommended as it presents additional concerns regarding potential interpretive inaccuracies as well as clear privacy concerns when discussing potentially sensitive personal material.

Cultural formulation. Culture can influence communication and therefore impact accurate diagnosis, formulation of symptoms and behaviors, and treatment planning, including referral to external resources for patients and families. A model of cultural consultation developed by Kirmayer and colleagues[33] provides a helpful list of considerations in the cultural formulation of patients in the consultation-liaison setting. In addition, the DSM-5[34] provides a framework of cultural formulation that may be helpful for beginning a culturally informed interview.

THE FIRST ENCOUNTER

Informed Consent

The process for introducing a patient to the role of the therapist, and to psychotherapy in general, is unique in consultation-liaison settings. It is often a patient's first encounter with mental health providers. You will need to provide information about the nature of your role and how it may benefit them.

We suggest that you review the following with new patients: the nature of the therapeutic role, the indications for why you are seeing the patient, description of the framework for therapy, goals and anticipated outcomes, and potential limitations. Here is what that would look like for Mr. R:

1. *The nature of the therapeutic role* (eg, "As a therapist here in the hospital, I typically speak with patients about topics such as stress about their health, as well as ways to help cope with these feelings").

2. *Indications for why you are seeing the patient* ("Your doctor asked me to see you because she was concerned that you might be feeling depressed regarding your new cancer diagnosis").

3. *Descriptions of the framework for therapy* ("Typically, therapy involves meeting together for several visits depending on your needs and goals for therapy").

4. *A review of goals and anticipated outcomes of treatment* ("We can work on developing coping skills to help manage your mood and find ways to feel less anxious about your pain and your upcoming procedure"), including

psychoeducation regarding the potential benefits on medical outcomes ("By managing your depression more effectively, it may help you feel more motivated to use the recommendations that your doctors are asking of you").

5. *Potential limitations to treatment* ("In this hospital setting, we may only have a limited amount of time to work together toward these therapeutic goals"). You should also include descriptions of any limitations to privacy in medical settings ("I want you to know that I plan to share a summary of what we discuss today with your doctor that referred you to me").

6. *Allowing time for questions about your role, the process of therapy, and any privacy concerns.* Frank discussions of limits to privacy and sensitivity to Mr. R's previous concern about staff "eavesdropping" on his statements indicating suicidal ideation would be particularly indicated.

In summary, you are in a unique position to provide patients with psychoeducation, including educating them about psychological symptoms, treatment options, and relationships between psychiatric comorbidities and their current medical problems. It is important to make sure that you bear in mind the initial referral question so that your introductions, descriptions, and psychoeducation may all be service of furthering the patient's care in the hospital or other medical setting.

Conducting Screening and the Initial Assessment

Screening and more in-depth initial assessment of the patient are the cornerstones upon which your subsequent recommendations and therapeutic work begins. As such, the importance of the initial evaluations cannot be overstated. Prior to your initial assessment of the patient, seek any data to inform the consultation from the patient's medical record, including any current and past hospitalization records. Sadock and Sadock[35] provide a detailed overview of the process for a routine initial psychiatric assessment, highlighting the identification of the chief complaint, evaluation of psychiatric history and treatments, history of the present illness, family history, and other biopsychosocial elements of the patient's personal history. Be sure to check with your supervisor to see if there are any available templates to help assist in your assessment and work to cover key components. Beyond the information documented in the medical record, talking with medical care providers (eg, nurses, physical therapists, case managers) and family members or friends (with appropriate patient consent) provides useful collateral data.

Screening for emotional distress is typically accomplished via brief sets of questions or questionnaires (eg, Patient Health Questionnaire or PHQ[36] and the Montreal Cognitive Assessment [MoCA],[37] among others). This is usually performed by non-psychiatric providers such as nursing staff or intake coordinators, but also by mental health providers at the bedside as part of the assessment. Screening is helpful to identify issues that need to be explored further by a more in-depth assessment. Following screening and identification of a particular concern, you may be asked by the medical team to assess patients for symptoms of psychological disorders such as depression, anxiety, cognitive problems, eating disorders, or other psychological factors affecting the patient's medical condition. With proper assessment, you will have set the stage for empirically supported therapy via accurate diagnosis.

10

Key components of a typical initial assessment in a hospital setting are similar to traditional diagnostic clinical interviews (see Chapter 2 in this book). However, the focus of the interview is usually focused on the immediate medical context, meaning exploration of the current impact of any psychologic distress on medical issues or vice versa. Be curious about the patient's response to their illness and hospitalization, and consider their current emotional status as compared with their reported baseline. During the initial assessment, help the patient begin establishing initial therapeutic goals, as the need for targeted goals is made even more important in consultation-liaison settings due to the typically time-limited nature of their hospital stay (and thus, of your time to work with them).

In the case of Mr. R, concerns from staff regarding his problems with information recall may spark a referral to you for evaluation of his cognitive status. A careful clinical history, including timelines of any memory deficits, medical comorbidities that may influence cognition, and cognitive screening (eg, via a formal mental status exam) will help you provide recommendations to Mr. R and the referring provider. These recommendations might include providing Mr. R with a written list of his medications in his preferred language, verbal as well as visual forms of education, and/or further neuropsychological testing if indicated.

Assessing Safety: Delirium, Suicidal Ideation, and Self-Harm

For all patients, not just those in an emotional crisis such as Mr. R, it is also critical to assess for safety, including delirium, suicidality, and self-harm at the initial visit (and subsequently whenever questions arise regarding self-harm, suicidal, or homicidal thoughts). This will help you inform the medical treatment team regarding any behavioral safety planning that will prioritize the patient's safety. You may need to divert from other goals in psychotherapy to address immediate patient safety concerns, as these need to be addressed prior to proceeding with implementation of other psychotherapeutic interventions.

Delirium. One patient safety issue that can go undetected or misdiagnosed as psychosis, mania, or even depression is altered mental status. Sometimes mental healthcare providers are able to detect and assess cases of acute altered mental status (also known as *delirium*) due to an underlying medical condition, because it is misperceived as another psychiatric condition. Any indication of delirium would require rapid communication to the team for a delirium workup, as untreated delirium can be extremely dangerous to the patient. While we typically think of suicidality as presenting an urgent patient safety issue, delirium is another condition that we must be vigilant for within medical settings and help the team identify and treat.

In addition, while delirium is by definition due to an underlying medical condition, there are specific behavioral interventions that can be helpful for the management of delirium. For example, frequent reorientation for the patient and promotion of effective sleep hygiene (eg, sleep routine, shades open during day and closed at night with television off). Also, if medically appropriate per the treating team, avoiding anticholinergic medications, benzodiazepines, and dose opioid medications to the minimal amount possible to control pain, as these medications may exacerbate delirium symptoms.[38]

Suicidality. Assessment for suicidality in medical settings is similar to assessment in other settings. Namely, you need to assess for any suicidal ideation, intent for suicide, or development of any suicide plan(s). Do not be afraid to ask direct questions regarding self-harm or suicidal ideation. Those questions have not been shown to "put the idea of suicide in their mind" as some therapists may wonder. Rather, it is an important part of your role to be clear regarding whether or not the patient is currently experiencing suicidal ideation, intent for suicide, or has developed a plan to enact suicidal action.

In addition, you should provide education regarding basic suicide behavioral safety planning, including efforts to help stabilize acute emotional distress, developing methods to help ensure safety such as utilization of the patient's social support, removing access to lethal means, practical problem-solving to help address sources of acute distress, and development of coping skills, such as relaxation techniques or other stress management approaches.

One difference in medical settings is that you have supportive resources around you that might not be available in other settings. For example, another intervention you may be able to recommend is that a "sitter," typically a nurse or other technician, remain with the patient for a period should you deem the patient presently to have acute risk of attempting suicide. Be mindful of potentially lethal objects commonly found in hospital rooms, including cords (due to risk of strangulation), sharp objects (eg, needles or syringes), or the patient's personal belongings. Alert hospital staff or police if available if you have imminent concerns regarding lethal objects in patient's personal home belongings.

It may also help to prepare the patient regarding any anticipated interventions that you will suggest to the team to help reduce any potential confusion or agitation. For example, you could say to your patient, "You've described to me that you have a specific plan and desire to harm yourself this morning, and in the interest of your safety I am going to ask for a hospital caregiver to remain present with you to help keep you safe. Do you have any questions about this plan?"

Your work as a therapist does not conclude when you are finished with your assessment. A critical step is to relay any concerns regarding patient suicidality to the medical team. Effective communication helps ensure patient safety by applying appropriate safety resources in a timely manner. Be mindful of your hospital, legal, and professional policies regarding confidentiality and sharing of information in the context of suicide risk concerns.

After follow-up assessment reveals that the risk for acute suicidality has subsided, maintain communication with the team and discuss plans to reinitiate the safety measures should the suicide risk elevate again. Should the patient remain at high risk for suicide yet otherwise be ready for discharge from the hospital from a medical standpoint, admission to a psychiatric facility may be warranted.

Self-harming behaviors. There are also situations where self-harm is of concern to the medical team, such as using sharp objects in the hospital room to superficially cut on the skin with a nonsuicidal self-injurious behavior. In addition to your assessment of suicidality, you should also assess for self-harm ideation, intent, and any potential plans for self-injurious behaviors. Be specific in your questions related to self-harm. For example, ask "Are you currently having any thoughts about harming yourself physically in any way?" rather than "Do you think you may ever do something to yourself?"

Following your therapeutic assessment, it is critical to relay any relevant concerns regarding the patient's immediate safety. Contact the referring provider to let them know any self-harm risk immediately, and also provide education if needed regarding the differences between nonsuicidal self-injury and suicide. Again, be familiar with the resources in your particular setting, be mindful of potentially lethal objects commonly found in hospital rooms, and familiarize yourself with the hospital, legal, and professional policies regarding confidentiality and sharing of information in the context of self-harm and suicide risk concerns.

Interventions to prevent self-harm are often short term in nature, using the least restrictive means possible. Similar to suicide-risk interventions, you should provide education regarding self-harm behavioral safety planning including efforts to help stabilize acute emotional distress, discussing methods to help ensure safety such as utilization of the patient's social support, removing access to self-injurious means, practical problem-solving to help address sources of acute distress, and development of coping skills such as relaxation techniques. The more collaborative the safety planning can be with the patient, the better "buy-in" is achieved.

Communicating Recommendations to the Medical Team

After your initial assessment is completed, you will always want to communicate any findings and recommendations to the referring provider(s). Physicians often carry heavy workloads and have limited availability, so be concise when describing your findings and specific recommendations. Do not assume that they are aware of all the therapeutic terminology that you use, as this may contribute to miscommunication about your important findings and recommendations.

Hospital settings are fast-paced environments, and rapid, accurate, concise communication and documentation is a necessary aspect of collaborative patient care. After seeing Mr. R, the psychology intern decides to tell the medical team about the nature of Mr. R's irritability, his concerns regarding certain communication patterns while hospitalized, and the therapy treatment plan that will focus on treating depression and anxiety. The intern also conveys the practical recommendations for the team to help address the immediate impacts of the patient's apparent memory problems on medical treatment adherence and then discusses the assessment and plan for any identified safety concerns. Finally, the intern documents the findings and simple recommendations in the medical chart on the same day, according to the standard of practice in the hospital setting, as another way to communicate with the medical team.

ONGOING PSYCHOTHERAPY IN CONSULTATION-LIAISON SETTINGS

Goal-Setting and Brief Interventions

Once the patient has been assessed, the therapeutic work may need to be time-limited, as patients will be discharged from the hospital when their acute medical issues have stabilized. Psychotherapy in hospital or other medical settings is typically considered short term and often includes solution-focused models with behavioral goals.[39] Thus, goal-setting is essential in forming the therapeutic framework and establishing reasonable expectations. Remember to work collaboratively with the patient in order to establish these goals.

Common goals for therapy in hospital settings include reduction of emotional distress, bolstering adherence to treatment recommendations, eliminating or adjustment problematic behaviors that interfere with medical care, and providing opportunities to process and develop insight into the impacts of medical illness on important domains of the patient's life. As a result, consider interventions that are solution focused, include adaptive problem-solving, and those that emphasize specific skills training (eg, relaxation techniques such as diaphragmatic breathing, communication skills training to help facilitate expression of patient needs). Additionally, learning and practicing specific behavioral coping skills like guided imagery, activity pacing, or mindfulness-based stress reduction exercises to help reduce anxiety. Biofeedback, diaphragmatic breathing exercises, hypnotherapy, distraction strategies, mindfulness practices, cognitive restructuring approaches, and progressive muscle relaxation can be used as approaches for the management of pain.[40] This may be particularly useful in situations where the patient is reporting pain despite medical intervention (eg, pain medications or medical procedures). Please see Chapter 5 (supportive psychotherapy) and Chapter 6 (CBT) in this textbook regarding the specific methods for implementing these types of interventions.

For Mr. R, the psychology intern suggests a problem-solving approach involving writing down questions for his doctors, including family members during discussion of the treatment plan (with his informed consent), and asking the medical team to provide him with written information (in his preferred language) about his treatment plan and medications. This may help address the impact of memory concerns on his ability to recall and understand his current medical regimen. Mr. R also expressed interest in learning relaxation skills to utilize when he is feeling anxious. The psychology intern responded with an explanation of technique rationale, instructions and demonstration of the technique, assistance with helping Mr. R practice the technique while in his hospital bed, establishing a plan for when to use or practice the technique, and inviting any questions from Mr. R about the technique rationale or process. This skill was revisited and developed during the next few brief psychotherapy sessions during Mr. R's hospitalization, as were additional skills surrounding communication.

Dealing With Interruptions

Earlier in this textbook, you learned about specific therapy methods to help provide emotional relief and behavioral change for patients. In this section, some of the unique challenges to implementation of these methods in consultation-liaison settings will be explored, along with suggested approaches to help address the challenges.

Those of us who work in hospital settings rarely enjoy the opportunity to perform a comprehensive initial interview or subsequent therapy sessions free of interruptions, within a quiet, stable, well-decorated therapy environment. Some interruptions are

10

medically urgent, and many are not, but most are unpredictable and unavoidable. Examples include the food service staff delivering lunch, the financial services office representative requesting insurance verification, and the radiology technician taking the patient to their scheduled imaging procedure. Attempts to predict more optimal times for psychotherapy sessions during hospitalization may help (eg, knowing the timing of meals in the facility, coordinating with nursing about the likely timing of tests or other procedures). In addition, you must remember that your patient is hospitalized for a reason. Your patient may experience distressing and distracting physical symptoms during an assessment or therapy session including shortness of breath, significant pain, drowsiness, gastrointestinal distress or vomiting, and bowel/bladder urgency. Keep in mind that an initial mental health assessment may require more than one visit to comprehensively gather information. It is helpful to acknowledge the shared "interruption" experience with your patient and maintain sensitivity to their medical treatment needs.

On a related note, needing to maintain boundaries as other individuals enter and exit the room is a required skill that you will also need to develop. We must be ever mindful of patient privacy and not assume that a visiting guest, family member, or medical provider is welcome to join in the midst of the patient's self-disclosure or therapeutic treatment planning. It is important to meet with the patient privately at first, even if it requires you to ask others to leave the room, thereby removing the onus from the patient. You might say, "I am going to be working with the patient for a period of time this afternoon. May we please have privacy while we do this?" Helpful statements at the beginning of an assessment might then include, "Some people prefer to speak with me individually, as I do ask several personal questions, although you are welcome to have your guest join us later if you'd prefer." You also may be able to prevent some disruptions by placing generic "Treatment in Progress" signs on the door when you are conducting psychotherapy, alerting staff to your presence prior to entering the patient's room, or politely requesting additional time for privacy upon entry to the room by unexpected guests.

For the case of Mr. R, the nurse who he felt was "eavesdropping" entered the room during one of your therapy sessions to give him his scheduled medications. Awareness of your surroundings and circumstances is key, in that you want to give Mr. R as much control over his privacy as possible. You might say, for example, "Why don't we pause for a moment, Mr. R, until you're done with your vital sign check and nursing assessment?" Given Mr. R's tenuous relationship with some members of his treatment team, this question is yet another way to give him control over privacy, without putting the onus on him entirely.

The Hospital Room Environment and Boundaries

Beeps. Alarms. Oh those beeping alarms! Hospital rooms are filled with various devices that are helpful in alerting to problems or mechanical malfunctions, but can also serve as distracting elements when engaging in psychotherapy. You will need to develop an ability to tolerate these kinds of potential distractions, and there may be times when it can be therapeutically beneficial to acknowledge with the patient the shared challenge of working together under distracting conditions.

You may also need to wear protective gear (ie, personal protective equipment [PPE]) such as a gown, mask, and gloves for both patient safety, as well as your own. Although a psychotherapist typically does not touch their patients like a physical therapist does, you are still in the treatment environment and required to follow all patient safety protocols. Make sure to check for any protective precautions or isolation status (as determined by the patient's medical team). There are times when it may be therapeutically useful to inquire what it feels like to have others wear protective gear when coming into their hospital room, as some patients may describe related feelings of emotional isolation or fears regarding contamination.

Also, there may be times when physical contact is requested by the patient (eg, "Can I give you a hug?" or "Can you tuck in my blanket?"). In reality, some patients struggle to navigate their physical environment in the hospital because of their health limitations and may request that you help them with a physical task, like picking up a sock on the floor or helping them reach (or use) their water glass, simply because you are in the room. Be familiar with hospital policies regarding physical contact, as well as your own personal reactions to these requests or to the unanticipated physical contact that can occur when maneuvering in tight hospital room spaces. If you deem the request inappropriate or would feel uncomfortable with the request for physical contact, you might say, "Thank you for asking, however, I've been in other patient rooms and I'd prefer to give you some space out of respect for your health," or "I appreciate the request, but I typically don't (hug/ make physical contact) in the way you're asking. Is there another way we could express that sentiment?"

Termination

Termination of therapy is often different in medical settings versus traditional outpatient therapy. One of the primary reasons for this involves the uncertainty of length of stay. Thus, it is important to identify the potentially time-limited nature of the therapy from the outset and acknowledge the uncertainties regarding anticipated duration of treatment. It is also important to be prepared with outpatient resources, in case the patient is discharged from the hospital earlier than you might have anticipated. This helps bridge the gap between short-term therapy interventions and additional outpatient therapeutic support once the patient has left the hospital. It always helps to be familiar with local counseling and psychiatric resources, and consider having a printed handout with counseling options to provide to the interested patient.

Sometimes therapy is terminated unexpectedly, either by patient choice or if they become unable to participate due to worsening medical problems or death. Make sure you establish the parameters of your continued follow-up during their hospital stay, including contingency plans should the patient's health deteriorate (eg, "I will continue to follow how things are going for you medically and can plan to return as soon as you are medically able"). For cases of termination by patient choice (eg, after patient feels they have achieved initial therapeutic goals such as crisis stabilization), consider discussing a follow-up "booster session" to help ascertain the degree to which the patient's therapeutic gains have been maintained after the initial termination.

10

In the case of your patient's death, you may experience a range of emotions including grief, anger, and fear. It is normal to have an emotional reaction, as these are individuals that you have worked with closely, often in an emotionally intimate manner. Be mindful of your own emotions and self-care in these situations, and it may help to reach out to colleagues, supervisors, and other sources of support. In some cases, you may want to consider engaging in your own personal individual therapy or grief support groups.

Sometimes it is not death that leads to unexpected termination, but rather the patient may be rapidly discharged from the hospital. You may experience this type of situation as not providing sufficient closure. Again, this is a normal reaction and yet a common experience in consultation-liaison settings. Consider talking with colleagues about how they deal with unexpected termination—you are not alone in this.

Returning to our case example of Mr. R, psychotherapy during hospitalization might provide a positive therapeutic experience that can help set the stage for his improved understanding of how therapy can be helpful for him, as well as increase the likelihood that he pursues appropriate therapy resources following his departure from the hospital. During his last day of hospitalization, the psychology intern chose to say to him, "Since you're going to be leaving the hospital this afternoon, it looks like our time working together in therapy will be ending. If therapy is something that you would like to continue doing as an outpatient after you leave the hospital, I would be happy to provide you with some outpatient therapy options." In the theme of ending the therapeutic work together, it may also be appropriate to share an expression of the positive nature of the therapy relationship such as "Thank you for letting me be part of your care, and I wish you well moving forward."

Conclusion

This chapter was focused on providing therapy in medical settings and is meant to provide a framework for effective conceptualization and considerations for the actual therapeutic process. Inherent challenges in hospital environments highlight the need for awareness of the dynamic relationship between physical health and mental health, as well as the specific kinds of therapeutic needs of patients in medical settings. Navigating healthcare systems, managing elements related to the hospital environment itself, psychological factors, and medical comorbidities collectively influence each patient's experience as they seek medical treatment. Whether in response to medical illness or related to the stress of a hospitalization or surgical intervention, therapists help support patients through a variety of services including therapy and serving as a liaison between the patient and medical providers. Accordingly, there is rich value in providing therapy to contribute to meaningful physical and emotional improvements for patients in medical settings.

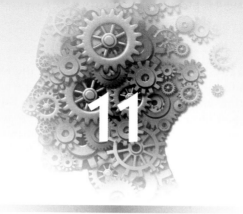

Psychotherapy in the Emergency Room/Crisis Clinical Encounter

ALEXANDER S. KANE, MD, ALISON E. LENET, MD, AND
DEBORAH L. CABANISS, MD

Case Study

Mr. R is a 38-year-old man who was born in a West African country, now living alone and recently working as a business analyst. He presents to the emergency room after experiencing intense suicidal thoughts to overdose on prescription opioids that were leftover from a recent oral surgery. The patient presents as distraught, tearful, and frightened by the intensity of his thoughts to harm himself. He tells the emergency medicine resident that he lost his job a few weeks ago after he found himself struggling to meet several important deadlines, and that he has since been "unable to keep it together."

INTRODUCTION

The emergency room may seem an unlikely place to conduct therapy. The pressures of rapid triage, diagnosis, and disposition, not to mention the oftentimes chaotic, loud, and disorienting environment, bear little resemblance to the steady pace and often tranquil confines of the outpatient office. What's more, patients who present to the psychiatric emergency room are, almost invariably, in some type of crisis—that is, their usual coping mechanisms and strategies have failed, and they do not know what to do. Patients often feel lost, hopeless, frightened, skeptical, and even angry.

Under these unfavorable conditions, trainees may find themselves understandably focused on simply gathering a coherent history, assessing symptoms, and making a diagnosis. After all, time and efficiency are of the essence. But far from being irrelevant in emergencies, a targeted psychotherapeutic approach can help us obtain the information we need to make a diagnosis and understand what interventions will be most useful to patients. Taking the time to consider how a person functions and how they came to be the way they are, even in a crisis, can help us build an alliance, accurately identify precipitants of crisis, organize their experience, and restore adaptive coping mechanisms.

HISTORY OF BRIEF INTERVENTIONS

Although it is true that the vast majority of psychotherapy is carried out in the comfort of consulting rooms over weeks, months, or years, Freud himself recognized the utility of brief psychotherapeutic interventions and carried out treatments that lasted only a few hours to days.[1] A few years later, in the early stages of World War I (WWI), it was noted that a segment of soldiers of the British Expeditionary Forces began reporting symptoms including confusion, panic, nightmares, and broader difficulties carrying out their duties. The term "shell shock" (now called posttraumatic stress disorder or PTSD) was used to describe these symptoms that were often found in the absence of physical injury and coined by soldiers themselves, linking these symptoms to their presumptive cause—the explosion of artillery shells.[2] By the end of WWI, many soldiers with shell shock symptoms would be given a few days of rest to recuperate and some brief treatment techniques were described. However, it was not until WWII that brief psychotherapy techniques were recognized broadly as a means of treating shell-shocked soldiers.[3]

Yet even as our understanding of mental illness has increased, the number of patients seeking care, the forces of deinstitutionalization, and the rise of community-based mental health care have together created a pressing need for specialized services equipped to manage the crises associated with decompensations of psychiatric illness. These include suicide prevention hotlines, mobile crisis services, and emergency psychiatry programs. The need for effective, time-limited interventions became increasingly clear, with this increased focus on management of mental illness and mental health emergencies in the community.

Contemporary research has demonstrated the efficacy of relatively brief, time-limited psychotherapeutic interventions across a broad range of psychiatric disorders, with depression being the most well studied. However, challenges in standardization, randomization, and identifying clear outcome measures have hindered the empirical study of psychotherapeutic interventions designed specifically for crisis situations. Despite these challenges, randomized controlled studies for a variety of therapeutic modalities (including brief psychodynamic psychotherapy, cognitive behavioral therapy [CBT], interpersonal psychotherapy [IPT], dialectical behavior therapy [DBT], and transference focused psychotherapy [TFP]) have shown significant acute reduction in depressive symptoms in as few as 6 to 8 sessions.[4-6] And while a single session of individual psychological debriefing has not proven to be effective in reducing distress or preventing PTSD in patients who have experienced trauma,[7-9] some randomized controlled trials of shorter courses (4-6 sessions) of CBT in the first month after trauma have shown significant reduction in PTSD symptoms at 6-month follow-up.[7]

There is some evidence that even single therapeutic encounters may have clinical benefit in crisis situations. For example, the safety planning intervention[10] is widely used in the management of suicidal thoughts and behaviors and draws on common psychotherapeutic principles such as building insight into triggers and engaging in joint problem-solving to identify coping strategies. Its adaptation for veterans has shown promise in the reduction of suicidal behaviors after a single in-person encounter before referral to other resources,[11,12] although further studies are necessary.

Thus, although more systematic empirical studies are required to quantify and understand the impact of psychotherapeutic interventions in crisis situations, the existing research in brief therapies, common factors, and clinical experience suggest a critical role for a psychotherapeutic approach for the crisis clinical encounter. Furthermore, the initial crisis encounter is not a circumscribed, comprehensive treatment for most patients. Rather, this encounter generally lays the groundwork and sets the tone for the potential longitudinal treatment to follow. As such, the goals of this kind of encounter are to create an alliance, contain affect, organize experience, support adaptive coping mechanisms, and facilitate transition to the next steps of care.

THE ER/CRISIS CLINICAL ENCOUNTER

What sets an emergency encounter apart from a routine office visit? How do these differences shape the contour of the encounter, and how does this alter the kind of psychotherapy we can offer?

The physical limitations of the emergency room, particularly regarding comfort and privacy, are perhaps what make a psychotherapeutic encounter here most different from one in an outpatient office. Clinicians may introduce themselves to patients who are resting on a gurney or draped in a hospital gown. There may be other patients nearby who are in acute pain, weeping, intoxicated, or shouting. There may be monitors beeping, medications being administered, or blood being drawn for laboratory testing. This discordant symphony of sights and sounds may be familiar to clinicians, but is likely to be strange, disorienting, and even frightening to patients.

The ER setting makes it necessary for crisis care clinicians to try to maintain at least some of the usual trappings of the psychotherapy encounter. For example, the interview should be conducted in a relatively private, quiet space with minimal interruption if possible. Both the patient and clinician should be seated and comfortable. Several studies have demonstrated that sitting with a patient can increase the patient's perception of time spent in the room[13] and enhance the patient's sense that the provider is listening carefully,[14] both critical elements in building a therapeutic relationship. When such an arrangement is not possible, acknowledging these limitations may help facilitate the development of a therapeutic alliance even in difficult circumstances.

11

The crisis encounter is also defined by its time-limited nature. Emergency evaluations force us to obtain a huge amount of diagnostic material within minutes from a patient we have likely never seen before and may never see again. What's more, our patients may be overwhelmed with sadness, fraught with anxiety, or in a state of shock—all of which may hinder their ability to provide a complete or accurate history.[15] This stands in stark distinction to longer-term therapies, in which a patient's history may unfold over the course of weeks, months, or even years. It is still critically important to think psychotherapeutically about our patients' conflicts, ways of relating, and patterns of thinking, feeling, and behaving. However, limited time means we have to limit our scope.

In order to focus our history as we gather information, keep in mind that the most critical question we must answer is "Why now?"[16] (see case conceptualization in Chapter 2 of this book). Although a patient's inability to form a secure attachment to a depressed and distant mother may contribute to their panic disorder, rarely will questions about infancy feel affectively pertinent to a patient in crisis. Additionally, the time constraints of the crisis encounter will rarely allow for such exploration. If we are able to answer the question of "Why now?" by identifying the patient's most relevant and immediate stressors during the initial encounter, current conflicts, patterns of coping, and symptoms, we will be able to begin the process of formulation (also known as conceptualization) in order to understand what interventions will then be most helpful.

FORMULATION IN THE ER/CRISIS CLINICAL ENCOUNTER

Emergency rooms or other crisis care settings are busy places where clinicians are pressed to make rapid diagnoses and decisions about disposition. Efficiency is essential and time is of the essence. Is this a place to think about formulation?

The answer is a resounding yes! Although trainees sometimes think about formulation as something that requires both long-term knowledge of a patient and time to construct, thinking about formulation is essential to taking care of patients in crisis care situations.

What Is a Formulation?

A formulation (also referred to as a *conceptualization*) is a hypothesis about how a person functions and how they came to be the way they are.[17] Formulations are based on knowledge about the patient and theories of causation. More than just a history, formulations offer ideas about why someone functions in a certain way. This knowledge is critical for being able to work psychotherapeutically, even in an acute situation. For example, it is hard to know what to offer someone psychotherapeutically if all you know is that they came into the emergency room with suicidal thoughts. However, knowing that the suicidal thoughts were, for example, in the context of a loss (amid several prior losses in the past) helps steer us toward a useful psychotherapeutic intervention.

Stressors and Vulnerabilities

We all experience stressors during our lives—losses, disappointments, conflicts with others, medical problems—yet we do not all experience them as crises.[18] Sometimes we do, and sometimes we do not. Understanding the "why" of the crisis often involves having a sense of specific vulnerabilities that turn certain stressors into crises. Formulating in ER/crisis situations thus involves having a sense of both common stressors and ways of thinking about vulnerabilities that may predispose a patient to experiencing those stressors as crises.

Common Stressors

Knowledge of the common stressors that often precipitate crises can help with history taking and pattern recognition. It is important to remember that people may or may not be aware that these stressors are linked to their crisis—it is often our job to put that together for them.

Loss—Attachment is a primary human need and thus loss often precipitates personal crisis.[19] This could be the loss of a person, either because of a death or a separation, or even the loss of a beloved pet. Loss of employment, physical health or capacity, or opportunities are also common forms of loss. Loss often presents as grief for what has been lost, which may linger for months or even years after the event.

Abandonment—While related to loss, abandonment is the sense that one has been actively left. It may be linked to feelings of betrayal. While people who have experienced loss may still feel connected, people who feel abandoned feel isolated and alone.

Trauma—This could be perpetrated by someone familiar or a stranger. It could be physical, sexual, or emotional. It could be part of a shared experience (eg, a natural disaster) or not (eg, rape). Difficult to contain feelings or impulses—extreme feelings of anger or anxiety can be nearly impossible to contain. The same is true of powerful impulses. They frequently lead to aggression, either toward oneself or others.

Common Ways to Conceptualize Vulnerability

In his classic paper, *Mourning and Melancholia*, Freud asked himself why loss precipitates crisis in one person and not another. He hypothesized that the difference had to do with whether one had unresolved (mostly negative) feelings about the lost person.[20] The idea that ambivalence about a stressor might trigger a crisis remains relevant.[18] But, other ideas are important as well. For example, the underlying level of function (sometimes called ego function)[21] plays an important role. Someone who has good reality testing, solid self-esteem, and the ability to think through problems might experience being fired as a difficult but manageable life event. However, this same event might precipitate a crisis in someone who lacks this high level of functioning. Personal or family history of major psychiatric illness, such as depression, bipolar disorder, anxiety, or substance use, as well as problematic core beliefs about oneself or insecure attachment, might also lead to vulnerability in the face of stressors. Social factors, including the level of emotional support provided by family and friends, financial resources, housing, access to appropriate mental

11

health care, immigrant status, and cultural attitudes toward the specific stressor may modulate a person's vulnerability to crisis (see Chapters 8 and 9 for more on these systemic concepts).

Focused Formulation in the ER/Crisis Clinical Encounter

Psychotherapeutic formulations of our patients generally rely on an understanding of their developmental histories and long-term patterns of relating and adapting to stressors. The time-limited nature of the crisis interaction means that we may not be able to generate the sort of detailed, exhaustive formulation that comes with months or years of outpatient therapy. But, even in crisis settings, having a sense of how people function, their patterns of coping, and their most relevant stressors will guide us as we consider what interventions will be most helpful.

Getting the information needed to formulate in the clinical crisis setting requires focus and efficiency. This is not the situation in which you have session after session to slowly understand the patient's underlying patterns and the precipitating problem. Rather, this needs to be done quickly and while simultaneously handling acute problems.

Generally, asking about someone's life history *in an empathic way* will help with engagement and make a person feel heard as an individual. Thinking about the common stressors listed above helps us to hone our questions and quickly recognize patterns in coping and vulnerability.

Example—Probing Stressors

In this setting, it is very reasonable to probe for the stressors mentioned above. You might use the following approach:

I see how upset you are and I'd like to understand it better. Has anything upsetting happened recently? Perhaps with someone close to you?

In addition, to get a sense of how people have handled stressors in the past, you might ask the following:

Has anything like this ever happened to you before? What happened then?

Once we have a sense of the stressor and potential vulnerabilities, we can learn something about them, but accept that the understanding will be fairly superficial given the constraints of the situation.

To think more about formulation in the crisis care situation, let us go back to Mr. R, the patient introduced at the beginning of this chapter—a 38-year-old man born in a West African country who presented to the ER after experiencing intense suicidal thoughts to overdose on painkillers left over from dental surgery. We have information about the presenting problem, but still remain far from being able to answer the question "Why now?" Below is an illustration of one way to identify the patient's perceptions of a recent loss, in the context of prior losses.

Case Study—Identifying Loss

Dr. G, the emergency room psychiatrist, is asked to consult on Mr. R. Dr. G learns that Mr. R has a history of mild depressive symptoms for which he took sertraline in his early 20s, but that Mr. R has not been in treatment since then. Dr. G tells Mr. R that he understands he recently lost his job. Mr. R responds, *"Yes—I used to take a lot of pride in my job—I was able to send a lot of money back home to my mother. When she passed away 6 months ago, at first it was helpful to distract myself with work, but as time went on it just got harder and harder to get out of bed. I guess I've really screwed this up."*

Knowing that loss is a common stressor, and hearing about this recent loss, Dr. G asks Mr. R about his relationship with his mother. Mr. R explains that he emigrated alone from a West African country at age 19 years for college in the United States, leaving behind his mother and his adoptive father. He says that this man, who died of cardiac disease 10 years ago, was physically abusive to both him and his mother. He explains, *"I've always felt so guilty about leaving, but she wouldn't let me pass up the opportunity. We spoke almost every day on the phone—I didn't visit as much as I should have, but we spoke all the time. It was so hard coming here and not knowing anyone. I knew I had to succeed for her sake."* Noting the patient starting to brighten somewhat as he talks about his mother, Dr. G says quietly, *"It seems like she was incredibly important to you."* Mr. R goes on, *"Yeah. I've had a hard time feeling connected to people in the United States, I've been sort of a loner. But, I knew I could always turn to her. When she was gone, I didn't have anyone to talk to, not really. I didn't see the point anymore."*

How Formulating Helps Treatment in the ER/Crisis Clinical Encounter

With just a few questions, Dr. G learns both about a recent loss (common stressor) and vulnerability (loss of an important attachment). This will help him to formulate and construct potential psychotherapeutic interventions. Having a sense of the "why" of the crisis helps us to engage the patient by enhancing our understanding of the situation, and being able to articulate this explanation to a patient in crisis can be very therapeutic. It also helps us to select the type of psychotherapeutic technique to use. For example, if we view the crisis as due to weakened function, we can try to bolster function through supportive techniques. However, if we feel that the crisis was precipitated by thoughts or feelings that are out of the patient's awareness, we might try to help the person become aware of them. Perceived abandonment might prompt a crisis family meeting, while extreme anger might require the formation of a temporary holding environment.

11

PSYCHOTHERAPEUTIC GOALS AND TECHNIQUES IN THE ER/CRISIS ENCOUNTER

As we have discussed, seeing a patient in a crisis setting is quite different than seeing a patient in the office. The physical setting, time frame, presenting complaint, and emergency clinician's role in the treatment all set the emergency encounter apart from "therapy as usual." What does this mean for how we conduct therapy in these settings? How do we adapt our psychotherapeutic technique and goals to meet the needs of a patient in crisis?

Common Factors

Some aspects of psychotherapy are critical no matter the setting. They are the heart of all psychotherapeutic interventions, including those in crisis care situations, and were covered in Chapter 4 of this book. Many of the fundamental therapeutic skills described previously translate well to the crisis setting. To review, these are generally referred to as common factors[22] and include the following:

Empathic listening—This involves helping the patient to feel that the clinician is trying to understand the patient's current experience of the world. It requires active techniques such as using comments like, *"What I hear you saying is…"* and *"It sounds like that was really difficult for you."*

Instilling hope—Therapy in the crisis care setting is not the moment for stone-faced neutrality. It is essential to say things like, *"I'm so glad that you came in. I really think that talking about this will help you. I think that we can even make a difference today,"* as long as these sentiments are realistic.

Offering a cogent rationale for psychotherapy—Everyone knows that psychotherapists talk to patients. But, patients want to know how and why this will help them. Saying something like, *"Often, locking feelings away is enough to put you over the edge—I think that you'll be surprised at how much talking today will help,"* explains why you think that talking is important.[21]

Areas of Emphasis in Crisis

Undoubtedly, at the foundation of psychotherapy in crisis are techniques and goals that are found in nearly all psychotherapeutic modalities. That said, the unique demands of the crisis clinical encounter will lead us to put particular emphasis on the techniques and goals below.

Safety

Perhaps the most important factor that differentiates the crisis care encounter is the explicit focus on safety. Patients in crisis are often driven to emergency care by intense feelings—fear, despair, anxiety, anger, or even agitation—coupled with a difficulty managing and containing those feelings. In this setting, patients are at an acutely elevated risk of engaging in actions that may cause harm to themselves and potentially others. As such, the safety of the patient, the clinician, and other patients in the milieu is always the first priority and should be assessed and monitored throughout the therapy. Some critical safety interventions include the following:

- Reviewing records prior to interview, with a focus on prior suicidality, non-suicidal self-injury, trauma, substance use, and prior aggression or violence, to better understand the patient's risk of acute dangerousness to themselves and others.

- Attending to the safety of physical surroundings, including removal of objects that may be used as weapons.

- Ensuring that patients who are at immediate risk of harm to self or others are maintained on an appropriate level of observation.

- Maintaining a safe distance from patients who are aggressive, agitated, or impulsive.

- Performing a thorough suicide risk assessment and documenting your decision-making process.

- Assessing if the patient is at risk of harm by others and identifying areas for intervention.

- Reviewing coping strategies that the patient may use to manage intense affects.

Safety in the ER Setting

It is important for providers entering a psychotherapy encounter in the ER to be mindful of environmental differences in this setting versus more traditional psychotherapy settings and to have strategies to maintain safety. These strategies include the following:

- Communicating with other staff (nurses, security personnel, physicians) who have interacted with the patients to see if they have safety concerns.

- Telling staff where you will be meeting with your patients so they are aware of your location.

- Maintaining a safe distance and positioning yourself closest to the door during encounters.

- Being aware of the environment, including comings and goings of other staff and patients, as well as noises and alarms in the environment.

- Avoid wearing accessories that can be used against you in an unsafe manner (neckties, dangling/hoop earrings, etc.).

- Following your instincts—if something about a patient's history or initial response makes you nervous, seek assistance/supervision and determine whether it may be necessary to enter the encounter with additional staff members present.

Case Study—Talking About Safety Concerns

It sounds like you have been having a really difficult time these past few months with your mother's death and your struggles at work. I am very concerned about the suicidal thoughts you have been experiencing and I would like to focus our conversation on ways you can keep yourself safe while you feel this bad. You mentioned that distraction is one technique you try when things are difficult. Let's take some time to think of other ways to help you cope with these distressing thoughts.

Alliance

Therapeutic alliance is among the best predictors of success in psychotherapy.[22] In crisis settings, the patient's affective bond to the clinician, ability to work collaboratively, and alignment of patient and clinician goals are critical. Developing a working therapeutic alliance and rapport in emergency conditions may be challenging, but, at the same time, the inchoate quality of an initial encounter with a patient in crisis offers unique opportunities for therapeutic intervention and growth.[23]

Case Study—Building Alliance

It was so important that you brought yourself to the emergency room today. It was a great start to turning things around. What was your goal in reaching out for help today? Knowing that will help us to focus our work together.

Containing Affect

Patients in the crisis care setting almost invariably experience intense panic, anxiety, sadness, despair, or anger in the setting of an acute stressor. In crisis, the usual coping mechanisms patients use to maintain their equilibrium and manage stress have failed—we can expect that our patients will often have difficulties managing these overwhelming affects. One of our core psychotherapeutic objectives will be to help lessen and contain affect, so that our patients can begin to mobilize their individual strengths and more adaptive coping mechanisms. Containing affect is the process by which a clinician helps keep a patient from being overpowered by strong emotions. We can contain affect by using supportive interventions such as naming emotions, providing reassurance, empathizing, and validating a patient's feelings.[21] By remaining calm, tolerating the intensity of the patient's emotions, and helping to put those feelings into words, we can help patients to translate overwhelming, chaotic feelings into something more concrete and promote self-reflection.

Case Study—Containing Feelings

You've just told me how difficult things have been these past few months. Taking into account what you have explained about your past, it sounds like these recent stressors have really intensified your feelings of guilt and anxiety and it has been really difficult to manage. Does that sound right to you? If it does, it can help us to understand your experience and to work on ways to cope with these feelings.

Organizing Experience

Patients in crisis often feel disoriented and unmoored by the chaos of stressors and their difficulties adapting to them. By organizing the patient's narrative and placing the current crisis within the broader context of the patient's life, clinicians can calm patients and help restore more helpful coping strategies. This technique may help the patient to make sense out of what otherwise may feel like a senseless situation, restoring some semblance of control and order to the patient.[24]

Case Study—Organizing Experience

It sounds like feelings of loss have been a major stressor for you. I have to imagine moving far from your family felt like a loss and played a role in your feelings of depression in your early 20s. With the recent loss of your mother, you are feeling understandably more isolated and sad.

Bringing Thoughts and Feelings to Awareness

There are many reasons that a patient may not have full awareness of their underlying feelings. Defense mechanisms often help push conflicts or more difficult feelings such as shame, guilt, and anger out of awareness. Feelings that are out of a patient's awareness can often influence the way they behave and react, especially during times of stress. When done with care, helping patients become aware of underlying feelings and conflicts can sometimes make an enormous difference in a crisis situation. It can help them understand their own reaction and help them feel more in control.

Case Study—Increasing Awareness

You know, it sounds like this job was more than just a job for you—it represents the type of opportunity you sought when you left your home country. You have also had a lot of complicated feelings about this job. While it allowed you to support your mother and stay connected to her in a way, it was also associated with the chronic guilt you felt in leaving her. When a crisis or tragic event happens, it tends to bring up some of these more difficult feelings.

Providing Structure and Encouraging Adaptive Coping

Although our formulation may take in broader aspects of the patient's history and life, our goals and techniques in the crisis encounter generally focus on the here and now. Helping patients to identify coping mechanisms that they can use immediately after discharge or providing structure for the hours and days until an outpatient appointment can be the most effective psychotherapeutic interventions for this setting.

11

Case Study—Encouraging Adaptive Coping

I know that you want to talk more about your mother, and I think unpacking your feelings about your relationship with her will be really important moving forward. For now, I would like to focus on how you can start to use your other supports. Who are the other important people in your life that you can reach out to now? Can we think together about what you might say to them when you are feeling this distressed and how they may be able to help you?

Bridging to Further Treatment

Often, the most important thing that we can do to help a patient in a crisis setting is to help connect—or reconnect—them to longer-term treatment. Sometimes, a patient will have had a connection to a previously helpful therapist or a clinic that they fear has lapsed. Talking to the patient about this and actually working to restore the connection can be lifesaving. When this is not the case, helping the patient to recognize that longer-term treatment is needed can be the crucial goal.

Case Study—Bridging to Further Treatment

I am so glad that you came in today to talk about these distressing thoughts and feelings you have been experiencing. This visit marks a beginning of your recovery. Let's think together about the best and safest setting to continue to work on these problems and help you start to feel better.

THE THREE-STEP APPROACH TO SUPPORTIVE PSYCHOTHERAPY IN THE ER/CRISIS CLINICAL ENCOUNTER

As we have seen in the above example, supportive psychotherapy interventions that are designed to help support weakened or faltering function are ideally suited to the ER/crisis clinical encounter.[25] Regardless of the diagnosis, the issues that generally bring people to a crisis clinical encounter involve problems with functions such as impulse control, coping mechanisms, relationships with others, self-esteem management, anger/anxiety management, and the ability to perceive reality.[21] Supportive psychotherapy helps bolster these functions. For some patients, this help is needed acutely (eg, a person in the middle of a major depressive episode), while for others, this help is needed on an ongoing basis (eg, a person who has a severe and persistent mental illness). If someone is completely unable to use one of these functions, we can supply them; if they have some capacity to use them, we can assist them.

Example—Supplying

Patient—I'm totally inept. I can't think of anything that I've ever done that was any good.

Therapist—You know, just coming to the ER was a really good move. So you're doing better than you think.

Example—Assisting

Patient—I don't know what to say to my friend about why I came to the emergency room.

Therapist—OK, let's think about 3 things you want to be sure to communicate. We can even role-play exactly what you might say.

Supportive psychotherapy for the crisis context is easily learned, and its techniques can be used in as little as one session. The Three-Step Supportive Psychotherapy manual, created by the chapter authors and included as an appendix, breaks down the technique of this important treatment into three clear steps:

Learning about the patient—particularly learning about the way that the person is functioning, current stressors, and history of coping in the past.

Setting realistic goals—working with the patient to think of goals for the therapy that could be attained quickly and could help right now.

Working together on those goals—setting the frame for the therapy (which could mean talking once in an emergency room!) and utilizing basic techniques to help improve function now.

Here is how this might sound for Mr. R:

Case Study—Three-Step Approach
Step 1—Learning About the Patient

Dr. G—Hello, Mr. R, I'm Dr. G, one of the doctors working in the psychiatric emergency room today. I understand that you've already spoken to one of our nurses, but can you tell me about what happened that led you to come in today?

Mr. R—Jamal brought me in—I don't know if I needed to come.

Dr. G—Why did Jamal think that you needed to come in?

Mr. R—I haven't been feeling too well since I lost my job. It's been rough.

Dr. G—That sounds rough. How bad has it been?

Mr. R—I'm running out of money—I had some, but it's almost gone, and it all seemed pointless.

Dr. G—Did you have thoughts of hurting yourself or of taking your life?

Mr. R—Not really—I might have said something like that—but I don't know.

Dr. G—Is Jamal a close friend?

Mr. R—Not really. I don't really have anyone here.

Dr. G—So you feel pretty alone.

Mr. R—Yeah—and my mom died this year.

Dr. G—I'm so sorry to hear that. So you don't have anyone here now? No family?

Mr. R—No one. That's the hardest part. Sometimes I don't think anyone would notice if I weren't here anymore.

Dr. G—Wow—it's tough to go through something like losing your job when you feel so alone.

11

Step 2—Setting Realistic Goals

Dr. G—It seems like it would really help things if you felt more connected. Do you think it would make sense for us to think together about how to make that happen?

Mr. R—You can't bring back my mother.

Dr. G—No, of course not, but what if we took some time to think about ways that you might feel less alone, particularly now?

Mr. R—Sure, we could do that.

Step 3—Working Together Toward That Goal

Dr. G—Let's take a few minutes now to really think about this. Why don't you take this piece of paper? If you can, write down the names of three people you've spoken to in the last few days.

Mr. R—There's my landlord, but he certainly doesn't know anything about my life. I guess that leaves Jamal and Cynthia.

Dr. G—Isn't Jamal the person who brought you in?

Mr. R—Yeah.

Dr. G—How do you know him?

Mr. R—We worked together. He left about 6 months ago—got something better. We're both from my country. Turns out his father knew my uncle back home.

Dr. G—Oh, interesting. How did he know that you were feeling so bad?

Mr. R—He called me when he hadn't seen me in a while. Wanted to know what was going on.

Dr. G—Hmm—that means that he definitely noticed that you weren't around.

Mr. R—That's true, but he's got his own issues—kids, Cynthia, his wife.

Dr. G—Maybe we could get Jamal to come back in today to talk some more. I have a feeling that he may be more connected than you think.

Mr. R—I just feel bad asking him for anything.

Dr. G—Well, maybe that's what we need to talk about together.

Mr. R—OK—but please tell him this was your idea, not mine.

Dr. G—You're right, it was—that's no problem. I'll see if I can get him on the phone.

Using the three steps allows Dr. G to quickly hone in on a problem that he and Mr. R can address right now—the feeling of being disconnected from other people. Using a collaborative technique helps them to realize that there is a person who is connected to Mr. R, and to propose an intervention. Role-playing, helping someone to express a feeling, collaborative problem-solving, helping to organize thoughts, and suggesting alternate ways to look at a situation are other supportive psychotherapy techniques that work in the crisis clinical encounter.

TIPS FOR SUPERVISION IN ER/CRISIS CLINICAL ENCOUNTERS

While working in the ER, trainees will need guidance from supervisors to focus their assessments and plan therapeutic interventions. The following are suggestions for trainees to optimize supervision in this setting:

- Conduct supervision in a space that maintains patient confidentiality and is as quiet and free from distraction as possible.

- Ask supervisors to focus on tangible items from the patient's history that contribute to a focused formulation.

- Ask supervisors to help you identify high-yield goals that are achievable during a brief encounter and convey optimism.

- Discuss the risk factors and protective factors with your supervisor to assess patient safety.

- Discuss your feelings and reactions to patients with your supervisors and learn how this may inform diagnosis, formulation, strategies for building an alliance, and techniques for containing affect while working with patients.

- Ask for tips from your supervisors for self-care in managing the emotional strain that can develop during work with acutely ill patients in crisis.

Conclusion

Crisis clinical settings, such as ERs, provide fertile ground for brief psychotherapeutic interventions that are firmly rooted in common factors and supportive psychotherapy. In this chapter, we covered

- how to use information gathered in a brief encounter to develop a focused and relevant formulation,

- common psychotherapeutic techniques and goals for a brief psychotherapeutic encounter in the emergency setting, and

- an easy-to-learn three-step approach to supportive psychotherapy in an emergency setting.

Focused formulations and realistic, collaboratively constructed goals can help patients face the here and now and bridge to longer-term treatments.

11

Self-Study Questions

1. What are the goals for psychotherapeutic encounters in a crisis setting?

2. What goes into a focused formulation, and how does it help you plan treatment?

3. What areas are emphasized during therapeutic encounters in the ER?

4. Thinking of a recent patient you have seen in crisis, name three examples of things you said that might have been supportive psychotherapy interventions.

RESOURCES FOR FURTHER LEARNING

See Reference List.

APPENDIX

THREE-STEP SUPPORTIVE PSYCHOTHERAPY MANUAL

Much of what we do with patients all day is psychotherapy. When we do things like help patients to make sense of their experience, set personal goals, feel better about themselves, cope with stress, and get along better with others, we are doing psychotherapy. So, it is probably just a new way to think about what you are already doing! And, it does not have to take a lot of time. Here is a three-step manual to help you make psychotherapy part of what you do in every patient interaction. You can do all three steps in a single encounter with a patient.

The kind of psychotherapy we are talking about is supportive psychotherapy, which helps people improve their functioning. It is very well suited for acute or short-term clinical situations, as well as for settings in which you are less likely to do intensive or long-term psychotherapy (such as community clinics). Most mental health providers are engaged in supportive psychotherapy with patients without even knowing that they are doing it. This short guide is designed to help you to more efficiently use supportive psychotherapy in your interactions with patients.

Before you start—consider—what is psychotherapy?

To be considered psychotherapy, you need:

- A patient
- A mental health provider
- Talking
- A frame (the parameters of the therapy, such as where you will meet, for how long, and what the fee will be)
- The shared goal of improving the patient's mental and emotional health

This can be easily done in these settings and can be enormously helpful to patients.

Step 1—Learn About the Patient

When you meet patients, you are going to learn about them. To best help them with their function, you want to learn:

- What is happening right now?
- What is causing them the most difficulty?
- How have they handled crises in the past?

11

Important functions to learn about include:

- Sense of self

- Relationships with others

- Ways of coping with stress and strong feelings

- Thinking and decision-making

- How they spend their time (working and playing)

Even while you are getting this information—which you can do in a short initial encounter—you are beginning the psychotherapy. Remembering these essential questions will help you learn about the patient:

- Who are the most important people in your life now, and how are you getting along with them?

- Tell me about a time that you feel like you handled a crisis well.

- What are the things that you are most proud of in your life?

- How can I most help you now?

After talking to the patient, take a few minutes to review the patient's functioning and to think about how you and the patient together could work to improve it.

Step 2—Set Goals

Find out what the patient wants to work on and help them create a realistic goal to work on right now. Although patients may have many goals, here are six basic psychotherapy goals that can be useful for patients in any setting and clinical situation:

1. Understanding one's own feelings and feeling understood by others

2. Making sense of what brought them to treatment

3. Mobilizing adaptive coping skills to deal with current problems

4. Maintaining self-esteem in the face of current problems

5. Getting along with other people

6. Planning for the short-term future (ongoing treatment and reentry to their lives)

Next, take a few minutes to choose together one or two goals that make sense and are meaningful for this patient now.

Step 3—Work Together to Take Action on the Goal

There are three basic skills that you need for any psychotherapy:

- **Making an alliance**—To conduct psychotherapy, the patient has to trust that you are trying to help them. You can help to develop this trust by introducing yourself and trying, from the first time you meet, to show the patient that you are interested, that you understand, and that you can see things from his/her point of view (empathy). Being friendly, restating things that the person tells you, making good eye contact, and instilling hope are all ways to do this. There is always a way to instill hope, even when the situation is dire; for example, you can help someone to view their voluntary admission as the start of better self-care, or to think about a serious illness as a moment to really connect to family members. You have information to get, but making good eye contact rather than writing notes is key.

- **Setting the frame and establishing boundaries**—No matter where you see patients, you need to set a frame together—this includes

  - *Where you will meet*

  - *When you will meet*

  - *How long your meetings will be*

  - *How many total meetings you will have*

  - *Whether there will be a fee*

The frame is different in different settings—it could be a 10-minute conversation in front of a nurses' station on an inpatient unit or a 15-minute conversation at the bedside on a medical service. Think about the best frame for this patient, considering the capacity and needs of the patient and discuss so that you can decide upon a mutually agreed upon plan.

- **Empathic listening**—Try to listen in order to understand the patient's point of view. This could be very different from your point of view. Periodically check that you are on the right track by saying things like, "So it sounds like what you're feeling is…" or "Let me see if I'm understanding what you're trying to say…"

Take a few moments to think about your strategies for making an alliance, what frame makes sense in this situation, and how to listen empathically.

Now you are ready to go! When you see the patient, talk together about:

- Goals—ask about what they would like to work on, share what you are considering and why, and reach a mutually agreed upon decision.

- The frame—discuss the frame that you have thought of so that the patient knows your recommendation about when you will be meeting and for how long. Discuss and reach a mutually agreed upon decision.

11

You can use the following basic psychotherapy techniques to help you achieve the six major psychotherapeutic goals for these settings:

1. **Encouraging the patient to talk about feelings**—Simply talking about feelings can be very therapeutic. You can also help people to name their feelings, validate their feelings, feel that their feelings are understandable, and begin to understand why they might be having those feelings.

2. **Helping the patient to tell the story of the current situation**—This is already part of what you do when you take a history. Restating it in a linear form can help the patient to make more sense of what happened. This can be very organizing and therapeutic to a patient in crisis.

3. **Encouraging the patient to discuss ways they have coped with past difficulties**—This can help you to encourage use of coping strategies that are already strong and to try to modify or discourage less adaptive coping strategies. Encouraging patients to talk about their lives, particularly things that they think that they have done well, can give you information about strengths that you might not otherwise see in the patient in acute crisis. Once you have some sense of these, you and the patient can think together about how to apply them to the current situation.

4. **Highlighting strengths and past accomplishments**—You not only want to hear about the crisis—you want to hear about the whole person, particularly things that the person has done well and is proud of. Reminding the patient of these strengths is key to maintaining self-esteem during the crisis. Praise and encouragement are important supportive psychotherapy interventions that can help you to achieve this goal.

5. **Learning about key relationships and role-play**—Learning about the key relationships in the person's life will help you to know (1) upon whom the person can rely and (2) strengths and challenges that the person has in interpersonal relationships. Problems with relationships—either with family members and/or with members of the treatment team—are often central to the crisis. Practicing new ways of relating to these key people during this time, including role-play with you, is a good way of addressing this. "Let's think together about how to ask for help from the nurse next time she comes…"

6. **Talking about next steps**—One of the most important roles for psychotherapy in these settings is connecting the person to ongoing treatment and helping the person to reenter his/her life. Helping the person who has burnt bridges save face is important, as is building a bridge to the outpatient treatment team. Simple techniques, such as carefully planning out the first day after discharge (writing a list together) can be very organizing. Focusing on short-term rather than long-term goals is key here.

7. Consider discussing your plan with a peer or supervisor.

REMEMBER—You are always a psychotherapist! Most of your work with patients in clinical settings is psychotherapy. Psychotherapy does not just happen in outpatient offices during 45-minute sessions. So, when seeing patients, take a few minutes to think about how patients are functioning and how you might help them improve their function in the face of current problems. Your patients will benefit, and you will be doing psychotherapy!

REFERENCES

1. Freud S. On the psychical mechanism of hysterical phenomena: preliminary communication from studies in hysteria. In: Strachey J, Freud A, Strachey A, Tyson A, trans-eds. *The Standard Edition of the Complete Psychological Works of Sigmund Freud.* Vol 2 (1893-1895). London, United Kingdom: Hogarth Press; 1893.
2. Everly GS Jr. Emergency mental health: an overview. *Int J Emerg Ment Health.* 1999;1(1):3-7.
3. Glass AJ. Psychotherapy in the combat zone. *Am J Psychiatry.* 1954;110(10):725-731.
4. Cluver J. How brief can effective psychotherapy be? *Prim Care Companion J Clin Psychiatry.* 2004;6(2):89-90.
5. Nieuwsma JA, Trivedi RB, Mcduffie J, Kronish I, Benjamin D, Williams JW. Brief psychotherapy for depression: a systematic review and meta-analysis. *Int J Psychiatry Med.* 2012;43(2):129-151.
6. Winston A, Winston B. Toward an integrated brief psychotherapy. *J Psychiatr Pract.* 2001;7(6):377-390.
7. Ehlers A, Clark D. Early psychological interventions for adult survivors of trauma: a review. *Biol Psychiatry.* 2003;53(9):817-826.
8. Flannery RB Jr, Everly GS Jr. Crisis intervention: a review. *Int J Emerg Ment Health.* 2000;2(2):119-125.
9. Rose S, Bisson J, Churchill R, Wessely S. Psychological debriefing for preventing post-traumatic stress disorder (PTSD). *Cochrane Database Syst Rev.* 2002;(2):CD000560.
10. Stanley B, Brown G. Safety planning intervention: a brief intervention to mitigate suicide risk. *Cogn Behav Pract.* 2012;19(2):256-264.
11. Bryan CJ, Mintz J, Clemans TA, et al. Effect of crisis response planning vs. contracts for safety on suicide risk in U.S. army soldiers: a randomized clinical trial. *J Affect Disord.* 2017;212:64-72.
12. Stanley B, Chaudhury SR, Chesin M, et al. An emergency department intervention and follow-up to reduce suicide risk in the VA: acceptability and effectiveness. *Psych Serv.* 2016;67(6):680-683.
13. Swayden KJ, Anderson KK, Connelly LM, Moran JS, Mcmahon JK, Arnold PM. Effect of sitting vs. standing on perception of provider time at bedside: a pilot study. *Patient Educ Couns.* 2012;86(2):166-171.
14. Merel SE, Mckinney CM, Ufkes P, Kwan AC, White AA. Sitting at patients' bedsides may improve patients' perceptions of physician communication skills. *J Hosp Med.* 2016;11(12):865-868.
15. MacKinnon RA, Michels R, Buckley PJ. *The Psychiatric Interview in Clinical Practice.* Washington, DC: American Psychiatric Publishing, Inc; 2006.
16. Sulkowicz KJ. Psychodynamic issues in the emergency department. *Psychiatr Clin North Am.* 1999;22(4):911-922.
17. Cabaniss DL, Cherry S, Douglas CJ, Graver R, Schwartz AR. *Psychodynamic Formulation.* Oxford, England: Wiley; 2013.
18. Glick RA, Meyerson AT. The use of psychoanalytic concepts in crisis intervention. *Int J Psychoanal Psychother.* 1980;8:171-188.
19. Main M. Introduction to the special section on attachment and psychopathology: 2. Overview of the field of attachment. *J Consult Clin Psychol.* 1996;64(2):237-243.
20. Freud S. Mourning and melancholia. In: Strachey J, Freud A, Strachey A, Tyson A, trans-eds. *The Standard Edition of the Complete Psychological Works of Sigmund Freud.* Vol 14 (1914-1916). London, United Kingdom: Hogarth Press; 1917.
21. Cabaniss DL, Cherry S, Douglas CJ, Schwartz AR. *Psychodynamic Psychotherapy, A Clinical Manual.* Oxford, England: Wiley; 2016.
22. Frank J. Therapeutic factors in psychotherapy. *Am J Psychother.* 1971;25:350-361.
23. Kardener SH. A methodologic approach to crisis therapy. *Am J Psychother.* 1975;29(1):4-13.
24. Viederman M. The psychodynamic life narrative: a psychotherapeutic intervention useful in crisis situations. *Psychiatry.* 1983;46(3):236-246.
25. Winston A, Rosenthal RN, Pinsker H. *Introduction to Supportive Psychotherapy.* Washington, DC: American Psychiatric Press International; 2004.

11

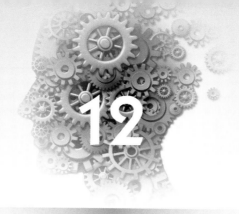

Psychotherapy on Inpatient Psychiatric Units

AMY S. BRENNER, MSW, LCSW AND ADAM M. BRENNER, MD

Case Study

Mr. D is a 35-year-old white man, married, with two young children. He held a good job as an upper-level accounts manager. This is his second hospitalization on the inpatient unit in the last 6 months. During his previous stay, he was diagnosed with bipolar disorder, due to the manic symptoms he was exhibiting—not sleeping, pressured speech, disappearing in the middle of the night, and the delusion that he was being followed by "men who want to hurt [him]." He had been stable on a mood stabilizer since the first hospitalization. This was prescribed to him by an outpatient psychiatrist he saw every 2 months for medication monitoring.

However, several weeks ago, he was fired from his job after a fight with his boss, when he yelled obscenities and threatened to kill him. He then disappeared for several days, during which time the bipolar symptoms were exacerbated. He was brought to the psychiatric emergency department (Psych ED) by the police, who found him wandering the streets of the downtown area, disheveled, talking to himself, and combative when approached.

The doctor at the Psych ED felt that Mr. D was too symptomatic to be discharged safely. Mr. D was still concerned about people following him, he was threatening in his approach to staff, and his pressured speech was often not completely coherent. He needed a period not only to restabilize on medications, but also to tease out whether there was more to the picture. During the initial ED assessment, Mr. D had casually mentioned he had nothing left to live for.

Collateral information indicated Mr. D's wife has become increasingly scared of her husband's behavior. After the first hospitalization 6 months ago, she thought about asking for a divorce. She was afraid Mr. D would hurt her or the children. However, because things settled down for a while, she felt disrupting the family dynamic would be too difficult on everyone. Several weeks ago, however, Mr. D started to seem worse. He was talking rapidly and incessantly, and he was not sleeping more than 1 to 2 hours a night. When she would ask if he had taken his medication, he would tell her he was fine and did not need it anymore. He called her from the office the day he was fired, incoherently telling her something had happened. He did not return home that night or the next. She filed a missing person report with the police because she could not reach him. She was notified by Psych ED staff 2 days later that Mr. D was being admitted to the inpatient psychiatric unit.

INTRODUCTION: THE UNIQUE NATURE OF INPATIENT PSYCHOTHERAPY

Often, the first place a trainee will work will be an inpatient psychiatric unit. Why start where the patients are at their most ill? This is a good question, but this setup is actually very fortunate for you. You will see a vast array of symptoms, many you have only read about up to now. Because of that array of presentations, you will also see a very diverse set of treatments.

Many inpatient units have a variety of treatment modalities that a patient participates in during the day. There are individual therapy and medication meetings. Often there are groups and individual treatment focusing on symptom and mood management, psychoeducation regarding illness, goal setting, stress reduction, and enhancement of coping strategies, with the idea that all of these decrease the current acuity and help prevent relapse. Depending on the robustness of the system, art and music therapy, occupational therapy, and physical therapy/body work may also be available.

Remember that you are part of a multidisciplinary team on the inpatient unit. It is important to be respectful of all team members, not just the attending physicians or supervising providers in your discipline. Each of the staff members on the unit will have therapeutic interactions with your patients all day in various settings, so getting to know their perspective is of great value. Also, a team where each discipline appreciates and respects the work of the others will combine to give the best care possible.

A great deal of psychotherapeutic work goes on in inpatient settings. And yet, you will sometimes hear people talk about inpatient stays as if psychotherapy was not central to the work of the unit. Why is this? We believe much of the effective psychotherapy that happens on inpatient units is simply overlooked because it may not be the stated purpose of the patient-clinician encounter. It is easy to appreciate that psychotherapy is at work when it is provided explicitly—for example, if a treatment team member is assigned to meet with the patient for psychotherapy sessions. However, experienced and effective inpatient clinicians often integrate psychotherapy into their administrative or medication management meetings with patients, as a great deal of therapeutic value can be provided even when you are not meeting for a specific "psychotherapy session."

Appreciating this broader view of how psychotherapy happens, we will next look at two specific ways that inpatient psychotherapy often differs from outpatient: (1) the degree of flexibility required of the clinician and (2) the unique challenges to the therapeutic alliance in inpatient work.

INPATIENT PSYCHOTHERAPY REQUIRES FLEXIBILITY

Psychotherapy on inpatient units often needs to be delivered with a much greater degree of variability of structure than in outpatient settings. In Chapter 4, we discussed that regular time and space provide a useful frame for therapy and add to the patient's sense of safety. However, during inpatient hospitalizations we cannot always provide that regularity.

However, inpatient psychotherapy rarely happens in uninterrupted 45- or 50-minute sessions. There are a number of reasons for this. First, you may not have enough time in your day to offer lengthy individual sessions to a single patient. Inpatient units can be busy places with rapid patient turnover. Your priorities for the day may involve safety assessments, assessment of medication response and tolerance, contact with families and outside treatment providers, diagnostic workups, reviewing abnormal lab work or imaging studies, and consulting with nonpsychiatric physicians about patients' medical problems. All of these make it hard to carve out the kind of extended, uninterrupted meetings that outpatient therapists are used to. In addition, you may get urgently called away from a meeting with a patient to respond to a crisis elsewhere on the unit. Similarly, the patient may get pulled away to attend a meeting or group session, or to receive some kind of other treatment.

Another reason for increased flexibility is that your patient may be too symptomatically distressed to tolerate a long therapy interaction. A 50-minute session might be too high a "dose" of psychotherapy for an acutely ill patient to tolerate. For these reasons, you may find your inpatient psychotherapy encounters are briefer overall, or even carved up into several briefer encounters through the day.

In regard to space, it may not be possible to meet with your patient in a completely quiet, fully private setting. The inpatient unit may be limited in the number of private treatment meeting rooms, which may be occupied. Or the patient may refuse to leave his room due to depression or paranoia and you will meet with him there, even though this means accepting interruptions when other staff members or roommates enter. Alternatively, the patient may have impulse control problems that make it safer for you to meet with them in an open, common area of the unit. You will need to be flexible, while at the same time doing whatever you can to help the patient feel that their privacy is being protected.

12

INPATIENT HOSPITALIZATION CAN CHALLENGE THE THERAPEUTIC ALLIANCE

One aspect of care that often makes inpatient work different from outpatient is the patient's feelings about treatment. Of course, patients are sometimes ambivalent about outpatient psychotherapy, but usually the patient and the therapist are at least in broad agreement about whether the therapy work is indicated (see Chapter 4 for a full discussion of the therapeutic alliance). This is often not the case for inpatients. Some inpatients did not want to come to the hospital and were involuntarily brought in by the police. Others came in on their own, but only because family or outside treatment providers put considerable pressure on them. Yet others presented fully of their own accord, but then decide they want to leave before the treatment team thinks this is safe. In all of these instances, the result is that the patient wants to go while the treatment provider wants them to stay.

The concept of ambivalence is also important in inpatient psychotherapy. Ambivalence means to hold two different and opposing opinions at the same time. For example, some patients who are suicidal simultaneously want to die *and* want to live. Patients with substance disorders may want to stop using the substance *and* deny that they need to stop. Patients may acknowledge that they have a mental illness *and* not feel that it is dangerous. In other words, the patient may agree with some aspect of the treatment team's goals, but adamantly reject others. As a result of this ambivalence, the therapeutic alliance (see Chapter 4) can be difficult to establish. Even when it is established, it can be put under a great deal of strain.

So how do you build a therapeutic alliance when the patient's goals and the treatment team's goals do not align, *and* when the patient is additionally ambivalent about their own goals? There is no easy answer, but transparency is a good first step. You begin by explaining to the patient why you feel it is not safe for them to leave the hospital, and you ask them to tell you at which points they see things differently.

Case Study: Transparency and the Therapeutic Alliance

Mr. D is seen upon admission by the inpatient psychiatry intern, Dr. F.

Mr. D: Why am I here? I would like to leave now. There is nothing wrong.

Dr. F: Why do you think you are here?

Mr. D: Like I said, it was a misunderstanding. The police were tricked into bringing me here. There have been some men following me. They want me out of the way. But I am fine! I just need to get home.

Dr. F: Unfortunately, we are not able to let you leave at this time. The doctor in the Psych ED thought you needed further assessment and treatment, which is why I am here. If we can talk more over the next several days and see what is going on, we can better understand how to help you when you go home.

> **Mr. D:** Several days? You understand they are monitoring my wife and kids right? Who is going to protect them? How old are you anyway? What are you ...like 12? Are there any adults around to speak with?
>
> **Dr. F:** (remaining calm) I understand that you are unhappy and scared. I also understand that you are eager to leave. But we have a protocol to follow when patients are brought in by the police to make sure you are okay and safe to go home. I can explain how we hope the next few days will go in helping to assess and treat you. I hope you will participate as much as you can so we can make decisions together about your safety and aggression that can set you up for success upon discharge.
>
> **Mr. D:** Fine, but it doesn't sound like "we" are doing any decisions "together."
>
> **Dr. F:** I know it feels that way, but I do want to hear your feedback and know what you want to do about your care, even if we don't agree.

It is not easy telling a patient that you are keeping them in the hospital against their will, or that you will be going to court to ask the judge for a commitment decision. Most of us are drawn to working in clinical mental health because we value relationships with patients and want to provide relief from their distress. But, if you have to go to court and testify in opposition to your patient's wishes, you are likely to have a patient who feels angry and betrayed. Particularly in the beginning of your career, it can be very painful to have your alliance with the patient damaged because your patient feels you have betrayed their trust and abused the power of your position.

Part of the difficulty is that there is a kernel of truth in their view—not that you have betrayed them of course, but that you have exerted your power against their will, to decrease their liberty. This is truly a profound thing for a clinician to do. This should always be undertaken with humility and from the understanding that it is the only way to prevent a far greater potential harm to the patient or others. Even when it does not change either the patient's position or your own, you should always listen to the patient carefully as they tell you why this is wrong, and you should try to explain why you feel involuntary hospitalization is necessary. Sometimes all you can do is "agree to disagree" and acknowledge that you cannot come together on this point. However, there may be other aspects of the patient's situation or symptoms that you both can agree to work on together. And sometime later, when the patient is no longer so acutely ill, they will hopefully remember that you listened and responded to them, which may help in repairing the ruptured alliance.

12

Perhaps less frequent, but not unusual, are patients who want to stay longer in the hospital, while the treatment team believes they are ready to leave. This should not be terribly surprising. If we succeed in creating an atmosphere on the inpatient unit that is safe and supportive, it will provide a patient with a respite from their own urges or from the stresses of their regular life. As with hospital stays for all kinds of medical and surgical conditions, sometimes the patient will feel they need more time before they are strong enough to take care of themselves outside of the inpatient environment. Finances can complicate this situation as well. If the patient has private healthcare insurance, the insurer may require review of necessity for inpatient care and may deny coverage before the patient is ready to go. Of course, if the treatment team does not think it is safe for the patient to be discharged, then they should not do so, regardless of the payment situation. But other times, it is actually safe for the patient to leave the hospital. In those situations, you will be helping the patient accept the disappointing reality that hospital care often is limited to what is absolutely needed for stabilization.

SPECIFIC THERAPEUTIC PRIORITIES DURING INPATIENT HOSPITALIZATION

Trauma-Informed Care

Trauma-informed care is also especially important on the inpatient psychiatric unit. This means that you as the clinician understand that many of your patients have been negatively impacted by trauma, violence, and victimization.[1] Some studies have found that up to 50% of psychiatric outpatients reported a history of trauma.[1] Part of our job is preventing the hospital stay from becoming an opportunity for retraumatization. You can think of this as analogous to our responsibility to prevent secondary infections in medically hospitalized patients.

This is critical if seclusion or restraints are necessary, particularly for patients who are disorganized, catatonic, or otherwise deeply impacted by delusions or hallucinations. Patients with these symptoms are not always aware of what is transpiring in the milieu around them. Additionally, they are the most fragile and vulnerable to retraumatization. Unfortunately, sometimes these patients also need seclusion/restraint while responding to internal stimuli, so being especially careful about preventing retraumatization is crucial. Remember, even if restraint is absolutely necessary, your patient is still experiencing other people taking direct physical control of their body against their will. That can result in understandable feelings of terror and rage.

We also have to be careful that patients are not retraumatized by other inpatients who are currently impulsive or aggressive. Group therapies and recreational activities on the unit must be closely monitored to ensure safety. For example, how are opposite sex patient interactions managed and monitored for inappropriate comments or touching? How is de-escalation of conflicts employed to prevent fighting and yelling that can be upsetting to patients?

Finally, trauma-informed care on an inpatient unit is not generally about exploring the past trauma or providing trauma-specific psychotherapies. That is often better deferred to a time when the patient is not acutely symptomatic and to an ongoing outpatient treatment provider who can provide a contained, continual therapeutic setting. Instead, our focus on trauma in the inpatient setting is about awareness and sensitivity to the context from which our patients present.

Coping With Psychotic Symptoms

As noted previously, some patients enter the hospital when their ability to cope with psychotic symptoms has overwhelmed them. This can be due to a number of factors, including medication nonadherence, a breakdown of supports, loss, trauma, or interaction with the criminal justice system.

Psychotic symptoms include hallucinations, delusions, and disorganized thinking and behaviors—all ways in which the patient's internal experience can become disconnected from external reality. Taking care of patients who have become so ill as to need hospitalization requires incredible flexibility, patience, and most of all kindness. Your first task is to listen as the patient tells you about the impact and affective experience of their psychosis. Many patients find their psychotic symptoms extremely distressing, as psychosis can be awful and terrifying. Your empathy needs to start there. Acknowledging this distress and fear with a patient is often a powerful alliance builder. In addition, because these patients are at their most vulnerable and frightening places—they need a therapist who will be able to sit in the "darkness" with them, hear what they have to say, and gently confront what is not real in a way that helps open up space for more than one explanation for the delusion or hallucination.

There are, however, other patients who experience their psychotic experience as benign or even comforting. This may be because they hear voices that simply comment on their daily activities and thus alleviate loneliness. Or this may include patients whose religious delusion helps them feel that they have a special, important, and even sacred role to play in the world. While the clinician must respect the patient's experience, you do not need to agree with the idea that hallucinations or delusions are positive. Symptoms that result in inpatient hospitalization are not a blessing, they are an illness. These types of symptoms usually are exacting a cost in the patient's life, even if they are not currently distressed by it.

So how can you help a patient with psychotic symptoms through psychotherapy? There are fundamentally two approaches—you help the patient change what they can about their experience, and/or you help them live with what cannot be changed. These two basic principles of change and/or acceptance can be found in different specific types of psychotherapy including cognitive behavioral therapy (CBT) for psychosis, acceptance and commitment therapy (ACT), and supportive therapy (Chapter 5).

There is also growing literature that attempts to define the essential elements of CBT for psychosis. It is a complex problem, because the treatment of a patient in recovery in the community would be different from someone in a more acute phase of the illness—such as an inpatient hospitalization.[2] CBT for psychosis in the acute phase includes an emphasis on exploring and gently debating the patient's beliefs about their symptoms, followed by considering alternative explanations.[3,4] This is very similar to the core ideas of reality testing.

One of the most valuable therapeutic interventions you will perform many times, regardless of the cause of exacerbation, is reality testing. This is the key ingredient in trying to change the patient's experience. Reality testing is the act of gently pushing back against the delusions and/or hallucinations a patient is experiencing,

12

helping them to see the disconcerting experience differently, and helping to lessen the emotional valence of the experience. Not only is this helpful to the patient in the moment, it helps teach them skills they can eventually apply themselves and start to self-regulate their reaction to these experiences.

Case Study: Reality Testing

The social work intern on the unit, Ms. J was assigned Mr. D's case. During their first intake meeting, Ms. J let Mr. D tell her what he thought the problem was. He began to ramble quickly about the police being wrong and stated they had been tricked by the men who were following him. The men had convinced the police to lock Mr. D up to keep him on "ice" while they staked out his family. He believed they were going to hurt his family eventually, but first they would kill him and were just waiting for an opportune time.

Ms. J: Tell me more about these men? Who are they? Why are they after you specifically?

Mr. D: I don't know—they are always different. There are many of them and they follow me, especially when I am downtown. I don't know what I did to them or why they are after me.

Ms. J: Can you think of any reason, anything you have done, debts you have, money you borrowed, someone you might have insulted, something having to do with drugs, or maybe the kind of work you do?

Mr. D: No. I don't owe anyone money. No drugs. My work was very boring, nothing high profile or involving the kind of money people would notice. I really can't think of any reason.

Ms. J: When they follow you, what do they look like? Do they approach you?

Mr. D: They have never approached me. They are all different. I have never seen the same one twice. They look like regular people walking, but I can tell they are different. Some have black clothes on, some wear hats, some are dressed in fancy suits.

Ms. J: This sounds quite distressing for you.

Mr. D: It is, I have never been more scared in my life.

Ms. J: You said they have never approached you. How do you know they have bad intentions?

Mr. D: In my head. I feel it in my head. It's like they send me signals. When I was at the hotel, I couldn't leave because I was getting the signals very strong—they were waiting outside. I finally went out and that's when the police came. It's like the men told them I was coming out and to get me then.

Ms. J: Is it possible the police came because the hotel called them?

Mr. D: No, it was because the men knew I was trying to leave.

Ms. J: How do you think they knew?

Mr. D: I don't know—it was the signals, I guess. They may have been able to read the signals in some way, to tell what I was thinking. Or maybe they were monitoring the room. What do you think? Do you believe me?

Ms. J: I really appreciate you telling me about this. I don't know what to believe yet. I know there are times people get caught up in things where they are followed or stalked by dangerous people. I don't think I know of times where this includes them sending mental signals. But I know it is very distressing for you, and I would like to talk about it more in our sessions while you are here. I hope we can meet again tomorrow.

Mr. D: Yes, that would be good.

Ms. J: Good—for our meeting tomorrow could you do one piece of homework? Could you think of any possibility that these men are not after you, some way in which the situation was misinterpreted or misread? That is not to say you are wrong, just to explore all possibilities.

Mr. D: I am pretty sure I am right. It has been going on for a while now. But, maybe I can think of one or two ideas.

Ms. J: That would be great.

Reality testing is not a magical cure-all, and some patients will need an even smaller task to help them learn how to look at other possibilities than their current reality. Many long-entrenched hallucinations and delusions may never respond fully to intervention. And, patients who are very disorganized will find reality testing difficult and possibly more agitating. So, it is important to go carefully, and allow yourself to be guided by the patient's reaction to your words. You should back off from the intervention when you feel a patient is getting agitated, but never be dismissive or condescending in your tone. The paternalistic statement, "Ok now, let's let you rest now," is better replaced with "This is hard work. Why don't we stop here for now?" Regardless, it is important to give a patient hope, even a small piece, as a respite from being terrorized. Even if Ms. J got Mr. D to entertain the idea that maybe there was more than one explanation for the men following him, he could hold on to that sense of hope after discharge. Reality testing, as you see, aims at helping the patient distinguish between symptoms and external reality. This can mean having insight into the experiences as symptoms of an illness, but still leaves the patient having to live with the presence of these symptoms.

This brings us to the second approach, which is focused on helping the patient live with psychotic symptoms that are not resolving with treatment. Some of these approaches to coping with psychotic symptoms are rooted in mindfulness techniques, such as ACT.[5] The idea of "acceptance" in this form of psychotherapy refers to learning that internal experiences such as these symptoms do not necessarily have to derail a patient's goals and desires. A patient learns to notice these symptoms (via learning skills such as mindfulness), acknowledge that they are present, and then work to be nonjudgmental about them. In addition, patients learn to separate experiences, such as thoughts, from who they are and what they choose to do

12

with their behaviors. The symptoms just "are" and do not have to derail the patient's overarching values, nor do these have to "become" the patient themselves. The goal is not to "overcontrol" or attempt to change these internal experiences, because patients often cannot.

It is not uncommon to work with patients whose hallucinations or delusions do not resolve fully or at all after medication therapy and psychotherapeutic interventions (although fortunately Mr. D's delusions did not fall into this category). A supportive therapy approach that uses gentle inquiry is one place to begin. Below are the kinds of things you might say to patients depending on their response to the experience.

To a patient who is being tormented by their symptoms:

- *"How can we work together to make these voices/thoughts less distressing for you?"*

- *"Can we practice noticing these voices/thoughts and just letting them be there, without you having to do anything in response?"*

- *"What strategies do you have to decrease your attention to these voices/thoughts? I would like you to make a list, and at what times they are helpful and not helpful. We will go over them in our next session."*

To a patient who finds these experiences benign or comforting and is not particularly distressed:

- *"Tell me more about how these voices/thoughts contribute to your well-being."*

- *"Can you help me understand how these voices/thoughts make you feel? Are you able to see how these might make others think that you are distressed or unsafe?"*

- *"Can we work together to come up with strategies for when it is appropriate to talk with other people about these voices/thoughts?"*

Treating Suicidality Psychotherapeutically

Many patients are admitted to inpatient psychiatric units because they have just attempted suicide, or to prevent them from making an attempt. When you work on an inpatient unit, this will be one of the most common problems you will encounter, and it will be one of your highest priorities. It is true that not all suicides will be preventable, although this is always our goal. Suicide assessment in its entirety is a topic beyond the scope of this chapter and includes systematic examination of an array of potential risk factors[6] (see also Chapter 5 on crisis response). We will not try to cover suicide risk assessment here. Instead, we will focus on those aspects of suicidality that have to do with the patient's internal, subjective experience and can be treated psychotherapeutically.

Some people may be so determined to die that they keep their plans to themselves and even avoid treatment altogether. But for the people we will see in clinical work, this is the rare exception and not the rule. The vast majority of people you see on the inpatient unit have fortunately had some degree of ambivalence about dying by suicide. They may experience this conflict directly, such as "a part of me wants to die *and* another part of me wants to live." Or they may be relatively unaware of one side of the ambivalence, insisting that their only wish is to die. The other side of what they feel may only have been expressed in the way the attempt left some room for rescue or a change of mind.

Here we want to focus on what the individual clinician and patient can do together in the hospital to decrease the risk of a future completed suicide. Can psychotherapeutic interventions make a difference in preventing suicide and relapses to suicidal thinking? Or is it the case that a person determined to kill themselves cannot be deterred?

Immediate Drivers of Suicide. In understanding what is driving the patient toward suicide, it is helpful to think about the following three questions.

First, *is the patient feeling intolerable psychic pain?* Many suicide attempts are driven by a need to escape from intolerable emotional states. Sometimes this is experienced as a definable specific feeling, such as shame or guilt or terror. Although all of us have experienced the pain of these feelings, any of them can be raised to a level of intensity that is felt to be unbearable. Guilt can be so overwhelming that the only possible course is to punish the self, to make the self pay the ultimate expiation for the alleged crime. Shame, and related feelings such as self-hate, self-contempt, or self-disgust, is often tied into an experience of the self as so ruined, grotesque, stained, or ugly as to be unworthy of living. Other times, patients will report that they cannot distinguish specific feelings and instead experience a flood or storm of undifferentiated emotional pain. This can be exacerbated by a general state of agitation, or overstimulation.

Second, *is there an aspect of attack or revenge to the patient's suicide?* Suicide can have a powerful interpersonal aspect. This does not mean that the patient is "manipulative" and not actually suicidal. It means that loss, disappointment, and other pain in the patient's most important relationships can be a part of what drives them toward suicide. This can have a variety of different meanings. Sometimes the suicide attempt is meant to punish someone. The patient may think "If I kill myself, I will rob my parents of their most precious possession" or "If I kill myself my ex-wife will feel guilty forever that she abandoned me." The motive may be more general: "If I kill myself, everyone will finally see how much pain they caused me." Alternatively, the suicide attempt may be meant to draw someone closer: "Maybe if I am dead, he will realize how much he has lost and love me again."

Third, *is there a fantasy of what will happen after death?* This might be a reunion with a lost loved one. Your patient may still be grieving the loss, or have been unable to grieve at all, and may hold beliefs that offer the comfort of finding this love again in an afterlife. Alternatively, some patients hold powerful fantasies of martyrdom. This means that they believe their death will result in some great benefit to those who are left behind. Perhaps this means simply lifting the burden of their illness from their family, or perhaps this means drawing attention to some political agenda they are committed to.

12

Problems of Grieving

As you know, many depressive episodes are triggered by a loss, and yet most losses do not lead to depression. Most losses are able to be mourned instead. One way to help the patient who is reacting significantly to a loss is to think about the things that can interfere with the normal grieving process. It is our experience that many inpatients have unexplored problems of grieving and/or loss, sometimes resulting in the suicide attempt and inpatient hospitalization.

Perhaps the patient has relied on the deceased to provide basic psychological functions, such as providing a sense of identity, self-worth, or relief from an over-powering sense of aloneness. It is harder to grieve someone when you have not only lost the things you loved specifically about them, but at the same time, have lost the capacity to hold yourself together psychologically. Other times, it is a pow-erful ambivalence that makes mourning hard. A patient might find that they can-not feel, and work through, the sadness of the loss because they are overwhelmed by their own anger or bitterness toward the deceased. Or they might not be feeling the sadness because they are numb, as they work hard to not feel angry or bitter.

The ways to help a patient grieve are not mysterious, and they are embedded in many different cultural rituals around death. First, it can be hard to grieve alone and so the gathering of support around the mourner can help. We can generally bear more pain and sadness together than we can in isolation. That support can come from a large religious community, but it can also be a small group of friends, or even a single dedicated therapist.

Second, healthy grieving involves a lot of remembering and telling stories. Stories bring the details of what was loved and lost back to life in the mourner's mind. This helps them connect with their sadness while also growing in perspec-tive of what the deceased meant in their life. It also means connecting with the ways they feel angry, disappointed, betrayed, or abandoned by the loved one. Feeling the bad is necessary in order to be in touch with the good. And this in turn helps consolidate the feeling that you carry something of the lost one with you still, in your memories and in your identity.

Remembering these tenets (grieving together instead of alone and being able to tell stories) will be extremely valuable when you address grief and loss with your patients during therapy. It may be that they are initially unable to address these feelings, but during the course of their inpatient hospitalization and as they tran-sition into outpatient care, there may be opportunities to acknowledge and assist with this process.

Addressing Suicidality During the Hospitalization. There is evidence that psychother-apeutic interventions can help suicidal patients. A variety of psychotherapies have been studied for suicidality and shown effectiveness, including CBT, dialectical behavior therapy, and psychodynamic therapies, including mentalization-based therapy. Unfortunately, most studies have been done with outpatients and there-fore there is not a very large evidence base for inpatient populations.[7]

However, one approach that has been piloted for feasibility in an inpatient setting is the Collaborative Assessment and Management of Suicidality (CAMS).[8] CAMS is not a specific psychotherapy, but is instead a system for organizing one's approach to the patient. It begins with use of the Suicide Status Form, which facilitates a joint assessment with the patient. This assessment looks at five negative states: (1) psychological pain, (2) stress, (3) agitation, (4) hopelessness, and (5) self-hate. Then, the assessment works to define the drivers of these states. The clinician and patient put together a crisis response plan to keep the patient safe, while working on understanding and decreasing the drivers. This leads to an examination of coping strategies, and eventually extends to larger questions of meaning, such as what would make for a life worth living. The CAMS approach shows that, regardless of the school of therapy we practice, a clinician has to start with understanding the patient's state of mind. To put this more directly, you need to help a patient tell you why they want or wanted to die.

In helping the patient tell us what makes them want to die, we want to learn how bad things can get at their worst. At the time of the interview, the patient may be feeling a fraction of the intensity that they felt in the middle of the night when they were closest to making a lethal attempt. You can help your patient connect with you by asking them to tell you whatever they can about those moments. You might say, "I know it can be very hard to find words for such overwhelming times, and that you may not want to revisit them. But I want to understand as best as I can how things are for you when you are hurting the most." A related question is whether the patient can feel any hope that things can get better. Hopelessness is also a fluid element and can be influenced by the intensity of the patient's pain and the availability of support.

As we discussed in Chapters 1 and 4, showing the patient you want to know the worst can itself be a powerful therapy. It can help your patient feel they are no longer alone with their suffering. It is important to establish this so that you can ask the patient about the part of their self that wants to live, without their feeling that you are trying to gloss over their pain. And it is important to talk about wanting to live, because any plan that you will make with the patient for treatment or suicide prevention will depend on allying with this part of your patient. It is important that this be an exploration, and not a coaching session. Your role is to understand what the patient might feel is worth living for; it is not to instruct them in the things you believe are worth living for.

Once you have helped the patient explore and express the various elements that drive them toward suicide, and those that protect them from suicide, it is important to remember that your goal as their inpatient treatment provider is not to eliminate or resolve these conflicting forces. This can take a long time and is not realistic for the time frame of an inpatient stay. Your goal, instead, is to thoroughly identify and articulate these forces and the situations in the patient's life that lend them strength, so that you can put together a suicide prevention plan.

A good suicide prevention plan identifies the events or situations that triggered the suicidality.[9] The plan may start with ways for the patient to avoid situations or experiences that are likely to make them more suicidal. But if that is not going to always be possible, then our plan moves on to monitoring. Together with the patient we define who, including the patient, will be looking for signs of danger such as symptomatic worsening or the recurrence of triggers. Sometimes the patient will be able

12

to self-monitor effectively. Other times we need to know that there are friends or family members who can recognize signs of a downward spiral and that they know how to call on professional help.

You may notice that we have referred to a suicide prevention plan and not a "contract." Contracts are binding agreements between persons, or other entities, that presume both the freedom to enter into the contract, and the ability to carry out the terms of the contract. Both of these presumptions are problematic. First, as we have seen, patients sometimes do not want to be in the hospital and feel a great deal of pressure to agree to plans or to tell clinicians what we want to hear. Second, and more important, is that the patient may have every intention to avoid suicide when they are surrounded by a supportive inpatient team during the light of day. That state of mind may no longer be the case when they are discharged and find themselves all alone in the middle of the night. Their capacity to follow through on their agreements can be compromised by overwhelming psychic pain such as panic or aloneness, by psychosis, or by intoxication, among other causes.

Case Study: Addressing Suicidality

As Mr. D's psychotic symptoms have been improving due to medications and daily therapy, he has started to feel more suicidal, exhibited by feelings of worthlessness and not wanting to be alive.

Ms. J: Tell me more about the worthless feelings. How bad do they get? What brings them on?

Mr. D: What is the point of all of this? I am going to lose my family. Everyone at work will know I am nuts. I'll be totally humiliated.

Ms. J: Sometimes the loss and the humiliation are overwhelming.

Mr. D: It feels that way. I just start spiraling into a really bad place. (He becomes tearful.) I'm going to end up just like my dad, alone and unloved. That's why he killed himself. No one would ever admit that, but that's really why.

Ms. J: That must have been hard on you.

Mr. D: It was, I was just a kid. I didn't really understand it. And, it's not like anyone talked about it. It's just something that haunted all of us.

Ms. J: And now you're afraid that will happen to you?

Mr. D: I can't lose my family. I will be all alone. My wife is the only person who gets me. Just thinking about it makes me panic. Everything we had planned together is just gone.

Ms. J: The thought that you may have driven your wife away is terrible. It sounds like you're afraid it's too late to repair things.

Mr. D: Can you talk to my wife; tell her everything will be ok?

Ms. J: I think it would be best for us all to meet. I think she would like to hear from you ways in which it will be better. I can help you in that meeting to talk about all of the work you have been doing here.

> **Mr. D:** That would be good. Yeah, let's do that.
>
> **Ms. J:** In the meantime, in our next few sessions, we will try to understand what brings you to your worst places. That way we can think about a plan to keep you from those times, and if they can't be avoided, we can make sure there are support people you can lean on and ways to cope to get past the scary moments.
>
> **Mr. D:** Ok, we can do that.

Finally, addressing the meaning of suicidality will sometimes lead to discussing spirituality and religion. Is this an appropriate topic for a therapist on an inpatient unit? The answer is yes, as long as it is clear that your task is to understand and not to instruct. Understanding what a patient might live for often means understanding their beliefs about questions of ultimate meaning. This is especially true if faith or spiritual practice is an important part of their lives. In times of crisis, such as when hospitalized, patients may ask us about our own beliefs. They may be seeking guidance or hoping to strengthen their bond with us through finding shared points of faith. It is important to remind the patient about the limits of your role. We find it helpful to say something like, "I understand why you are interested, but I'm not an expert in spiritual (or religious) matters. My role is to understand how your spirituality (or religion) is impacting your mental health (or suicidality)." It is generally wise practice, especially during training, to not disclose your own beliefs even when it seems that this might strengthen the alliance and be a source of comfort to the patient (see Chapter 8 for more on this topic).

Working on Self-Esteem and Worthlessness

Patients admitted to psychiatric units often suffer from feelings of worthlessness and very poor self-esteem. There are numerous reasons. Sometimes these are prominent symptoms of a major depressive episode or persistent depressive disorder. Other patients may have grown up in harsh and unloving environments and have been suffering from low self-worth all their lives. Yet other patients may have suffered repeated losses in function and social standing, as sometimes occurs in the progression of a psychotic illness, resulting in damage to their view of themselves. It would be foolish to think we can repair all these problems in the brief time in the hospital, but we can often make a dent. And that small dent can leave a patient feeling more hopeful and more motivated to continue in psychotherapy treatment as an outpatient. In this section, we are going to talk about how this can happen.

You may find it helpful to remember how self-esteem develops in a relatively healthy childhood. What does the average parent do that results in a typically solid sense of self-worth? There are three major elements.[10]

First, parents provide unconditional love, and acceptance of their children. This is how children develop the sense that they are valuable and matter in the world. This is very powerful, and throughout life we seek to find other close relationships that can leave us feeling similarly embraced.

Second, parents provide praise and appreciation. But for praise to lead to solid self-esteem, it cannot be unconditional. Praise needs to be connected to actual growth and achievement. Healthy self-esteem develops through learning that with effort, we can become better at all sorts of things.

Third, parents believe in the child. They have a vision of what the child can do and that is an important gift. It conveys a sense of confidence that more is possible and inspires the child to put in the effort to grow.

When we meet patients as adults and try to help them with problems of self-worth, we work in these same veins of unconditional acceptance, conditional appreciation, and belief in their capacity to grow. We cannot, of course, provide the love of a parent, but we can provide an atmosphere of empathy and compassion that genuinely accepts the patient for who they are right now. As an inpatient clinician, you will try to remember that each patient you are meeting is very often at a low point in their life, and that they have arrived at this point while nonetheless doing the best they can. No one growing up envisioned a future for themselves that included hospitalization for mental anguish or destructive behavior. One of the beginnings of change in self-esteem can be meeting a clinician who sees the patient as a person like all of us, who was dealt a hand of cards in life and has played that hand the best they can, equipped with the brain, family, and social environment they were born with.

At the same time, you will also be aware that you need your patient to work with you to get better. It is very rare for the recovery of a psychiatric inpatient to not require their active participation! When it comes to building or rebuilding self-worth, this is actually fortunate. The patient's efforts in the hospital can provide many opportunities for honest appreciation, rooted in the actual difficult things you are asking the patient to do. It is important to be genuine in doing this. Here are some of the kinds of things you might say that reflect actual work during a hospitalization:

- *"I can see that you're working hard with me to make sense of a long, complicated treatment course. This will help me make better recommendations of next steps."*

- *"I know I've asked you to talk about some painful things, and I appreciate that you've been brave enough to do that today."*

- *"It isn't easy to reach out for help from family when you have so many painful and conflicting feelings about them. That takes some strength."*

- *"Going to the group session yesterday and talking about your experience of recovery was a real support to the other patients."*

Patients with psychiatric illness may have had losses that make them feel ineffective and insignificant in the world. These kinds of comments help convey that you do not see them as just an ill person who needs help, but as a collaborator and partner in a process of healing. This can lead, in small steps, to the patient's growing confidence that they can try to take control of the rest of their lives as well.

So far, we have been talking about issues of self-esteem and worthlessness from the perspective of what the patient is lacking (a sense of themselves as valuable, effective, and competent). However, feelings of worthlessness do not only result from what is not there inside the patient, but also from what is. Some patients view themselves with hatred, contempt, and disgust, with accompanying emotions of intense shame and guilt. Attempts to help a patient's self-esteem without taking into account the shame or guilt they carry are doomed to fail.

Self-hatred or contempt, which may have incubated and developed over many years, is unlikely to be resolved in a brief inpatient hospital stay (and as noted previously, can be a driver for suicide attempts). That is going to be the work of months or years in outpatient psychotherapy. But you can still do something profoundly important in the hospital—you can help the patient feel that they do not need to be alone with their guilt or isolated in their shame. You do this by inviting the patient to tell you the painful truth of what they live with, and you simply listen to them. Over time, you will hear stories of childhood sexual abuse, adultery, addiction, the trauma of war, betrayal of principles, and irreversible acts of neglect or violence that caused great harm.

Your willingness to hear the story of what they have done, and what they believe they have consequently become, will not magically erase the effects. But two very useful things can begin to happen in the hospital. First, as we have said, you will be chipping away at the idea that their experiences have rendered them fundamentally ruined, unacceptable, or unforgivable. Second, in listening to a patient, you are also helping them learn how to listen to themselves. This means having one part of the mind able to critically reflect on other mental experience (such as memories, feeling states, fantasies, etc.). This capacity of the mind to reflect on itself is called mentalization and it is very valuable.[11] Many patients experience their mental states as defining them and as unchangeable realities. It is as if the guilt the patient feels is who they are and indeed is proof of their crime. Developing the mental ability to observe and reflect on our own minds opens up entirely new ways of understanding things, and this can begin with learning to listen to oneself.

Impulse Control

Some patients are admitted to inpatient psychiatry units out of concern for safety that is not related to suicidality. This includes the following:

1. Patients whose behavior is aggressive or frightening.
2. Patients who are putting themselves in danger due to recklessness.
3. Patients who are homicidal.

Often, hospitalization itself is the first step in treatment, as it directly blocks or contains whatever the dangerous behavior might be. A patient on a locked inpatient unit is now physically prevented from driving recklessly or seeking someone out to exact revenge. Because there is often a part of the patient that has been alarmed and frightened by the behavior, or possible behavior, just being admitted to a restricted setting is a relief. However, there are other kinds of behavioral problems that can recur on the ward. A patient with a volatile temper that led to physical confrontations or assaults brings that same temper into the hospital with them.

12

How do inpatient units provide a safe environment for these patients? We will briefly discuss each of the following necessary components: (1) Decreasing stimulation and de-escalation of conflict, (2) Forming an alliance with the part of the patient that wants to remain in control, (3) Fostering a community that values impulse control, and (4) Planning and rehearsing for challenging moments.

Inpatient units provide an environment that is less provocative and stimulating than the outside world. An inpatient psychiatric unit offers a regular schedule, a quiet environment for sleep, and a group of staff people who are themselves calm and trained in de-escalating confrontations. De-escalation protocols and techniques are variable and may differ from one hospital to another. It is critically important to not attempt to engage in de-escalation of a potentially violent patient unless you have been trained and approved for this by the institution you work in. Your supervisors in inpatient settings will orient you to the processes used on their units and when, if at all, you will be involved.

Nonetheless, there are some general characteristics that de-escalation protocols tend to share.[12] Generally, the clinician works to remain calm (or at least appear calm) and to approach the patient with a mild and unthreatening posture and tone of voice. The goal is to engage without the patient feeling their personal space is violated or intruded upon. The clinician inquires and attempts to empathize with whatever is provoking the patient, and often aims to provide choices or options for the patient. Every attempt is made to help them reclaim any sense of lost respect or dignity.

When de-escalation is unable to contain a volatile patient, the treatment team then considers acute medication options and, as a last resort, physical restraint. Fortunately, verbal de-escalation very often succeeds in defusing tense situations and this has great value on several levels.[13] First, it avoids a potential physical restraint that involves physical danger to both patient and staff, as well as often being a traumatic experience for all involved. But beyond this, the staff's use of verbal de-escalation is a demonstration to the patient of socially appropriate ways of managing confrontation. Patients who grew up in violent or chaotic environments may have had little chance to see this kind of coping; other patients may have learned to see physical aggression as the only way to not "lose face" or be targeted as a potential victim. In order to prevent future difficulty with the law, or future hospitalizations, the patient will need to learn new skills. The staff's demonstration of verbal de-escalation is a powerful learning opportunity.

A second component is to form an alliance with that part of the patient that wants to control impulses. Manic behavior, for example, can be both exciting and gratifying, yet also frightening and costly. You have to appeal to the part of the patient that is aware of the negative aspects to convince them that treatment will be a good idea in the hospital. However, this alliance will be exponentially more important when the patient has left the hospital and does not have the staff around to remind them of the possible consequences of nonadherence. Hopefully the patient will have strengthened the rational and deliberative parts of themselves while in the hospital, and this, combined with a sense of ongoing alliance with hospital clinicians, can help the patient maintain the goals of behavioral restraint and inhibition.

Third, you want to help the patient be part of a community that is working toward the same goals, a community that is going to use positive peer pressure and to support control of impulses. The opinion of one's peers is usually a more powerful incentive than the opinion of authority from above. This is especially true when the patient has learned from experience, or from other peer groups, to be distrustful of authority. This is part of the reason why group therapy, and other group interventions, on inpatient units is so important. The group can provide a community of peers that values and validates expressing feelings in words and not actions. Also, the patient will have the opportunity in groups to provide this same reinforcement to others, and being helpful to others is a good way to begin repairing the damaged self-esteem that many patients bring to the hospital. When the patient has experienced the value of the inpatient group, it can be much easier for you to explore with them how they can find a similarly supportive group of peers outside the hospital.

Finally, you help the patient learn strategies to use when frustration is rising. You might help the patient learn meditation techniques that they can use to help calm themselves. You can also help the patient learn more effective ways to respond to interpersonal stressors. Some of your patients will have a limited repertoire of responses, perhaps because they have grown up in chaotic environments or perhaps because their illness has interfered with the development of their social learning. You focus on whatever kind of situation tends to provoke the loss of control. Perhaps this is about being disappointed by someone important, or perhaps it is about being disrespected or insulted. You can help your patient plan out ways to put this experience into words, rehearse what they might actually say the next time it happens, and finally how to remove themselves from situations that are not improving.

Many of these strategies will be taught and strengthened through psychoeducation and problem-solving while on the unit (more on that in the next section). In the case of Mr. D, this psychoeducation focused on helping him understand that bipolar disorder might lead to being more irritable. His inpatient therapist, Ms. J, strategized with him about what he could do next time he felt himself being irritable at work. They discussed in detail the events leading up to his fight and outburst with his boss and identified different points where Mr. D could have kept the situation from escalating.

Psychoeducation

Psychoeducation has long been used on inpatient units to help patients come to terms with not only their diagnosis, but what life is like managing a chronic, and sometimes unrelenting, illness. Psychoeducation occurs in several settings: individual, group, and family therapy. One of the most crucial ideas in educating patients and their family/supports is that becoming ill was not their fault. Through some combination of genetic predisposition and environmental stressors, this illness has come about. Of note, some family members often blame themselves for passing along "bad genes," so this is another helpful area for psychoeducation that genes are not purposefully passed along or withheld by parents. Furthermore, the patient has the right to get help, to get better, and is not trying to manipulate the family/support unit with their illness. It is also crucial to expect of the patient that they want to get better through participating and making informed decisions in their treatment.[2]

Next, helping patients identify symptoms is a priority. You will see patients who do not acknowledge that they have a mental illness. The experiences you identify as

12

symptoms are explainable to them in other, seemingly rational ways. Where you see pressured speech, a patient might say they are just excited to tell you the whole story. Where you see tangential or tangled thought patterns, they see a coherent story that you are just unable or unwilling to understand. Some patients may never accept your explanation of their symptomatology, but gently offering alternatives to their explanations can be helpful.

For patients who can already identify their symptoms, they may need assistance talking about them. The stigma in our society against mental illness is so strong that many people are reluctant to talk about hallucinations and delusions. They might be afraid of what a diagnosis means for their future. Allowing patients the time to speak about what is happening to them, without judgment or disdain, can be an excellent step. It can be a relief just to be heard, and then to be informed that though the symptoms are distressing, they are typical for the illness.

Often inpatient clinicians have to discuss a diagnosis with the patient. Sometimes this is for the first time, while other times it is to reinforce previous discussions held with other treatment providers. In the case of severe illness such as bipolar disorder, schizophrenia, schizoaffective disorder, or treatment-resistant depression, it is never easy to tell someone that they have a diagnosis that can likely become chronic and affect their ability to live their regular life. It does not make it easier that some of the medications used to treat these illnesses come with a host of unpleasant side effects that may make the patient want to stop them. It helps to maintain a recovery mindset (see Chapter 9) that maintains hope while realistically setting expectations and aspirations with the patient.

Next, you often teach the patient about how to manage their illness. You may need to explain that there is real evidence supporting the medications we are asking them to take, and that these medications will not work effectively if they are not taken consistently. You might also identify ways to cope with their symptoms. Try first asking a patient what they have typically done to cope and how these strategies became ineffective or overwhelmed. Concretely listing previous coping strategies can be a good place to assess where a patient is now, what needs to simply be reemphasized, and what new ideas need to be taught. Using techniques from the aforementioned CBT for psychosis or ACT can be helpful here as well.

Sometimes it is crucial to address ADL (activities of daily living) issues. These include issues such as showering, laundering, wearing clean appropriate clothes, grocery shopping, cooking or otherwise procuring prepared food, keeping the home clean, meeting transportation needs, taking medications as prescribed, ambulatory needs, and toileting/continence issues. You will need to assess how the patient has been functioning in these areas and if there were setbacks prior to hospitalization. These functions then become goals for the multidisciplinary treatment team to address.

Lastly, helping patients organize their non-hospital life and environments can be of great use. Often known as "disposition planning," this phase of treatment tackles a multitude of concerns for a patient, such as where the patient will live, what benefits need to be or have been applied for, and coordination with outside supports, treatment providers, and any agencies that can provide patient support.

Case Study: Psychoeducation

Mr. D was in group therapy on the unit. The discussion that day focused on ways to identify bothersome symptoms early, before a patient became so ill as to need the hospital. Mr. D identified that sleeping less and less often was a sign that he was doing poorly. However, he also noted he got a great deal of work done during these times, so sometimes it was hard to give in and try to sleep. Even when he did try to sleep, sometimes sleep never came.

Mr. R (psychology intern): It can be hard in the middle of a regression of the illness to identify symptoms, and that is normal. Can we as a group think of ways to identify this particular symptom, of insomnia and trouble sleeping, and offer some ideas for how to manage it?

Ms. M (patient in group): I agree, these are some of my most productive times. I get so much done. My house gets cleaned top to bottom and I can work on my art. But, soon after, I crash, and things quickly go downhill. I try to keep a sleep journal of how many hours I am sleeping. I also try to go to bed at the same time each night.

Mr. B (patient in group): I call my doctor as soon as it starts. He can sometimes adjust my medications over the phone. Sometimes, I also take something for sleep. I find the sleeplessness makes me more anxious. I cannot do my work well the next day, and it just becomes a spiral of negativity. It did not work this time, so I am here working out my medication situation.

Mr. R: Thank you both, those are very helpful ideas. It is also helpful for all of you to share your points of view, and to realize that you are not alone in these experiences.

ENGAGING AND STRENGTHENING THE PATIENT'S SUPPORT SYSTEM

One of the most useful things you can do as an inpatient clinician is to help the patient connect with support outside the hospital. Sometimes this means referring the patient to treatment or support groups such as AA, but often it means helping the patient reconnect with family or optimize the support from family. It also can mean helping the patient and their outpatient clinicians make the most of their ongoing treatment.

Consultation With Outpatient Treatment Providers

It might seem very strange for us to suggest that you will be able to provide valuable consultation to outpatient therapists. We are used to thinking of consultation as something that flows only from the more expert to the less knowledgeable, and you may in fact be much less experienced than the outpatient therapists that are

12

treating your patients. In fact, depending on the structure of your training program, you may be working in inpatient settings before you have done any outpatient psychotherapy at all.

However, you can often be very helpful, not as an expert in psychotherapy, but as a clinician who can provide a different perspective. You can think of your role as offering observations and insight about the treatment and as supporting the patient by taking seriously their observations and insight. These observations and insights can be grouped in two categories.

First, there is the issue of why the patient is in the hospital now. Even though you have only known the patient briefly, you may be in possession of insight into causes of their distress that have not been apparent to the outpatient therapist. This is because you will have had the experience of seeing the patient when their pain is at its worst and/or when their defenses are at their weakest or most broken. In these circumstances, the suffering person will be in touch with things that they may otherwise be able to keep out of awareness, or at least out of communication. It is not uncommon during a patient's first day in the hospital to hear about, for example, fear and anger that a loved person will reject them, or shame about an old trauma that the patient has carried alone, only for these topics to recede when the patient has settled in and been symptomatically stabilized. Sometimes in the acuity of the crisis and the containment of the inpatient unit, the patient will open up a window onto something very important. Helping the patient remain in touch with this material and supporting them in bringing this into their outpatient psychotherapy can be very useful.

Second, you may also learn something about what is and what is not working in the outpatient psychotherapy. It can be very hard for patients to tell their therapists that they are angry with them, or disappointed by them. People often expect that their therapist will respond to criticism as other people in their life have—for example, as a personal attack that triggers retaliation. You can help the patient by reminding them that it is part of our job as therapists to listen to difficult things, even or especially when it is about us. Their therapist should welcome this input and be curious about what it means. They should consider whether they made an error that they should acknowledge or if there is some change in technique that would be more useful for the psychotherapy. If neither is the case, the therapist might simply help the patient tolerate that they have negative feelings for someone who is important to them. Because we all have feelings of hurt or anger with the people we most depend on and are closest to, simply learning to tolerate this in psychotherapy can be a great help!

As you can see, much of your consultation's impact will come through helping the patient share more of the difficult parts of their experience with the outside clinician. But it is also often a good idea to talk with the outpatient therapist yourself. You can learn a great deal at the beginning of the hospitalization about why the patient is doing poorly and what this means in the context of the outpatient treatment plan. And at the end of the hospital stay, you can make a real contribution by conveying to the outpatient therapist what you have been working on in the hospital and any thoughts about how this might be built upon after discharge.

Case Study: Consulting With Outpatient Treatment Providers

Dr. F is speaking to Dr. Z (Mr. D's outpatient treatment provider, prior to Mr. D's discharge).

Dr. F: Since Mr. D gave me permission to speak with you about what we have been working on, I wanted to update you on how he has been progressing during the hospital stay. He discontinued his medications, which led to an exacerbation of his symptoms. The police picked him up wandering the streets downtown. He was delusional, feeling that people were following him and wanting to harm him. His speech was pressured, he had run off from home for several days, and he had not been sleeping. Here he has started taking his mood stabilizer again and also a low dose of an antipsychotic medication. As he started to improve, however, he voiced ideas of wanting to harm himself. These seemed to stem not only from a fear of losing his family, but from some earlier losses, including his father, who had died by suicide when Mr. D was younger. It sounds like that loss was traumatic and has never been really dealt with. The team is feeling he could use some additional support upon discharge. We were thinking he could go to the intensive outpatient program for the 6-week program there.

Dr. Z: That is a good idea. That's a good program. I am concerned that every 2 months visits are not enough. I can start seeing him weekly, for a hybrid medication/psychotherapy appointment. Coupled with the IOP, weekly meetings could start to address some of the issues with suicidality. He never mentioned specifically how his dad died, so that's helpful for me to be aware of.

Dr. F: That sounds great. I will make sure that you get my final discharge note and that he has an appointment made with you within a week of his discharge.

Working With the Family

Psychoeducation interventions for families and other support people in a patient's life are often helpful while a patient is on the inpatient unit. Some families have been through a grueling cycle of hospitalization, improvement, discharge, noncompliance, and relapse that has led to problems in the family/support dynamic. Or, possibly, the patient is having a first episode of mental illness after much unexplained difficulty in daily living. Intervening with the family/support system not only helps them manage their expectations going forward, but also helps them to be the "right" kind of support to the patient. Both of these can be useful tools in discharge treatment compliance and engagement. It also helps the patient with on-going symptom management and care.

As with psychoeducation of the patient, it is important to educate the family/support system about symptoms a patient might experience with their diagnosis, and also to explain how their current symptoms impact their daily living skills. It is important to reiterate:

1. This is no one's fault—neither the patient's nor the family members'.
2. The patient is ill, not malingering or manipulating people or trying to avoid obligations.

12

3. The difficulties the patient has been having are a direct result of the symptoms of the illness.

4. There are unique stressors in dealing with a major mental illness and it is important to help the patient lean on their coping strategies when having symptoms.[2]

The feelings of loss and anger that the patient is going through are often mirrored in their family members. Parents and spouses had a mental picture of the way they thought life would be, just as the patient had ideas about how life would play out for them. This loss of an idealized future can be destructive to all involved. As a therapist, helping everyone involved process this loss is important. Of equal importance, however, is helping all involved start to see a new, different, but possibly equally fulfilling future with the management of the patient's symptoms under control. Turning the dynamic from a conflictual one to a "we are all on the same team" one can be profoundly reassuring to the patient and give family/supports granular ways to be of assistance. See Chapter 8 for further input on how to involve family members in individual psychotherapy treatment.

Case Study: Working With the Family

Ms. J meets together with Mrs. D and Mr. D, to discuss plans to have in place for Mr. D's discharge.

Ms. J: Thank you for joining us today. I wanted to start by opening our discussion up to any issues that need to be addressed before Mr. D returns home.

Mrs. D: Well, honey—don't get mad, but I am very nervous about you coming home. Before you ran off last time, you were so angry and yelling all the time. It was very scary.

Mr. D: But I told you—I thought the men were after me. I am feeling a little better, I feel less scared about them. I have been working hard to get better here.

Mrs. D: I don't think anyone is after you.

Ms. J: Often when patients are suffering with bipolar disorder, they can have thoughts that may not make sense to others, but make sense to them at the time. This is part of the illness, as was some of the agitation you experienced. You are right to be scared, and to seek help. I understand your concerns about your husband returning under those conditions.

Mr. D: I have been very calm here in the hospital. I have been taking my medication and feeling better. I have been going to groups and having therapy every day.

Mrs. D: Yes, but last time things were going well, and then you stopped the medicine, and here we are. What will prevent you from stopping the medication again?

Mr. D: Well, Dr. F spoke to Dr. Z and he will be seeing me weekly now, instead of every 2 months. I am also going to be going to the intensive outpatient program for 6 weeks when I get out. There is also a group meeting I can attend for weekly support after that.

Mrs. D: That all sounds good, but what if you don't go? What happens then? The kids can't live like this, with so much stress in the house. I can't do it either. I can't walk on eggshells all the time.

Mr. D: Do you think I want to be like this? In the hospital, worrying about strangers following me? I did not see life going this way either.

Ms. J: It can be very hard to worry that the future you saw for your family will not come to pass. However, many people go on to live fulfilling lives with this illness, with the right support. It has been hard for both of you. Dealing with a mental illness is just like dealing with any other medical illness. It is important to have the right kind of support, to take medications as prescribed and to be on the same team. Additionally, Mrs. D—perhaps you could use your own support? I can give you referrals for a support group or for individual counseling. Attending one of those might help you both have your own avenues for discussing the stressors for you, but also give you some hope about how the future can work out.

Mrs. D: Thank you, yes that would be helpful. Can I meet with Dr. Z at my husband's next outpatient appointment?

Ms. J: Mr. D, how do you feel about that? It is not unusual for family members come to initial appointments to help express their support, and learn from the therapist what can be of value.

Mr. D: I am good with that.

Using a Recovery Frame to Inform Discharge Planning

If you are going to convey a message of hope and recovery in your treatment, you must be willing to not only enlist the patient as a partner in their care, when possible, but to keep all care as patient centered as possible (see Chapter 9 on recovery models of care). You will need to think about how principles of patient collaboration and choice fit into each of your treatment planning and therapeutic interactions, and this is especially important for discharge planning. You and the patient need to be on the same page about what the steps are to the ultimate goal of getting discharged.

When thinking about the word "recovery," think about alternatives to the idea of regaining lost ground. Your patient might not ever recover fully in a premorbid medical sense, but new ground can be covered, new ideas about what life should look like can be formed. The emphasis of the recovery movement is to help patients reintegrate with society in a way that empowers them, allows them to be as independent as possible, and allows them the same opportunities as everyone else. It is an idea that rejects the disabled role or victim role and embraces optimism for the future through continued support by both professionals and peers/family. Patients need to be involved in all aspects of their care and to help make decisions about their treatment and/or their desire to not accept treatment.

12

Given the emphasis on keeping lengths of stay brief, our treatment planning tends to be symptom focused—that is, how do I decrease the disruptive or painful symptoms so this person can return to the community? This is not a bad place to start, and it may feel like all you have time for. However, as you have seen throughout this chapter it is possible to integrate a more "holistic" view. You have been treating a whole person, with a whole world that you have been learning about.

As you work through discharge planning, make sure you also acknowledge and integrate strengths. For example, what are the patient's coping mechanisms, and what is the quality of their family and outpatient supports? Reflecting on this with your patient is important in preventing them from having a relapse and coming right back to the hospital. Taking the time to think more fully now can have a great reward for the patient later, and actually decrease their overall use of hospitalization by preventing readmissions. The more focused you are on including the patient in the process of setting goals for discharge, the better the outcome will be.

Conclusion

We have looked at the special therapeutic interventions you might need to implement on an inpatient unit. Flexibility in your role is a vital part of being a good therapist in this setting. Focusing on specific priorities, such as alliance building, trauma-informed care, suicide assessment, and helping patients build self-esteem can go far in helping your patients thrive. Helping patients cope with psychotic symptoms and impulse control can provide lasting assistance posthospitalization. Family/support members, as well as patients, need specific psychoeducation to help build and maintain coping strategies for ongoing management of the illness. Lastly, providing messages of hope and recovery to patients and family members gives them the motivation they need to continue to focus on symptom improvement and sustainable healing after discharge.

Self-Study Questions

1. What are some of the unique challenges to forming a therapeutic alliance on inpatient psychiatric units?

2. How can you use "reality testing" effectively to help a patient cope with acute psychotic symptoms?

3. List three questions that will help you organize your understanding of the forces driving your patient toward suicide.

4. How does self-esteem develop during childhood? How can this inform helping patients with feelings of worthlessness during a hospitalization?

5. What are some important aspects of psychoeducation that patients and families will benefit from during a hospital stay?

RESOURCES FOR FURTHER LEARNING

Chiles JA, Strosahl KD, Roberts LW. *Clinical Manual for the Assessment and Treatment of Suicidal Patients.* 2nd ed. Washington, DC: American Psychiatric Publishing; 2019.

Fenton WS. Evolving perspectives on individual psychotherapy for schizophrenia. *Schizophr Bull.* 2000;26(1):47-72.

Lonergan BB, Duchin NP, Fromson JA, et al. Skills-based psychotherapy training for inpatient psychiatry residents: a needs assessment and evaluation of a pilot curriculum. *Acad Psychiatry.* 2020;44(3):320-323.

12

REFERENCES

1. Butler LD, Critelli FM, Rinfrette ES. Trauma-informed care and mental health. *Dir Psychiatry.* 2011;31:197-210.
2. Fenton WS. Evolving perspectives on individual psychotherapy for schizophrenia. *Schizophr Bull.* 2000;26(1):47-72.
3. Morrison AP, Barratt S. What are the components of CBT for psychosis? A Delphi study. *Schizophr Bull.* 2010;36(1):136-142.
4. Byrne RE. CBT for psychosis: not a 'quasi-neuroleptic'. *Br J Psychiatry.* 2014;204(6):488-489.
5. Gaudiano BA, Herbert JD. Acute treatment of inpatients with psychotic symptoms using Acceptance and Commitment Therapy: pilot results. *Behav Res Ther.* 2006;44:415-437.
6. Chiles JA, Strosahl KD, Roberts LW. *Clinical Manual for the Assessment and Treatment of Suicidal Patients.* 2nd ed. Arlington, VA: American Psychiatric Publishing; 2019.
7. Brown GK, Jager-Hyman S. Evidence based psychotherapies for suicide prevention – future directions. *Am J Prev Med.* 2014;47:S186-S194.
8. Ellis TE, Green KL, Allen JG, Jobes DA, Nadorff MR. Collaborative assessment and management of suicidality in an inpatient setting: results of a pilot study. *Psychotherapy(Chic).* 2012;49:72-80.
9. Stein MB, Jacobo MC. Brief inpatient psychotherapeutic technique. *Psychotherapy(Chic).* 2013;50:464-468.
10. Loewald H. *The Essential Loewald: Collected Papers and Monographs.* Hagerstown, MD: University Publishing Group; 2000.
11. Fonagy P. *Attachment Theory and Psychoanalysis.* New York, NY: Other Press LLC; 2001.
12. Price O, Baker J. Key components of de-escalation techniques: a thematic synthesis. *Int J Ment Health Nurs.* 2012;21:310-319.
13. Spencer S, Johnson P, Smith IC. De-escalation techniques for managing non-psychosis induced aggression in adults. *Cochrane Database Syst Rev.* 2018;7:CD012034.

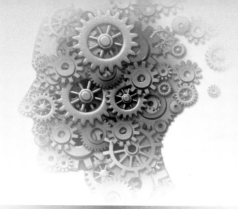

Section 4

FURTHER DIRECTIONS IN LEARNING PSYCHOTHERAPY

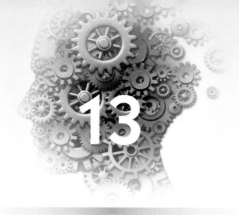

Integrating Medication and Therapy

MATAN WHITE, MD AND HEIDI KOEHLER, PhD, ABPP

Case Study

Ms. A is a 17-year-old Hispanic female who was referred to her current therapist by a school counselor. Her academic performance has declined over the past year, and her school counselor became more concerned when she began skipping classes. Her school performance and attendance had been excellent prior to her parents' divorce 16 months ago. Initially, she did not want to see a therapist outside of school, but with her mother's encouragement, she began weekly individual sessions.

Ms. A has been participating in individual therapy for the past 6 weeks. She and her therapist, a licensed psychologist in private practice, have developed a good working therapeutic alliance. Her therapist has been addressing Ms. A's symptoms of depression using a cognitive behavioral therapy (CBT) approach. Through their work, Ms. A has become more aware of the depressive themes in her thinking and how her thinking specifically impacts her emotions and actions. However, despite her adherence with her CBT action plan assignments, which have included daily monitoring of her activities and thoughts, symptoms of depression (depressed mood, poor concentration, insomnia, fatigue, and loss of appetite) have not improved. Moreover, Ms. A also reported that she was reprimanded by several of her teachers after missing important college application deadlines. Afterward, she felt she might be better off dead. It was at this point that her therapist recommended Ms. A make an appointment to see a psychiatrist.

INTRODUCTION

There are times when neither psychotherapy nor psychotropic medications alone are sufficient to provide our patients with satisfactory care. We must then determine if our patients' particular set of symptoms and circumstances might best be treated by a combination of medications and psychotherapy. In situations where both modalities are indicated, it is helpful to understand the potential implications and complications of one provider integrating both treatment arms versus having the two treatments provided by two different individuals.

In our example, Ms. A was referred to a psychiatrist for medication management by her therapist, meaning that she will have two mental health providers working with her. This chapter will look at some of the methods and challenges to effective collaborative care. One caveat—although "psychiatrist" is used to represent the medication management specialist throughout the chapter, please recognize that the approach in this chapter could also apply to collaborating with a primary care provider who is prescribing psychiatric medication.

Alternatively, Ms. A could have presented to a provider that is able to provide both therapy and medication management simultaneously. This chapter will also explore what unique challenges would arise in a situation when the prescribing provider is also providing psychotherapy.

EFFICACY OF COMBINED PSYCHOTHERAPY AND PHARMACOTHERAPY FOR SPECIFIC DISORDERS

Numerous studies have looked at the combination of psychotherapy and pharmacotherapy for specific disorders, and some have concluded that combination therapy is more effective in certain cases than monotherapy. Below we will describe some of the literature that exists regarding the use of combination therapy, specifically for mood and anxiety disorders, as these are the two disorders on which the bulk of the combination therapy research is conducted.

Mood Disorders

A meta-analysis from 2011 by Cuijpers et al. found that combination therapy was significantly more effective than pharmacotherapy or psychotherapy alone in the treatment of depression.[1] Another added benefit to combination therapy may be that it improves compliance with and completion of therapy.[2]

As for which type of psychotherapy, CBT and interpersonal therapy (IPT) are two of the more frequently studied therapy modalities when combined with antidepressant pharmacotherapy, but there have also been studies indicating that psychodynamic psychotherapy may also be beneficial when combined with pharmacotherapy[3] and that supportive psychotherapy in combination with medications may have an advantage over pharmacotherapy alone.[4]

There are relatively fewer studies regarding the effectiveness and use of combined treatment for bipolar disorder. However, the data indicate that there is a role for combined therapy in preventing relapse and improving function. A 2008 review looked at family therapy, interpersonal therapy, CBT, and psychoeducation, and found that in 17 of the 18 studies, when therapy is used as an adjunct to medication, there is some benefit to patients struggling with bipolar disorder.[5] In fact, when the American Psychiatric Association created a workgroup to establish treatment guidelines for bipolar disorder, these same therapy modalities were recommended as useful adjuncts to treatment.[6]

Anxiety Disorders

The treatment for anxiety disorders with the most randomized control trial evidence is CBT, though there is also a small evidence base for psychodynamic therapy. CBT addresses symptoms through a process of learning to recognize, challenge, and effectively change faulty cognitions while encouraging the practice of new behaviors that then constitute a form of corrective exposure. The goal of CBT is to create a shift in both thinking and actions that results in a reduction in anxiety symptoms (this is addressed more fully in Chapter 6 on CBT). However, despite the advances in CBT with augmentations to the original model for specific patient populations (eg, dialectical behavior therapy [DBT] for patients with pervasive affect dysregulation), some anxiety disorders remain difficult to treat. For example, a patient suffering from symptoms of panic disorder with agoraphobia may have difficulty adhering to a treatment plan involving only outpatient individual therapy sessions, such as missing sessions, arriving late for sessions, or not completing homework assignments given by the therapist to be performed before sessions (thought records, activity monitoring, etc). The panic attacks a patient may experience with just leaving home to attend a therapy appointment may be so overwhelming that the therapy itself, while wanted by the patient, may be avoided altogether.

An important part of sound clinical practice is the modification of the treatment plan when a current therapy is not effective in reducing the symptoms of anxiety.[7] The modification can take the form of adding a new therapy approach shown to be effective in treating a specific set of symptoms or the addition of psychiatric medication. In one study with primary care patients diagnosed with generalized anxiety disorder, panic disorder, posttraumatic stress disorder (PTSD), and social anxiety disorder, an improvement in anxiety symptoms was noted following the addition of CBT to standard pharmacotherapy.[8] Similarly, adding pharmacotherapy to a patient in therapy can be of great benefit. For example, the addition of pharmacotherapy to patients struggling to make significant progress in CBT may provide enough symptom relief (by reducing the intensity of the anxiety or improving sleep quality), so that a patient then has the resources to apply the skills learned in therapy.

As research has not produced a clear formula for the combination of CBT and pharmacotherapy for specific anxiety disorders, the need for consultation between a therapist and psychiatrist is paramount to the success of treatment. Each patient presents with a unique set of needs and personal circumstances that can either contribute to or hinder the progress of treatment. Therefore, a patient's treatment providers must be willing to collaborate with one another with a focus on creating a treatment approach that satisfies both the parameters of evidenced-based treatments like CBT and standard pharmacotherapy, while addressing the specific needs of the patient.

13

What if I Don't Prescribe?

Nonprescribing psychotherapists should learn the basics of clinical pharmacology as well. Because a therapist will likely engage in collaboration across disciplines with psychiatry and other prescribing providers for some patient care, it is important in professional development to integrate clinical pharmacology concepts into practice and case conceptualization. For example, the American Psychological Association Clinical Practice Guidelines for the treatment of PTSD list both recommendations for psychological and pharmacological interventions. Specifically, therapeutic effectiveness for PTSD can be enhanced with a knowledge and understanding of medications being prescribed to a patient being treated with a psychotherapy intervention such as cognitive processing therapy or prolonged exposure.[9]

In addition, patients will often ask your opinion about medications they are, or believe they should be, prescribed. As a nonprescribing provider, there are specific limitations on your boundaries of competence to comment on and/or make recommendations about medications. However, a basic knowledge of psychopharmacology is essential for your own understanding for patients who are taking psychiatric medications. You can learn concepts about medications for specific psychiatric disorders by reading books or articles on psychopharmacology, as well as through routine consultation with psychiatrists. Additionally, there are continuing education companies which offer a variety of learning modalities such as live workshops (single- or multiday) and webinars on the topic of psychopharmacology. These companies offer continuing education credits for multiple disciplines including LPCs, LCSWs, LMFTs, and psychologists. It is recommended that you check with your state licensing board and scientific and professional organizations affiliated with your discipline (eg, The American Psychological Association for psychologists and National Association of Social Workers for social workers) for guidance concerning appropriate and approved continuing education.

REFERRALS FOR MEDICATION MANAGEMENT

Psychotherapy has limitations, and a patient may continue to exhibit symptoms despite adherence to a therapy protocol that is provided by a competent provider. When considering a referral to a psychiatrist for an initial psychiatric evaluation, a therapist must first take into consideration both clinical indications and patient factors.

Clinical Indications

It is important to remember that the course of psychotherapy can change over time and new issues arise as a therapist and patient work together. A therapist, for example, may increase the frequency of therapy sessions to address a new crisis or loss that occurred as the therapy focused on a much different issue. As the intensity of the treatment changes, there can be short-term fluctuations in symptoms. However, despite any planned or unplanned changes, some type of gradual progression or improvement is expected by both the therapist and the patient. When there is a lack of progress in treatment (eg, inadequate symptom relief), you should first consider possible issues within the therapy itself. For example, the therapeutic alliance may have unaddressed conflicts (see Chapter 4), or the treatment approach itself may be inappropriate (see Chapter 3). It is only after these possible causes have been ruled out can a therapist make a clinically sound recommendation for the patient to consider a referral to a psychiatrist.

The following clinical situations may *specifically* prompt referral for medication evaluation:

1. Worsening of symptoms.

2. Lack of improvement in symptoms, even with appropriate application and frequency of psychotherapy (eg, mood remains as depressed as it was at the start of therapy).

3. New symptoms emerge (a client reports chronic insomnia, drastic changes in appetite, anxiety, psychosis, or symptoms suggestive of an addiction).

4. The patient's safety or the safety of others is of significant concern.

In our case example, Ms. A has been working with her individual therapist for several sessions using CBT to help reduce her symptoms of depression. While Ms. A developed a strong working alliance with her therapist and demonstrated adherence with her CBT homework assignments, her mood, concentration, sleep, energy level, and appetite have not improved. Furthermore, Ms. A's admission to having morbid thoughts prompted her therapist to increase the level of care with a referral to a psychiatrist. While beyond the scope of this chapter, Ms. A's therapist would need to complete a suicide risk assessment prior to making the referral to the psychiatrist and determine if Ms. A's thoughts constitute morbid thinking or reflect suicidal ideation. The information gained from the risk assessment would be used to create a revised treatment plan, including a referral to see a psychiatrist.

Patient-Specific Preferences

Clinical factors are not the only factors to take into account—you must also assess patient-specific preferences regarding psychotropic medications and referrals to another mental healthcare provider. Before making a referral to another provider for medication management of psychiatric symptoms, you should begin the process by first talking with the patient. This discussion offers the patient an opportunity to take an active role in treatment decision-making, which will enhance treatment adherence.[10] The discussion about a psychiatric medication referral needs to include the following steps.

First, it is important to talk with the patient about the lack of progress in psychotherapy alone. You may want to communicate to the patient that a worsening of symptoms does not mean the therapy is not progressing well, or that they have somehow failed the therapy protocol.

Second, the therapist needs to fully understand the patient's beliefs about medications and, in particular, beliefs about psychiatric medications. Some patients believe

13

that taking psychiatric medications indicates psychological weakness or impairments that are permanent.[11] Some patients may also believe psychiatric medications are addictive and to be avoided at all costs. A host of cultural factors also impact perceptions of psychiatric care (see Chapter 8). Therefore, it is very important to understand the patient's worldview and belief system, and provide an empirically supported point of view to consider a consultation for psychiatric medication management.

Third, if a patient is willing to accept the referral, you may need to reassure the patient that psychotherapy will continue with the agreed upon schedule of sessions. This can reassure the patient that the therapeutic alliance will not be in jeopardy of a premature termination if the patient also receives psychiatric care.

Fourth, you must anticipate and assess any practical barriers to psychotropic treatment access, including the cost to your patient of seeing another provider, psychiatrist availability, and potential impact of medication costs. Sometimes, this means the psychotropic prescribing provider will be a readily available primary care physician (PCP) or Ob-Gyn, with whom the patient already has ready access. Or, you may know that generic medications may be the only option for your patient, due to cost.

In our case example, Ms. A's therapist would need to take the important step of discussing plans to make a referral to the psychiatrist prior to making the actual referral. The therapist, working within the limits of the therapeutic alliance, would need to discuss the need for the referral due to lack of improvement with compassion and validation. Specifically, the therapist could acknowledge the development of insight along with overall compliance with the CBT homework, while, at the same time, communicating a rationale for the change in the treatment plan with a possible addition of medication. It would be in this context that the therapist would allow Ms. A to voice her concerns or fears about medication and even about the course of therapy itself following the referral. You would need to discuss the reasons for the referral and the referral process using age-appropriate language and take into consideration her resources to both attend added psychiatry sessions and the potential costs of any medications prescribed. Finally, given Ms. A's age, it would be recommended to include her mother in the discussion and allow her to ask any questions prior to making the referral. Reassurance that therapy will continue after the referral is important to emphasize to both Ms. A and her mother.

The following is an example of how the therapist would approach Ms. A with a recommendation to see a psychiatrist:

> **Therapist:** For our session today, I have a couple of items to add to our agenda before we get started. Are there any items you want to make sure we cover today?
>
> **Ms. A:** Not really. I guess everything is okay.
>
> **Therapist:** Well, I wanted to talk with you first about your progress in treatment. You have been working hard on your CBT homework and I can see from your responses that you are making positive gains in terms of your awareness of

depressive themes in your thinking, and how those thoughts negatively impact your emotions. How do you feel about your progress?

Ms. A: I do notice how I talk to myself. I'm pretty hard on myself and my thinking is repetitive. I mean I tell myself how "dumb" I am or "why did I do this or that…that was really dumb." I also notice I feel really sad and lonely when I think others do not want to be around me.

Therapist: I think you are taking some important steps in understanding your thinking and how these thoughts impact your emotions and ultimately your actions. I noticed that you continue to experience a depressed mood, poor concentration, insomnia, fatigue, and loss of appetite just based on the symptom inventory we use you typically completed prior to the start of our sessions. What are your thoughts about these ongoing symptoms?

Ms. A: Well, I didn't want to say anything, but now that you mention it, I'm still feeling pretty lousy. I didn't want you to think I was not trying or I didn't want to keep coming back to see you.

Therapist: I do see how hard you are trying and honestly, I'm glad we can talk more openly about how you are feeling, not just about your symptoms, but also about our work together. I think that the treatment is working and at the same time we may need to add to your treatment. From our understanding of depressive symptoms, the research suggests that medications might help improve them. What are your thoughts about talking with a psychiatrist to discuss the possibility of taking an antidepressant?

Ms. A: I'm not sure. Can we ask my Mom to come into the session now?

Therapist: Absolutely. I agree that your Mom needs to be part of this discussion. I wanted to let you know first what I was thinking before we talked with her about this.

(Mom joins the session and the therapist provides a summary of what was just said.)

Ms. A's Mom: I do have some questions about how all this will work. First, does this mean my daughter will no longer have sessions with you?

Therapist: No, not at all. She and I will continue to have our individual therapy sessions. My commitment to working with your daughter does not change because I'm referring her to a psychiatrist. The psychiatrist she would see would need to first determine if a psychiatric medication is needed and if so, talk with you both about the options. If medication is recommended, the psychiatrist would work with you on scheduling follow-up appointments that would be separate from my appointments with your daughter.

Ms. A's Mom: What is the cost of these medications? And will you and the psychiatrist talk with one another about my daughter's care?

Therapist: These are really good questions and I want to provide you with the best guidance. There may be additional costs with seeing another mental health provider like a psychiatrist and so I would recommend checking with your

13

insurance carrier. Once you select a psychiatrist, I would get your written permission for myself and that provider to communicate with each other about our treatments. In other words, you must give your written consent to allow us to share information about your daughter's mental health care.

Ms. A: If I take a pill for my depression will I become addicted to it? Some of my friends take drugs and they are just not the same. I don't want to be like them or turn into a zombie.

Therapist: I understand taking a medication for depression may seem really scary, especially if you have had friends in the past take medications or "drugs." While I cannot speak to specific side effects of these medications or make a recommendation for a medication, because that's beyond my scope of practice, I can tell you that medications used to treat symptoms of depression are typically non-addictive. The psychiatrist can definitely give you more detailed information once you meet. It is important you ask your psychiatrist questions about the medications recommended and provide any feedback about side effects you are experiencing after you begin taking your prescription.

Ms. A: I'm willing to see a psychiatrist if it is okay with my Mom.

Ms. A's Mom: Yes, I am willing to take her to see someone. Do you recommend anyone?

Therapist: Great, I'm glad to hear you are both in agreement. I think this will be a helpful step in your care. I do have a list of colleagues I can recommend.

PSYCHOTHERAPY INITIATION WITH A TREATING PSYCHIATRIST

Alternatively, a patient may express a preference for treatment methods that primarily use psychotropic medications and seek psychotherapy only if they are unsatisfied with the results of medications. If a psychiatrist is already providing medication management, the following situations might lead the psychiatrist to consider adding psychotherapy:

1. The symptoms are not remitting with medications alone.

2. The patient has an interpersonal or environmental conflict impacting their mental well-being.

3. The patient describes patterns of problematic behaviors that are affecting them in a negative way and are amenable to psychotherapy.

4. The patient seems interested in and curious about their own contributions to their mental health and would like to take a more active role to build new skills and/or insight.

5. The patient has the physical and emotional capacity to participate in emotionally challenging conversations.

In the case above, had Ms. A seen a psychiatrist for medication management first, it would have quickly become clear that her behavioral patterns (eg, skipping class, withdrawing from her support system, dropping grades, etc.) need to be explored and addressed. If, after getting to know her, she seemed to be physically and emotionally in a space where she was ready to discuss these things, it would have been beneficial for her psychiatrist to discuss with her the idea of concurrent therapy, either during their sessions or with another provider. In this discussion, Ms. A and her psychiatrist could discuss different types of therapy and the amount of therapy that might be useful but also feasible for Ms. A to attend as a busy student. Then, if those were possible within the confines of their current treatment arrangement, therapy could be added to their sessions. If not, they could discuss therapist referral options with Ms. A that might be a good fit.

An example of such a conversation is as follows:

> **Psychiatrist:** Now that your sleep and appetite are improving with your medication, I am wondering what your thoughts are on exploring things like your school performance and relationships in talk therapy?
>
> **Ms. A:** My mom suggested that I try something like that, but I am not sure how that would even help.
>
> **Psychiatrist:** Well, there have been studies that have shown that sometimes pairing psychotherapy with medications can actually improve depressive symptoms more than medications alone. And while several of your symptoms are improving, you have mentioned that there are still several things that you are doing that are not usual for you, like missing classes and pulling away from your loved ones. I think it would be beneficial to spend some time thinking about how these changes came about and how they are affecting you.
>
> **Ms. A:** I guess I can see how that would be important, but I don't really want to tell my story all over again. Is this something that we could do in our sessions?
>
> **Psychiatrist:** Now that we are not needing to make medication changes very often, it is. However, we would need to meet more often, probably every week at first, and for a longer period of time for each session.
>
> **Ms. A:** I would be willing to give it a try.
>
> **Psychiatrist:** Great, let's plan to spend the first few minutes of our next session reviewing your medications, and then we will dedicate the rest of our session to psychotherapy that would focus on thinking through these recent changes in your life.

PSYCHOTHERAPY REFERRAL FROM A TREATING PSYCHIATRIST

13

When a provider (eg, a psychiatrist) is technically able to provide both psychotherapy and medication management, there are still scenarios that may lead them to consider an outside referral for psychotherapy and therefore a split treatment approach. Here are some examples of when a psychiatrist might choose to *refer out* to someone else for psychotherapy:

1. The patient would most benefit from a type of therapy that the psychiatrist is not competent in or trained to provide.

2. The patient needs more intensive or more frequent therapy than the psychiatrist is able to provide.

3. The medication management is sufficiently complex that it would dominate a significant portion of appointments, shortchanging time for therapy.

An example of such a conversation is as follows:

> **Psychiatrist:** In response to your question about whether or not we would be able to add psychotherapy to our sessions here, I think it would actually be best for me to refer you to one of my colleagues who specializes in cognitive behavioral therapy (CBT). I find that this approach to talk therapy helps us identify some of the thought patterns that might be playing a role here. I do not provide this type of therapy in my clinic, but I do have a colleague who I think that you would work really well with.
>
> **Ms. A:** I am kind of nervous about meeting someone new. Are you two going to communicate with one another?
>
> **Psychiatrist:** I think that would be very helpful, and if you and your mom are okay with it, I would like to collaborate with your future therapist in order to provide you the best possible care. If all of this sounds okay to you, we can have your mom sign a release of information form at the end of our visit today, and I can call your new therapist to tell them a bit about what we have been working on and also hear about their thoughts and plans.
>
> **Ms. A:** Well, if you think this therapist would be a good fit for me, I am willing to give it a try.

IDEAL COLLABORATION BETWEEN PROVIDERS

Once a decision has been reached by the patient and the therapist to refer to a psychiatrist or other prescriber for psychotropic medication treatment, it becomes imperative for the therapist to facilitate the process of incorporating the other professional in the therapeutic relationship. In some situations, the therapist may know the prescriber through a personal relationship or may routinely refer to a prescriber who works in the same outpatient clinic.[12] Whatever the preexisting nature of the professional relationship between the therapist and the prescriber, the process of forming a professional collaboration between the two to address a specific patient's needs must be the goal.

Although many therapy providers can prescribe psychotropic medications (and in fact, do), we are going to focus on the relationship between the therapist and a psychiatrist, specifically. While these recommendations are going to be useful for all collaborations with prescribing providers, these types of issues more readily emerge when both care specialists are trained mental health providers.

The collaboration between a therapist and psychiatrist offers a unique opportunity to approach a patient's mental health concerns from different perspectives. More specifically, the decision-making process involving the therapist, the psychiatrist, and the patient needs to be integrative in nature, allowing the patient's values and preferences to be considered as much a part of the process as the expert contributions of the providers themselves.[13]

The collaboration between the referring therapist and psychiatrist can be strengthened with following agreements (see Thase et al.[12]):

1. *Information sharing:* A patient needs to be informed that information will be shared between the therapist and the psychiatrist for optimal treatment outcomes. A patient or guardian needs to give consent prior to the sharing of information. Your supervisor will guide you in what specific processes or forms you will need to complete and sign with your patient.

2. *Expectations of specific medications:* A referring therapist should never promise a patient that a particular type of medication will be prescribed by the psychiatrist. Such a promise would be outside the scope of practice for the therapist, might demonstrate a lack of respect for the clinical judgment of the psychiatrist, and can set the patient up for disappointment.

3. *Emergency plans:* An emergency can be addressed with greater effectiveness if a response plan is determined ahead of time so that if such an emergency occurs, such as a need for hospitalization due to suicidal behavior, action can be taken quickly to address the patient's needs.

It is also important to keep the psychiatrist informed of the treatment details and progress. The session structure, symptom monitoring, and indicators that the therapy is effective or ineffective are all important points to communicate to the psychiatrist. By the same token, a psychiatrist should keep the therapist informed concerning medication side effects and expected results. A clear process of sharing (within the limits of a patient's written consent) of the electronic medical records should include up-to-date progress notes and weekly treatment updates, along with regularly scheduled consultation calls. This will benefit both providers and keep an open channel of communication. The rate of exchange of information between a therapist and psychiatrist would depend on the needs of the patient or changes in the treatment offerings. For example, if a psychiatrist changes the medications or the therapist changes a course of psychotherapy, such as adding a group therapy to an existing individual therapy schedule, patient care and professional courtesy would direct that this change be openly communicated between providers. This will help strengthen the patient's sense of security and the providers' reciprocal respect across disciplines. Ultimately, the patient will benefit from the strength of the collaboration by having a comprehensive treatment approach that addresses symptoms from mutually beneficial treatment modalities.

13

In the case of Ms. A, she may be informed that the psychiatrist works in the same clinic or is perhaps someone in the community with whom you have a long-standing professional relationship. Further, you would explain to Ms. A how information would be exchanged between the two providers, with her verbal assent and the written consent of her parent or guardian. The basic message given to Ms. A is that the goal of the collaboration between her providers is to work for the benefit of recovery from symptoms. This assurance adds stability and trust to the treatment process. Finally, the therapist, working in the role of an information sharer, can monitor Ms. A's compliance with any medications prescribed by her psychiatrist by conducting routine medication adherence checks at the beginning of therapy sessions and facilitate the use of problem-solving strategies if Ms. A experiences problems with the medications. These problem-solving strategies could function as guides for how to approach her psychiatrist with these concerns.

The following is an example of how the therapist would communicate sharing information with Ms. A's psychiatrist:

Therapist: So, how are you feeling since you've been on the medication prescribed by your psychiatrist?

Ms. A: I'm feeling better. Has she called you?

Therapist: Yes, we spoke just the other day about your progress. Remember you and your Mom signed those forms allowing your psychiatrist and me to talk about your treatment and progress.

Ms. A: Good and maybe you can call her and tell her I've been having some weird stuff happening when I forget to take the medicine.

Therapist: We can add this question to our session agenda for today. Before I answer your question, I need a little more information. How many times have you missed a dose of the medication and what happens when you do?

Ms. A: I'm not sure how many days I missed last week. I just noticed that I get these chills. At first, I thought I had the flu.

Therapist: That sounds really uncomfortable and I can see why you would worry. Have you called your psychiatrist?

Ms. A: No, I'm a little nervous about telling her I forgot to take the pills. I don't want her to get mad at me. Can you tell her for me?

Therapist: I understand you are worried about talking to her because you think she will get mad at you. I can tell her you have not been consistent in taking the medication, but I think it would be important for you to tell her as well. While I can't jump to conclusions about her reactions because that would be a thinking error, I can tell you that we are both concerned about your well-being. It would be important for you to communicate with her directly about forgetting to take the medication and the physical effects you've experienced when you missed a dose.

Ms. A: Why is it so important I tell her?

Therapist: She can provide you with an explanation about missed doses and the likely side effects. More importantly, you will receive helpful information disconfirming some of your thoughts connected to your fear. For example, you have the thought, "If she expresses anger or annoyance towards me that means I'm a bad patient."

Ms. A: I just don't know what to say. I feel as though I don't make any sense when I'm talking to her.

Therapist: We can role-play the conversation and I can offer you strategies on how to adjust your thinking and communication style. Plus, the role-play would give you the opportunity to practice keeping your anxiety better contained so you can clearly state your thoughts and feelings. What do you think about doing a role-play in our session today?

Ms. A: Okay I'll give it a try.

Therapist: Great! And afterward we can talk about when would be the best time to reach out to her.

Managing Provider Disagreements

The patient now has two different providers for the same problem, and occasionally, there may be a disagreement regarding diagnosis, approach, treatment plan, or prognosis. Disagreements should be managed in a way that maintains collaboration and with the patient's best interests always in mind.

The first step should always be to explore and clarify each provider's understanding of the situation as soon as either provider becomes aware of a potential disagreement. It is helpful to also clarify the specific treatment goals in the situation and try to reach a consensus on how to achieve it. After the facts—and each provider's interpretation of them—are understood, it is important to explore any discrepancies in how the patient is relating to each of the two providers as this too may influence what information is shared and how it is understood. However, there are times when even collaboration and understanding do not allow two providers to come to an agreement on the best course of action. In these cases, the two providers should explore whether they are able to disagree on this topic without affecting the patient's care or clouding the collaborative relationship. If the answer is no, supervision or consultation should be sought. It is *never* appropriate to explore your disagreement with the other provider in the patient's therapy sessions.

For example, in Ms. A's case, her psychiatrist may disagree with the diagnosis of major depression after meeting with her. In this event, the psychiatrist should contact the therapist to explore what symptoms and signs led to the previous diagnosis and share what information was uncovered during the psychiatric assessment that may have differed. This would preferably occur in person or over the phone rather than over email or text messaging. While text methods may seem faster

13

and more efficient, they also make it difficult to truly gauge the other person's responses and can introduce uncertainties in tone. In addition, there are issues with communication confidentiality when using unsecured methods such as email and text.

An example of such a conversation is as follows:

> **Psychiatrist:** Thank you so much for calling me back. I met with Ms. A, and she consented to my speaking with you. I just wanted to let you know my initial impressions and also hear what your thoughts are.
>
> **Therapist:** I am so glad that you reached out; she also signed a consent form in my office allowing us to discuss her care, which we faxed to your office last week. I have been encouraging her to seek out a psychiatrist for quite some time, and I am really happy that she finally did so.
>
> **Psychiatrist:** It sounds like she has been really depressed for quite some time. She told me that you two have discussed a diagnosis of major depressive disorder. I wanted to share with you that she mentioned that a few months ago she experienced some unusual symptoms. She stated that she was unable to sleep for several days and was extremely energetic during that time. She was also more impulsive and irritable and spent much more money than usual that week. I am wondering if she may actually have bipolar disorder.
>
> **Therapist:** I was actually wondering the same thing when I saw her that week. However, when I asked her about it, she reluctantly shared that she was using some of her friend's Vyvanse that week in hopes that it would help her focus on her final exam studies. After admitting this, she agreed to stop using the Vyvanse, and those symptoms immediately improved.
>
> **Psychiatrist:** That is really helpful to know. She didn't share the part about the Vyvanse with me.
>
> **Therapist:** Yes, in our sessions she has usually been hesitant to open up about things like this, but as we got to know one another, she has begun to trust that she can share more in our sessions.

At times like these, it becomes clear that the patient has disclosed different information to the two providers either inadvertently because the conversation took a different turn, or purposefully and because she is more comfortable with her therapist given their longer relationship. As a result, she left out significant pieces of information about her symptoms during her psychiatric assessment, leading her psychiatrist to doubt the previous diagnosis and/or misunderstand the situation and diagnoses.

As above, after noting the discrepant diagnosis, the psychiatrist should always contact the therapist (with appropriate patient permission) to review one another's understanding of the patient. After uncovering a difference, it is worthwhile for the two providers to explore what factors may be contributing to the discrepancies. If Ms. A is resentful of one or both providers or is idealizing one provider over the other, it may be worthwhile to address this discrepancy with Ms. A and hopefully deepen both treatment relationships. Likely, this shared information will help everyone come to a better understanding of the patient's issues.

However, if this is not possible, both parties should discuss whether the disagreement can be reconciled and potentially seek supervision or consultation if necessary. For example, if after the psychiatrist and therapist discussed the diagnosis, the psychiatrist still felt that Ms. A has bipolar II disorder, but the therapist did not agree, they would need to discuss how they were going to handle this. The psychiatrist might suggest that Ms. A meet with one of her colleagues for another psychiatric assessment or they could agree to both watch for an agreed upon set of symptoms for a set period of time before coming together again to discuss the diagnosis once more.

Issues With Treatment Overlap

At other times, providers may agree to repeat the same treatment-related information to the patient. In some cases, it is beneficial for a patient to be hearing the same thing in two places and striving for the same goal with two different providers, as this can provide the patient with increased support and works to reinforce important concepts.

For example, Ms. A may benefit from exploring her struggles at school with her psychotherapist via CBT on a weekly basis, as well as from brief supportive psychotherapy from her psychiatrist during medication management sessions. This approach can even be synergistic as long as both providers are aware of their roles and are consistent in their approaches.

On the other hand, there may be situations as above where Ms. A shares her struggles with one of her providers and doesn't want to repeat herself to the other provider. For example, she may have disclosed her recent Vyvanse abuse to her therapist but then not mentioned it to her psychiatrist, feeling that she has already discussed it with "a treatment provider." As above, this could pose a problem for her treatment plan, as substance use could very well contribute to her recent mood and behavioral issues and may impact her symptoms. In this situation, if the two providers are sharing important updates with one another, the therapist could inform the psychiatrist of this new development and the psychiatrist could explore this further during their next session, deepening everyone's understanding of the issues at hand.

Another potential issue can arise when providers use significantly different therapeutic approaches. For example, Ms. A's therapist may be working diligently with her on decreasing avoidance, but when Ms. A discusses her discomfort in difficult situations with her psychiatrist, the psychiatrist might recommend using distraction to cope. This results in giving Ms. A mixed messages about how she should be approaching distress. In this case, we recommend again that the

13

therapist and psychiatrist talk directly and come to a consensus about the treatment approach.

An example of such a conversation follows:

> **Therapist:** Great talking to you again. I have been working with Ms. A on decreasing her tendency towards avoidance, I wanted to share with you what steps we are taking toward this and see if you could help me reinforce some of these techniques.
>
> **Psychiatrist:** Absolutely. I would love to hear more. Just yesterday she was sharing with me how distressed she feels when she starts to think about her dropping grades. We discussed that after she has finished studying for the day, and there is nothing more to do, she might try doing a crossword puzzle to distract herself from her distress so that she can fall asleep. But it sounds like that might be the opposite of what you are doing.
>
> **Therapist:** Yes, that is a perfect example. In those situations, what we are working toward in therapy is for her to sit with the distress and journal what she is feeling. I want her to then bring her journal entries to session so that we can process what she was feeling in those moments.
>
> **Psychiatrist:** Thank you for letting me know. I would be happy to encourage her to do this next time we discuss a similar situation.

MEDICATION MANAGEMENT AND PSYCHOTHERAPY IN A SINGLE SESSION

Some prescribing providers, such as psychiatrists, may be able to provide both medication management and psychotherapy in a single session. Any provider trying to provide both pharmacotherapy and psychotherapy in the same session will need to balance both psychotherapeutic and pharmacologic issues by making sure that enough time and energy are spent on each, as well as be flexible enough to shift between modalities.

This balanced approach starts with the very first session, where the appropriate techniques must be employed to gather information about both psychotherapy and pharmacotherapy needs. In addition to discussing past medical history, family history, previous medication trials, and a relevant review of systems, the psychiatrist will also explore behavioral patterns, key relationships, and current interpersonal conflicts. The process continues through each subsequent session to identify the combination of pharmacological and psychological factors at play. The ratio of each of these components in a given session is dependent on several factors, including the etiology and severity of symptoms, relevant standard of care, patient preference, and acute needs.

Benefits of Doing Both

Assuming this balance is achievable, there are several potential advantages to being able to provide both treatments in one session. For the patient, this may be more convenient and feasible in their otherwise busy schedule, as only one visit and payment is required. For the psychiatrist who does both, there is the ability and discretion to titrate the ratio of medications to therapy as they see fit to meet the patient's needs at any given time. Psychiatrists in these situations also have the opportunity to gain a deeper understanding of the factors impacting medication efficacy. Just like any other part of the patient's life, their interaction with medications can be ripe for exploration, and discussing their feelings and thoughts about the meaning of this part of their treatment may actually deepen the psychiatrist's understanding of the patient.[14]

Complications of Doing Both

Medications and therapy may take on new meanings for both the patient and the therapist when both are utilized by the same provider. For example, in the eyes of a patient, medications provided can signify a loss of control or an indication that their mind/body is somehow biologically broken, rendering them passive participants with a lack of ownership.[15]

Alternatively, patients may consider medications to be a special gift from their psychiatrist, which may complicate their acceptance of pharmacotherapy depending on their feelings about their psychiatrist and about gifts in general. For example, if a patient mistrusts their psychiatrist or has had negative experiences with receiving gifts as a form of manipulation, medication may be viewed negatively, and medication adherence may be affected. On the other hand, a patient who feels positively about their psychiatrist might feel that they are being given the medication because they are special to the psychiatrist and might feel badly refusing it even if they are struggling with significant side effects. Such a situation would be especially exacerbated if this patient has a fear (conscious or subconscious) of disappointing others.

The effects of medication management on therapy are complex and can also take on new meanings to the provider. In the eyes of the therapist, medications may represent a potential hindrance to uncovering the unconscious[16] or promote chronic avoidance,[17] which can render a psychiatrist less likely to prescribe certain medications that could otherwise be useful, out of a fear of preventing therapeutic progress. Anxiolytics are a common example of this phenomenon, as some providers feel that in order to fully process one's anxiety, it is important to actually experience it. However, it is good to remember that while a little anxiety can promote learning and growth (as in our professional development), too much anxiety is paralyzing and shuts down progress.

Other psychiatrists may feel the opposite, viewing a medication prescription as a way to rescue a patient or take control of the situation.[15] For example, a psychiatrist making little progress with a patient in therapy may begin to feel an overwhelming urge to break out their prescription pad. However, this urge should be explored in consultation or supervision to make sure that the psychiatrist's own

13

countertransference is not prompting the urge and that there are actual medical/biological reasons for the prescription (see Chapter 7 for a more in-depth discussion of countertransference).

Given the complexity of these issues, one can see that there are also advantages to splitting up medication management and therapy to two different providers, especially if there is not enough time to think about and address complications that may arise. Another drawback to combined treatment is that one runs the risk of providing too limited of a dose of psychotherapy if the patient actually needs weekly or biweekly therapy, and it is not feasible to meet more frequently with the psychiatrist.

In Ms. A's case, if she was not already seeing a separate therapist and merely presenting for the first time for medication management, a combined approach from a psychiatrist would be a consideration, as she had initially expressed some ambivalence about starting therapy. In that case, it would mean she would only have to share her story with one provider and attend one type of session, which might appeal to her and seem less daunting. The ability to engage in therapy could then be further assessed during already scheduled appointments. Furthermore, there are clearly situational stressors such as her school performance and college applications that need to be explored. Adding therapy sessions would likely provide her psychiatrist with a better understanding of Ms. A's condition and complicating factors. However, should the psychiatrist realize that there is a need for more intensive or frequent therapy than can be provided in a combined session, Ms. A may need to be referred to a separate therapist. Again, as noted previously in this chapter, it will be important to engage Ms. A in those discussions, assess her view of treatment type(s) and cultural background, and ensure that she does not feel discarded to another treatment provider.

Conclusion

The integration of medication and psychotherapy should be a process of providers working together to facilitate psychological healing in a shared clinical case. Each provider must take into account the needs of the patient first and be willing to seek out assistance from trusted colleagues. Furthermore, nonprescribing psychotherapists need to be informed about psychiatric medications, while remaining firmly within the limits of their competence, leaving recommendations for medications to the judgment of the psychiatrist.

When differing clinical opinions arise, each provider must work to address their differences, maintaining a mutual respect for the contributions each is making for the benefit of the patient. While many cases can be successfully treated with medication or psychotherapy alone, cases where both forms of treatment are needed afford providers with a unique opportunity to develop an ongoing collaboration that transcends disciplines and brings new perspectives to the patient's care.

Self-Study Questions

1. What are some clinical indicators that might lead you to refer for an evaluation for medication management? What are some patient-specific preferences to consider when referring for medication management?

2. What are some situations that might lead a psychiatrist to initiate psychotherapy as part of medication management? What situations would leave a psychiatrist to refer to another provider for psychotherapy?

3. Imagine that your patient has recently started seeing another provider for medication management. They present to your weekly session, stating that their diagnosis has been changed by the new provider, but you are not sure that you agree with this. How might you handle this situation?

4. What are some of the benefits and complications of attempting to balance both psychotherapy and pharmacotherapy in a combined session?

5. Do opportunities exist for mental health providers who do not prescribe medications to learn more about psychopharmacology? If so, what are those opportunities?

6. What arrangements do a referring therapist and psychiatrist need to make with one another to help strengthen their collaborative relationship?

RESOURCES FOR FURTHER LEARNING

Powell AD. The medication life. *J Psychother Pract Res.* 2001;10(4):217-222.

Shoemaker SJ, Ramalho de Oliveira D. Understanding the meaning of medications for patients: the medication experience. *Pharm World Sci.* 2007;30(1):86-91.

Spencer J, Goode J, Penix EA, Trusty W, Swift JK. Developing a collaborative relationship with clients during the initial sessions of psychotherapy. *Psychotherapy.* 2019;56:7-10.

Thase ME., Riba M, Safer DL. *Integrating Psychotherapy and Pharmacology: Dissolving the Mind-Brain Barrier.* New York, NY: W.W. Norton; 2003.

13

REFERENCES

1. Cuijpers P, Andersson G, Donker T, van Straten A. Psychological treatment of depression: results of a series of meta-analyses. *Nordic J Psychiatry*. 2011;65(6):354-364.
2. Jonghe de F, Kool S, Aalst van G, et al. Combining psychotherapy and antidepressants in the treatment of depression. *J Affect Disord*. 2001;64:217-229.
3. Jakobsen JC, Hansen JL, Simonsen E, Gluud C. The effect of adding psychodynamic therapy to antidepressants in patients with major depressive disorder. A systematic review of randomized clinical trials with meta-analyses and trial sequential analyses. *J Affect Disord*. 2012;137(1-3):4-14.
4. de Maat S, Dekker J, Schoevers R, et al. Short psychodynamic supportive psychotherapy, antidepressants, and their combination in the treatment of major depression: a mega-analysis based on three Randomized Clinical Trials. *Depress Anxiety*. 2008;25, 565-574.
5. Miklowitz DJ. Adjunctive psychotherapy for bipolar disorder: state of the evidence. *Am J Psychiatry*. 2008;165(11):1408-1419.
6. Hirschfeld R, Bowden C, Gitlin M, et al. *Practice Guideline for the Treatment of Patients with Bipolar Disorder*. 2nd ed. Washington, DC: American Psychiatric Association; 2010. Retrieved December 6, 2019, from https://psychiatryonline.org/pb/assets/raw/sitewide/practice_guidelines/guidelines/bipolar.pdf.
7. Pollack MH, Otto MW, Boy-Byrne PP, et al. Novel treatment approaches for refractory anxiety disorders. *Depress Anxiety*. 2008;25:467-476.
8. Campbell-Sills L, Bystritsky A, Byrne PP, Sullivan G, Craske MG, Stein MB. Improving outcomes for patients with medication-resistant anxiety: effects of collaborative care with cognitive behavioral therapy. *Depress Anxiety*. 2016;33:1099-1106.
9. American Psychological Association (APA). *Clinical Practice Guidelines for the Treatment of Posttraumatic Stress Disorder*. 2017. Available at https://www.apa.org/pstd-guideline/.
10. Spencer J, Goode J, Penix EA, Trusty W, Swift JK. Developing a collaborative relationship with clients during the initial sessions of psychotherapy. *Psychotherapy(Chic)*. 2019;56:7-10.
11. Aikens JE, Nease DE, Klinkman MS, Schwenk TL. Adherence to maintenance-phase antidepressant medication as a function of patient beliefs about medication. *Ann Fam Med*. 2005;3(1):23-30.
12. Thase ME, Riba M, Safer DL. *Integrating Psychotherapy and Pharmacology: Dissolving the Mind-Brain Barrier*. New York, NY: W. W. Norton; 2003.
13. Chong WW, Aslani P, Chen TF. Shared decision-making and interprofessional collaboration in mental healthcare: a qualitative study exploring perceptions of barriers and facilitators. *J Interprof Care*. 2013;27:373-379.
14. Powell AD. The medication life. *J Psychother Pract Res*. 2001;10(4):217-222.
15. Shoemaker SJ, Ramalho de Oliveira D. Understanding the meaning of medications for patients: the medication experience. *Pharm World Sci*. 2007;30(1):86-91.
16. Cabaniss DL. Shifting gears: the challenge to teach students to think psychodynamically and psychopharmacologically at the same time. *Psychoanal Inq*. 1998;18(5):639-656.
17. Hayes SC, Strosahl KD, Wilson KG. *Acceptance and Commitment Therapy: The Process and Practice of Mindful Change*. 2nd ed. New York, NY: Guilford Press; 2012.

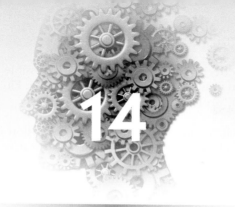

Using Psychotherapy Supervision in Training and Beyond

SALLIE G. DE GOLIA, MD, MPH AND MEGAN E. TAN, MD, MS

Case Study

Dr. X is an incoming second-year resident who is starting an outpatient psychotherapy rotation. He has no experience with psychotherapy, other than his own brief personal experiences during medical school, and what he has learned in residency didactics thus far. His residency program has assigned Dr. C (an outpatient psychiatrist) as the supervisor. He knows very little about Dr. C, other than what a few advanced residents have said about working with Dr. C in supervision. She has been described to Dr. X as a supervisor with "high expectations" for learning psychotherapy, presenting to weekly supervision prepared, and frequently reviewing tapes of sessions in supervision itself. As Dr. X has never completed a session as a psychotherapist, he finds himself very anxious about how he should even prepare for the first supervision session. He begins to reread a few basic psychotherapy books but is still concerned he will not be able to "perform" psychotherapy adequately.

INTRODUCTION

For the beginning therapist, supervision is how we learn to do our trade. It is a unique, relationship-based teaching modality where we learn the nuanced skills of working with our patients. Supervision is where we sort out the complex issues our patients share with us in order to provide the most appropriate treatment. The primary goal of supervision is patient care—to ensure that you as a trainee are providing the most effective and appropriate care possible to the patient. A secondary goal is for you to learn how to make this happen. Finally, supervision is also where we develop our professional identities as therapists.

Despite the many well-documented benefits of supervision for trainees, new therapists often report feeling apprehensive about starting supervision or simply confused about the parameters. This is understandable—psychotherapy supervision is a complex process. It is notably different from any other kind of didactic teaching or learning experience you may have participated in up to this point in your training.

Thankfully, the seemingly mystifying process of psychotherapy supervision can be more easily grasped by breaking it down into four chronological phases: Preparatory, Introductory, Working, and Termination Phases.[1] Throughout this chapter, we will use clinical vignettes to explore each phase of psychotherapy supervision. The goal of the chapter is to aid early trainees in understanding how to approach and understand psychotherapy supervision, regardless of modality. See also *Table 14.1* below for basic "Dos and Don'ts" to help get you started.

TABLE 14.1 Dos and Don'ts for Therapy Supervision

Dos	Don'ts
• Get to know your supervisor • Be clear about your goals and objectives • Discuss any discomfort in supervision early on • Let your supervisor directly observe the therapy whether through in vivo, one-way mirror, audiotape, and/or videotape observation • Try out a variety of learning modalities (video review, transcripts, role-play, etc.) • Try to articulate what you understand about the patient, even if you are uncertain • Practice being autonomous in your clinical decision-making • Suggest potential interventions and troubleshoot potential consequences • Self-assess and ask for feedback often	• Do not show up late or cancel supervision at the last minute • Do not take your supervisor for granted • Do not expect to know everything on day 1 (if you already knew how to be a therapist, you would not be in a training program!) • Do not hesitate to let your supervisor know when you are lost or confused • Do not become defensive if your supervisor points out a blind spot. Learning how to identify our own common blind spots is an important part of the process of becoming a skilled therapist • Do not treat supervision as individual therapy

THE PREPARATORY PHASE

The Preparatory Phase takes place *before* you even meet with your supervisor for the first time. As you prepare for psychotherapy supervision, it is useful to reflect upon the following questions:

1. What should I expect in psychotherapy supervision?

2. What is the clinical setting in which I will practice?

3. What do I hope to get out of the experience?

4. How do I select a supervisor?

Recognize the Scope of Supervision

Many beginning trainees are uncertain about what to expect in psychotherapy supervision. This is complicated by the fact that supervision has many moving parts. Depending on the patient and clinical context, you may be expected to learn a wide variety of skills, theories, and/or techniques. At the same time, interpersonal dynamics frequently come into play, bringing up complex questions about power dynamics, boundaries with patients *and* supervisors, and countertransference, among other issues. Supervision is a place for discussion and exploration of all these topics and more. It is also where you will develop a deeper understanding of the utility and meaningfulness of psychotherapy, as well as develop your identity as a psychotherapist.

Many beginning therapists wonder how much to disclose about oneself to their supervisor. This question may be particularly anxiety-provoking, given your supervisor also has an evaluative role. Supervisees also often have concerns about whether supervision will feel like personal psychotherapy. Let us strongly emphasize this point here—psychotherapy supervision *is not* individual psychotherapy. However, there may be moments where it begins to push up against this fine line. Remember—the goal of supervision is to help you provide effective care for your patient while developing skills, knowledge, and attitudes associated with a given modality. That being said, much of the practice and "art" of doing psychotherapy depends on the therapist having insight around their own feelings and behaviors in response to the patient. It is, therefore, incumbent on your supervisor to help you assess what might be driving your feelings and behaviors *in relation to your patient* and to help you address these matters so that you can provide appropriate and effective therapy. Your supervisor might suggest you consider working through some of these issues in your own personal psychotherapy, while using supervision to explore *only* those aspects necessary to help with patient care. In short, supervision will require a developing therapist to self-reflect—but it is *not the place* to work through your personal issues in depth.

Understand the Specifics of Your Clinical Setting

Before you start supervision, be sure to understand the clinical environment. Are there specific clinic requirements and/or expectations of you as a trainee? If audiovisual equipment is required, do you know how to use it? Have you used the outpatient electronic medical record format before? Hopefully, your training program has an orientation to help you consider all these various parts of the supervisory process before supervision begins.

In addition to these logistical considerations, educate yourself about the type(s) of therapy you are expected to learn and the resources available to you. Depending on the type(s) of psychotherapy in which you will be supervised (eg, supportive, cognitive behavioral, dynamic, couple's therapy, or group psychotherapy), you might need to seek out a variety of resources for learning. For example, you may be expected to help your patient develop new ways of thinking (cognitive behavioral therapy [CBT]), practice deep breathing techniques (mindfulness-based stress reduction), or probe unconscious conflicts around identity, agency, and self-worth (psychodynamic psychotherapy). Although there are common factors that cut across all types

14

of therapy[2] (see Chapter 4), each psychotherapy modality also involves different and specific approaches. Consider reaching out to senior trainees or recent graduates of your program for advice about good books and online resources. Once you begin supervision, your supervisor will no doubt be able to direct you to additional learning materials. However, the more prepared you are in advance, the more you will get out of the supervisory experience.

Reflect on Your Motivation to Learn Psychotherapy

Even before entering the supervisory experience, take some time to reflect on your motivation for learning psychotherapy. Most likely, you are starting supervision in a particular psychotherapy modality because it is required by your training program. For many, this is an exciting opportunity. For others, learning a particular psychotherapy modality may be viewed as unrelated to your long-term career goals. Particularly if you are in this latter category, take some time to consider how you might make this experience useful and engaging to you. How might learning this type of psychotherapy augment your personal growth and/or future endeavors? For example, if you are hoping to become a medical director of a community clinic, consider how practicing specific communication techniques within psychotherapy supervision might help you manage employees effectively in the future. The more you can identify (or conjure up) your own motivation and personal interest in the material at hand, the more you are going to learn from and enjoy the experience.

Select a Supervisor

Selecting a supervisor is not always so straightforward—if this choice is even available to you. Some programs assign supervisors without input from the trainee. However, if you have the option to select a supervisor, you will want to consider three factors: (1) your identified learning needs, (2) a supervisor's efficacy,[3] and (3) whether or not the supervisor would be a "good fit" (aka, the supervisory alliance).[4]

In reflecting upon your learning needs, consider both the modality of therapy you are learning as well as your own learning style. Are you able to select a supervisor with expertise in the kind of psychotherapy you want to learn? Are you more comfortable with a directive, "hands-on" supervisor? Or do you prefer a supervisor who approaches the process as a consultant, allowing the learner to be more autonomous? You might also consider the supervisor's approach to teaching (eg, emphasis on use of role-play, transcripts, self-reflection, etc.). Finally, depending on your own personal preference and clinical interests, you may want to consider other aspects such as gender, race, and awareness of economic, cultural, spiritual, and/or sexual diversity. You may also want to consider training location and the opportunities that working with a specific supervisor would afford you. Have you been able to experience providing therapy within a community clinic setting, a health maintenance organization, or a rural or urban setting? Over time, it will be important to have worked with a diverse set of supervisors and modalities.

Next, you will want to identify an "effective" supervisor. *Table 14.2* lists several of the qualities that are ascribed to a "good supervisor."[5-7]

TABLE 14.2 What Makes an Effective Supervisor?

Effective	Less Effective
Empathic, genuine, respectful, supportive	Authoritarian, critical
Prepares for and is involved in session, enjoys supervisory role	Lacks time to prepare or frequently cancels supervision
Self-discloses in the service of supervision	Limited self-awareness, not accepting of feedback
Adheres to ethical guidelines	Engages in discriminatory behaviors, microaggressions, stereotyping, cultural insensitivity, or violates boundaries
Communicates goals and expectations clearly	Unclear agendas, sets vague expectations, or changes expectations without warning
Adapts to supervisee's learning needs, style, and character (flexible)	Prescribed supervisory style (rigid)
Avoids providing psychotherapy during session	Conflates supervision with psychotherapy
Provides appropriate and timely feedback	Confrontational approach to corrective feedback; ascribes blame; provides limited or no feedback
Facilitates the supervisee to further understand the patient and keeps to the material presented within the session	Digresses into topics that are not particularly relevant to the task at hand
Encourages the supervisee to speculate about clinical material	Uses solely didactic approaches, rather than interactive learning opportunities
Allows the supervisee to tell their clinical narrative	Dominates the sessions
Attends to supervisee's concerns when addressing relationship either between the patient and supervisee and/or supervisee and supervisor	Avoids important affective cues brought into the supervision sessions
Avoids jargon and is concrete	Uses jargon, is vague, and gives convoluted explanations
Consistently tracks most immediate aspect of supervisee's affectively charged concerns	Fails to identify and follow what supervisee is concerned with and misses important affective cues

Adapted from Carifio MS, Hess AK. Who is the ideal supervisor? *Prof Psychol.* 1987;18:244-250; Hubregsen JJ, Brenner AM. How to select an individual psychotherapy supervisor: a practical guide. In: De Golia SG, Corcoran KM, eds. *Supervision in Psychiatric Practice: Practical Approaches Across Venues and Providers.* Washington, DC: American Psychiatric Association Publishing; 2019; Ratliff DA, Wampler KS, Morris GH. Lack of consensus in supervision. *J Marital Fam Ther.* 2000;26:373-384; and Shanfield SB, Matthews KL, Hetherly V. What do excellent psychotherapy supervisors do? *Am J Psychiatry.* 1993;150:1081-1084.

14

As with therapy, the alliance between a supervisor and supervisee is foundational to a good supervisory experience.[4,8,9] You will want to find someone with whom you feel comfortable, safe, respected, and engaged. Finding the "right fit" supervisor is important but sometimes difficult to determine in advance. If your clinical environment provides you with a list of supervisors, try to find out as much as possible about each one before selection. Consider talking to senior trainees or graduates about their experiences with specific supervisors. Finally, if your program allows it, consider meeting with a couple of supervisors to see how it feels. Remember, this is an important working (and learning) relationship that may last for months to a year or longer. Just like mentorship, you will want to be able to work with someone who is a "good fit."

How to Select a Supervisor

- Identify personal needs

  - Seek variety in supervisors—gender and other cultural group diversity (eg, LGBTQ/sexual and gender minority, spirituality, race)

  - Seek variety of supervisory techniques used (role-play, transcript, video, etc.)

  - Identify personal preference regarding supervisory style (directive, hands-off, flexible)

  - Determine the therapy modality in which you need more practice

- Learn qualities of an "effective supervisor"

  - See Table 14.2

- Consult with other peer colleagues, faculty, or graduates regarding their experience with a supervisor

- Informally interview potential supervisors, if appropriate, to consider the relationship "fit"

THE INTRODUCTORY PHASE

This phase takes place during the first few sessions of supervision. It involves establishing a working alliance, setting the frame for supervision, and identifying learning objectives.

Establish a Working Alliance

Building a solid *working alliance* in supervision is critical. Research shows that the relationship between a supervisor and supervisee is the foundation of how supervision works.[10] It is the quality of this relationship that predicts the willingness of supervisees to disclose,[11,12] a supervisee's satisfaction with supervision,[13] and supervisory outcomes based on supervisee ratings.[14] A strong supervisory alliance has also been shown to decrease supervisee burnout and enhance job satisfaction.[15] Finally, although no studies have clearly linked supervisory outcomes to patient outcomes, Patton and Kivlighan[16] suggest an inferential link between the quality of supervision and patient outcomes.

Thus, it is important to spend time during the Introductory Phase developing a good working relationship with your supervisor. By investing in the creation of a safe and respectful environment, you will be more likely to admit vulnerabilities, concerns, fears, and mistakes, with reduced shame and anxiety, thereby facilitating greater learning.

Case Study

Dr. X is an incoming second-year resident who is about to start working in an outpatient psychotherapy clinic for the first time. His program has assigned him a supervisor, Dr. C. At their first meeting, Dr. C welcomes Dr. X to supervision and asks how his training is going. What has he liked most about his training so far? What has surprised him? Does he have a favorite "type" of patient to work with? Dr. C listens actively, empathizing and reflecting back what Dr. X expresses. They banter a bit about the residency program.

A bit later, Dr. C inquires as to how Dr. X became interested in medicine and, in particular, psychiatry. She wonders, have there been any particular successes or challenges in terms of learning experiences? Dr. C observes that Dr. X is somewhat less forthcoming than other residents with whom she has worked. She encourages him to be as open as possible during supervision but appreciates any space he may need.

In the example above, Dr. C has expressed interest in Dr. X, but she also respects his need for space, thus facilitating a safe environment. During the Introductory Phase, pay attention to how you feel toward and with your supervisor. If your supervisor facilitates a trusting and effective working alliance, this will help you feel more comfortable seeking help and integrating feedback.[17]

In contrast, if you are feeling unheard, unsafe, or disrespected by your supervisor, you may want to address this directly with your supervisor and/or seek guidance from your peers, process group, or even your program director. This can be an enormous challenge for the supervisee because of the inherent power differential that exists between the supervisee and the supervisor. See the section "Navigating Moments of Tension or Discomfort With Your Supervisor" for a more detailed discussion of this topic.

Set the Supervisory Frame

In addition to establishing a working alliance, the Introductory Phase also includes setting the supervisory frame. While individual supervisors may vary in some of their specific "ground rules," there are several universal features of the supervisory frame.

Your supervisor will be juggling numerous roles—often at the same time. Some of these supervisor roles include being a manager, clinician, educator, and mentor. It is helpful to be aware of these roles in order to understand the parameters of supervision. You might engage your supervisor in a discussion about these various roles and responsibilities—in relationship to you, your patient, and your training program. Discussing these roles may also help you form goals for supervision.

In the *manager* role, your supervisor should explain the logistics of the psychotherapy clinic, if these have not been explained elsewhere. This might include scheduling, how to write a psychotherapy note, and how to bill appropriately. As with most kinds of therapy, supervision typically occurs once a week, at a regularly scheduled time. Be punctual. It is important to inform your supervisor as soon as possible if you are not able to attend supervision.

As the *clinician (or attending)-of-record*, your supervisor is legally and ethically responsible for ensuring patient safety and effective treatment. Your supervisor is your go-to person for any emergency or other baffling clinical issue that may arise in the therapy. During the Introductory Phase, you should obtain your supervisor's contact information, including an emergency number. Conversely, your supervisor should have all your contact information in case of any clinical issue that might arise outside of supervision or in the event the supervisor is unexpectedly unable to attend a supervision session. Finally, you should discuss general plans for supervision cross-coverage should you or your supervisor go out of town. You must *always* have a supervisor available for consultation should your supervisor be away *and* a clinician who covers your patients' care in your absence.

As an *educator*, your supervisor may use a variety of teaching methods to help you learn the essentials of your particular modality of psychotherapy. The supervisor will explain how to obtain patient information for review (eg, video recording, transcripts, etc.) and how to present such information within the supervisory sessions. Although being directly observed may feel anxiety-provoking, particularly for the new supervisee, direct observation provides your supervisor with more accurate information about the session. As a result, your supervisor will be able to deliver more precise feedback that allows you to improve as a therapist.[18]

A supervisor will also evaluate your performance and hopefully provide frequent feedback to help you improve. But here is the challenge: the trainee, on the one hand, is encouraged to be as open as possible and vulnerable about their work in psychotherapy, yet, on the other hand, the supervisor has the mandate to inform the training program should issues in competency or safety arise. This can be confusing. By virtue of the supervisor's role as an evaluator, specific limits to confidentiality are imposed on the relationship. If a supervisor is particularly concerned about your competence, or a health issue that may be interfering with your patient care duties, the supervisor may contact the program director to confirm concerns and/or request guidance. Should the issue go unresolved (persistent poor performance despite feedback), it is incumbent on the supervisor to inform the program director. The best approach is to talk frankly about these limitations to confidentiality so that you understand early on how they will be enacted should a problem arise. Hopefully, your supervisor will discuss with you any problems they perceive and at what point they may need to engage with the training leadership for guidance or resolution. Ideally, there should be minimal surprises around these issues.

Finally, as a *mentor*, your supervisor is available to help you navigate how to become an excellent therapist within the training program and beyond. They may also be open to helping you construct a healthy work/life balance, manage training-related frustrations outside the direct supervisory context, and/or think about a specific career path.

Another part of setting the frame involves clarifying the difference between psychotherapy supervision and psychotherapy, the so-called *"teach/treat" boundary*. Ideally, your supervisor will preemptively clarify the difference between these two domains during the Introductory Phase and how the supervisor intends to pay attention to these boundaries throughout supervision. This may go a long way to relieving your anxiety. Again, supervision is NOT personal psychotherapy.

Psychodynamic psychotherapy supervision in particular can place a supervisee and supervisor at particular risk for blurring the boundary, given the nature of countertransference discussions. These types of discussions require a certain amount of vulnerability on the part of the supervisee to disclose personal feelings, thoughts, and behaviors in response to patient material. Any material that relates to the work with a patient is part of supervision; however, a supervisee's personal life and problems unrelated to this material are not part of the supervision. If you feel your supervisor is entering into personal territory that seems to go beyond how your behavior, thoughts, or feelings impact the therapy you are doing with your patient, your supervisor may be engaging in psychotherapy with you. This is complex terrain and one that may require you to speak up directly with your supervisor or seek guidance from a trusted colleague, peer, and/or training director. You certainly may grow personally and learn a great deal about yourself within the process of supervision, but the personal focus and deep work occur in your own psychotherapy.

Finally, it is not uncommon to have multiple relationships with a supervisor (eg, working together on a committee, coauthoring a paper, etc.), particularly if the supervisor has an active role in your training program. Although ideally avoided to limit the potential of a boundary transgression, these multiple relationships are not necessarily problematic.[19] However, they should be directly addressed at the beginning of supervision, given the evaluative role of the supervisor and the increased risk for boundary transgressions. As long as the supervisor's intent is not to exploit the trainee or benefit from their engagement, but rather provide opportunities to enhance the education and career development of the supervisee, such relationships are generally not forbidden.

Establish Learning Objectives

Your supervisor will help you establish your learning objectives during the Introductory Phase. For many new supervisees, this is easier said than done, as explored in our clinical vignette below.

Case Study—Establishing Learning Objectives

    Towards the end of their first supervision session, Dr. C asks Dr. X about his goals for their supervision work together. In a rather awkward manner, Dr. X admits he is unclear about his goals for supervision. Having just begun his first psychotherapy didactic class last month, the material is all brand new to him, and he feels rather unprepared to begin working as a therapist.

14

Dr. C is grateful that Dr. X can admit this and normalizes his comments by acknowledging the fact that he is a novice to psychotherapy and this type of supervision. It is understandable to have difficulty identifying specific goals at this time. Dr. C explains that the primary purpose of supervision is to try to help Dr. X provide the best care for his patient while concomitantly learning the principles and skills of psychotherapy. She describes a few of the key skills identified as being most helpful across nearly all types of psychotherapy—active listening, developing a nonjudgmental approach, and building a solid working alliance with a patient.

Dr. C discloses that, when she was a resident, she often turned to the educational program guidelines and evaluation forms and/or her profession's regulatory organization's guidelines to help create and think about learning goals. She suggests Dr. X might take a look at the program guidelines. In addition, she encourages him to reflect on his work with inpatients and whether there may be specific, relevant issues that might translate well into a goal for this type of therapy. Finally, she encourages him to consider his long-term career goals. How might the present experience support or be relevant to his future and can he extract some goals from that reflection? Dr. X agrees that this makes sense and feels achievable. They make a plan together for him to review the program guidelines and reflect on his past clinical experiences and future career aspirations before their next session.

At their next meeting, Dr. X explains that as a budding researcher, and someone who probably would not be providing psychotherapy in the future, he would like to keep his eye on those psychological concepts that might be relevant to his eventual work running a large lab. He recognizes that improving his interpersonal skills would be quite useful, as he currently feels somewhat lacking in this area. As such, he identifies three goals: being able to actively listen better, allowing the patient to have the space to talk freely without interruption, and working on use of facilitating and empathic comments.

Not all trainees are passionate about psychotherapy nor eager to learn as much as possible about a given modality. Others may be more interested in psychopharmacology, neuropsychology, school psychology, neuroscience, or policy work. Know what you want out of this learning experience. Think hard about what is important to you, the modality you are learning, your career goals, and your past clinical experiences. These reflections might lead you to identifying some specific goals for the psychotherapy supervision. Finding relevance and collaborating on goals will increase your motivation and engagement in the learning process.

THE WORKING PHASE

The bulk of supervision occurs in the Working Phase. During this phase, you and your supervisor will juggle several roles, often simultaneously: providing clinical care, learning basic therapeutic skills and techniques, managing potential or real ruptures in the supervisory relationship, attending to issues of diversity, evaluating your work, and learning from feedback. In addition, many trainees turn to their supervisors for career mentorship over the course of the Working Phase. We will address each of these topics in the following section.

Provide Clinical Oversight

Ideally, your supervisor's clinical oversight will include direct observation either through a one-way mirror room, cotherapy (when the supervisor and supervisee are in the room together doing therapy with the patient), or through audio or video review (most common). The goal of clinical oversight is to ensure patient safety and quality of care. Although many trainees and supervisors rely on simple session recall or written process notes, this approach is suboptimal, as it necessarily includes the supervisee's unique biases and blind spots. Providing your supervisor with direct access to objective session data—most easily done in the form of video, audio, and/or verbatim transcripts—is highly recommended. If something particularly concerning or perplexing occurs during the course of your therapy work, it can be useful to review the recordings with your supervisor. In some situations, it may be necessary for the supervisor to meet with the patient or sit in a session with you to clarify what is happening.

Consider Learning Strategies

The Working Phase of supervision is where you will learn the theories, skills, and nuances of interpersonal behaviors, as well as the interplay of culture and diversity within psychotherapy. But what do you as a supervisee need to do to help facilitate an optimal learning environment?

Supervision is a collaborative process, so *come prepared*. Unlike traditional lecture-based learning, in which trainees may be expected to simply listen, supervision requires your full and active engagement as a learner. Be prepared to bring in questions you have for your supervisor or even an agenda for the session.

How to Come Prepared for Supervision

- Have your session documentation completed before supervision (if possible)
- Send the audio or video clip/transcript to your supervisor *before* supervision, with a specific question you want help with
- If you have multiple patients with a given supervisor, bring an updated patient log to supervision, complete with information about no-shows and cancellations in the past week
- Bring an agenda of issues and questions you would like to discuss
- Provide your supervisor with objective data (eg, transcript, video)
- Seek feedback often
- Ask for readings—particularly on something you are having difficulty with
- Incorporate feedback you received from supervision
- Practice a skill you learned in supervision session before your next session

14

This advice sounds straightforward, but many beginning therapists wonder, "*What questions should I even be asking my supervisor?*" The questions may focus on some aspect of the theory outlined in a didactic, an interaction observed within your clinical experience, or a feeling you have about your patient that you find confusing. You might also select a portion of a video (or audio) recording where you have felt "stuck," confused, sad, or angry, or one where you had an "ah-ha!" moment and want to share it with your supervisor. You may also want to ask for supplemental learning materials to help clarify a concept. Or you might ask your supervisor to role-play an exchange to help you practice articulating your thoughts, providing a particular intervention, or thinking on your feet. Do not leave the responsibility of teaching solely to the supervisor—come to each session engaged and prepared!

Because doing psychotherapy requires a broad range of knowledge and skills, learning psychotherapy requires a variety of teaching strategies. High-quality teaching within clinical supervision has been shown to impact a trainee's clinical competence.[20] We have highlighted a few of the most common teaching strategies that particularly involve your input as a learner in *Table 14.3*.

TABLE 14.3 Common Teaching Strategies in Supervision

Domain	Teaching Strategy
Objective observation	• Video review • One-way mirror • Transcript review
Practice	• Role-play • Deliberate practice
Self-reflection	• Working with countertransference • Reviewing process notes • Self-assessing performance
Didactic	• Lectures about theory or technique • Case presentations/formulations • Independent readings

The use of *self-reflection* can be a highly valuable source of learning during supervision, particularly with regard to understanding countertransference (defined as a supervisee's conscious or unconscious response toward the patient). Understanding your feelings toward the patient is a normal part of supervision that allows us to better recognize patient dynamics and determine effective approaches to care. Through such a process, you may sometimes feel quite emotional, which can be perplexing and, at times, overwhelming. This may be a result of complex interactions of unexamined experiences within you that the patient evokes and/or a result of the patient's unique interpersonal behaviors. Should this occur, bring these feelings and thoughts up during supervision. Even though it may be embarrassing, shameful, anxiety-provoking, or simply confusing at times, engaging in self-reflection within a secure supervisory relationship is a powerful learning tool.

Case Study—Self-Reflection in Supervision

After watching a video clip, Dr. X. spontaneously notes that working with a patient whose parents are divorced has unexpectedly brought up some strong feelings related to his own parents' divorce 5 years ago. He notes that listening to his patient talk about the holidays makes him feel frustrated and withdrawn. Dr. C. comments that there seems to be a variety of threads worth attending to: the patient who is starting to get in touch with some deeper feelings that have been blocked for a very long time, the emotional experience that this touches off in Dr. X., and the subsequent impact of Dr. X's countertransference on the therapist-patient relationship. She encourages him to reflect on these various aspects.

Dr. C notes that it may be useful to explore these multiple feelings with the intent of understanding their impact on the course of the patient's therapy. Dr. C asks Dr. X if he wants to talk about the incident and how it might play into the current therapy, with the caveat that he does not have to discuss the matter if it makes him uncomfortable. Dr. X notes he is aware he has some unresolved emotional wounds from his parents' divorce that may block him from exploring the depth of his patient's pain, for fear that his pain may deepen and become overwhelming. Dr. C praises his insight and asks if Dr. X has any ideas about how he wants to move forward from this point.

Dr. X notes he does not want his own unresolved conflicts to impact negatively on his approach to treatment and thus resolves to bring up the issue in his own personal therapy in order to work through it more fully.

In this vignette, Dr. C encourages Dr. X to reflect on his experience with the patient and related matters; however, she also is quite aware of pending boundary concerns—particularly around difficult countertransference material. Some modalities, such as psychodynamic psychotherapy, will focus on unconscious dynamics and the countertransference engendered by the patient's dynamics. These feelings and dynamics can be important to understand in the context of how they may impact patient care. These may also inadvertently lead us to avoid therapeutic interventions or cause us to "act out" with patients, resulting in damaging consequences. In CBT supervision, the supervisor might want the supervisee to pay particular attention to personal body language and language choices, as they may reflect the supervisee's own automatic thoughts and/or conditional or core beliefs. Should these issues arise for you, a reasonable approach is to consider seeking your own therapy to help understand your unique issues. An attentive supervisor will be cognizant of entering into particularly vulnerable territory and may ask your permission and/or encourage you to work through some of these issues in your own therapy. However, the depth in which you choose to reveal anything within supervision is entirely up to you. It will also depend on the nature of your alliance with your supervisor. It is best to be cognizant when self-reflecting and choose cautiously how you want to proceed. As we have noted before, should you feel your supervision is transgressing into therapy with you, it might be the time to address this with your supervisor directly or discuss the matter with a trusted faculty member or training director.

14

Reviewing *transcripts* is a useful, objective learning tool. Although this may be time-consuming for you to prepare (at least initially), the process immerses you back into the therapeutic experience, allowing you to further process what transpired during a session. When discussing case material, Miller et al.[21] found that use of objective methods was shown to increase therapist competence. By revisiting the session content word for word, or even by just reviewing a video, you may recognize aspects of the interaction you did not notice at the time of therapy. Transcripts will also allow you to annotate your work by easily keeping track of questions you might have, feelings that were evoked, or alternative responses you might consider—all useful to bring into supervision. They also provide a quick way for your supervisor to review a therapy session prior to supervision, allowing the supervisor to identify important teaching points in advance.[22] Ideally, transcripts would be paired with the video segment to incorporate nonverbals, intonations, and other components of a dialogue that would be otherwise lost in the written word alone. In addition, it is not necessary to create a written transcript of an entire therapy session—10 minutes is often sufficient. Transcripts that focus on a specific section or skill (eg, agenda-setting or other self-identified growth areas) can be quite helpful.

Another powerful objective teaching strategy is the use of *video or audio recordings* in psychotherapy. Like transcripts, a video provides the supervisor with objective data, rather than relying on trainee self-report. Reviewing a video with your supervisor will allow you to reflect upon, problem-solve, and analyze what has transpired in the session. This also provides the stimulus to consider new conceptualizations and/or interventions arising from the experience. It also provides concrete information about a trainee's actual clinical skills, thereby enabling the supervisor to better understand and target a trainee's competency gaps. Finally, it is a way for your supervisor to see exactly what transpired in a session, thereby allowing them to provide you with more accurate feedback.

If your program uses video recording, consider asking your supervisor to role-play the consent process. If setting up the equipment is confusing, seek help from a chief resident, clinic director, or IT specialist. Do not hesitate to ask for help when you need it: you want to decrease as many barriers to audio/video (AV) use as possible. However, if video and audio recordings are not officially part of your program, *you should not record a patient without authorization by the training program.* There are significant legal considerations and technical procedures related to data encryption that are necessary in order to protect patient confidentiality.

One simple way to integrate video review into supervision is to select a short (10-minute) section of a session in advance of your supervision. Review the section on your own time and come up with reasons for its selection and how your supervisor might help you with the segment. For example, you may feel "stuck" in the section, wonder why the patient responded in a certain manner or exhibited unexpected nonverbal behaviors, or you might wonder if it is an example of transference or a core belief. You also might feel proud of an intervention you made that you had been practicing for some time, or you might want to review a section where you tried to integrate your supervisor's feedback.

Working With Audio- and Videotapes

- Make sure video recording is authorized by your program

- If it is not authorized, but you are interested in video recording, meet with your clinic director

- Ensure audio- or videotapes are made on an encrypted device, transferred to supervisors, via encrypted thumb drives if appropriate, and, again, where appropriate, stored for a very limited time period in an encrypted, secure server that has been authorized by your institution

- Obtain your patient's consent with a program-approved form and process

- Set up the equipment before your patient walks in the room

- Try to capture *both* yourself and your patient in the camera view

- If the patient is uncomfortable, switch the camera focus onto you or turn off the video

- Review the video before supervision to identify areas for discussion in supervision

- Select a 10-minute segment to share with your supervisor with a question

- Consider selecting clips involving:

  - Where you experienced feelings, thoughts, and behaviors that may have surprised you

  - Patient nonverbal communications that surprised you

  - Examples of various concepts in psychotherapy (patient core beliefs, automatic thoughts, transference, strengths)

  - Places where you did not think your comments "worked"

- Delete tapes promptly following supervision

Condensed from De Golia SG. Videotapes: learning through facilitated observation and feedback. In: De Golia SG, Corcoran KM, eds. *Supervision in Psychiatric Practice: Practical Approaches Across Venues and Providers.* Washington, DC: American Psychiatric Association Publishing; 2019.

Finally, an effective but underutilized approach to supervision is the use of *deliberate practice*. This approach focuses on actual skill development and behavioral rehearsal (role-play). With your supervisor, identify an area of difficulty you are having. First, break down a perceived difficulty into the smallest behavioral components. Then, practice each component repeatedly until you experience mastery—like learning an instrument! By providing incremental learning that is just beyond your ability, deliberate practice aims to enhance your "microskills." This supervisory technique has been shown to be more effective than traditional methods of training.[23]

14

Case Study—Role-Play and Deliberate Practice

Dr. X brings in a video of a patient he is convinced will soon drop out of therapy. He tells Dr. C he does not know how to prevent it. After reviewing the segment, Dr. C suggests that there may be an issue with the alliance. She asks if Dr. X notices anything interesting about the patient and Dr. X's engagement in this clip. Sheepishly, Dr. X notices that he may have interrupted the patient. Dr. C agrees that she also noticed this and that, at times, Dr. X tended to speak over the patient. She wonders how the patient may have felt during that exchange. She also wonders how Dr. X may have been feeling during this segment.

After exploring Dr. X's reflections, Dr. C invites Dr. X to role-play with her. She suggests that he try to notice when he has the urge to interrupt or talk over her. She suggests that, at that moment, Dr. X could practice waiting 5 seconds before responding. She also encourages him to simultaneously reflect on any complex feelings or anxiety he may have at that moment. They repeat the role-play a few times until Dr. X understands the approach. Dr. C then suggests that he practice this approach for 10 minutes, three times a week, working with the most recent video session until he feels more comfortable with the skills. She instructs him to identify when he tends to interrupt and/or speak over the patient, then replay the video and, "speaking to the video," try the behaviors she suggests—waiting 5 seconds while being mindful of his internal process. She also asks him to report back on any feelings he was having during these episodes. Dr. X agrees to the homework suggested.

After they discussed the homework at the next session, Dr. C invites Dr. X to consider alternative behaviors he might employ when engaging with his patient. Dr. X has been successful at eliminating most interruptions and talk-overs but is not quite sure what to do aside from saying nothing. Dr. C suggests he might leave more space for the patient by considering the use of silence, use more facilitative expressions ("go on," "uh-huh"), or perhaps reflect on the patient's experience and/or consider asking the patient to explore more thoughts and feelings. She now invites him to try these various alternatives with his patient in their next session and report back to her.

By utilizing deliberate practice, you will not only become more mindful about your behaviors and feelings, but through targeted practice, you may be able to improve your skill base more quickly and consistently.

How to Work With Deliberate Practice

- Identify a behavior with which you are having difficulty
- With help from your supervisor, deconstruct the behavior into two to three microskills
- Practice microskills with your supervisor (role-play)

- Spend 10 minutes two to three times per week reviewing your video to identify similar difficulties and practice the microskills

- Notice your feelings, thoughts, and behaviors when you practice the skills

- Implement new skills in the therapy

- Report back on the implementation at the next supervision session

Navigate Moments of Tension or Discomfort With Your Supervisor

As in any relationship, tension may arise within the supervisory relationship. This is often complicated by the power differential that exists within the supervisory dyad—compounded by the fact that your supervisor is evaluating you. Depending on your training milieu, your supervisor might also serve in multiple roles within the program, further complicating the dynamic.

Ideally, your supervisor will preemptively address the potential for disagreement and tension within supervision and might ask for your input as to how you prefer to navigate such moments, if and when they arise. However, not all supervisors discuss these topics in advance, and even those who do may not identify ruptures when they arise. Therefore, it is useful to consider how you might address uncomfortable moments or topics within supervision. If you disagree with a clinical approach your supervisor has recommended, or if you feel uncomfortable within the supervisory sessions for any reason, try to speak up. But how?

It is not uncommon for a trainee to respond to tension in the supervisory relationship in one of two ways: through confrontation or withdrawal.[10] You may feel comfortable directly addressing your dissatisfaction with your supervisor about something that occurs within the supervisory relationship. This allows your supervisor to engage directly around the rupture and ideally work to repair and resolve the situation. However, this can be uncomfortable for many trainees. Instead, they may disengage from supervision when tension occurs, manifested by asking fewer questions, or by being less responsive or less involved in the process. Trainee withdrawal, in contrast to confrontation, can be more difficult for the supervisor to quickly identify.

If you are not comfortable directly expressing disagreement or discomfort within supervision, you may want to seek advice from a trusted colleague, peer, and/or previous supervisor *before* you talk to your current supervisor. Set aside time to process your concerns and clearly identify the issue at hand. An outside perspective is invaluable in these situations. Next, consider how to present the conflict in a respectful and mutually beneficial manner. For example, you might start by explaining how you have felt within the supervision and by commenting that you recognize the supervisor's goal is to create the best learning environment possible. You might ask if it would be possible to reflect on how to help you feel more comfortable and engaged in the process, as you want to get as much as possible from the experience. If your supervisor is not able to respond in kind or the situation persists, you should discuss the problem with the director of your training program.

14

In rare cases, a supervisory relationship may become harmful, exploitative, and/or lacking in adequate supervision (eg, the supervisor never discusses the case at hand despite your redirecting the discussion, does not seem to know what to do, or behaves unethically). If you have attempted to correct the situation without success, it may be necessary to terminate supervision. If you are at this point, you have no doubt already alerted your training director. If not, now is the time to meet to discuss what has taken place in the supervision. The training director might encourage you to have a final session with your supervisor to say your goodbyes and part amicably. If the situation is highly toxic, your training director might choose to alert the supervisor to the termination.

At other times, it might be the supervisor who is not able to work with a trainee based on a personality conflict, professionalism issue (eg, a trainee fails to show for supervision), and/or a concern about significant competency deficits where the supervisor is legally responsible for patient care and does not have the time to remediate the trainee in order to provide adequate care. The supervisor should be direct and clear with the trainee about their concerns and explain that they will need to discuss the situation with the program director. In this situation, the supervisor might opt to terminate supervision. It is up to the program director to determine the next steps with the trainee *and* the patient.

Attend to Issues of Diversity Within Clinical Supervision

Navigating issues of diversity and inclusion is an essential skill for therapists. However, evidence suggests these topics are often avoided within psychotherapy supervision—by trainees and supervisors alike[24,25] (see also Chapter 8). In the clinical vignette below, we explore common themes that emerge within supervision related to cultural differences: power differentials and avoidance of cultural factors. After exploring the unique features of the supervisory relationship in this context, we offer some practical strategies for bringing up issues of culture and diversity with your supervisor. It is important to remember: cultural differences are generally present in *all* supervisory relationships—not only when the supervisor and supervisee appear to be from different cultural backgrounds.

Case Study—Diversity Issues in Supervision, Part I

Towards the end of a supervision session, Dr. X presents a video of a new patient to his supervisor, Dr. C. The patient is a 32-year-old Latinx woman who works a high-profile job in the insurance industry. Her chief complaint is depression and chronic feelings of inferiority at work relative to her peers. During the video, the patient says she has been looking for a therapist for the past 3 years but cannot find a good match. When the trainee asks about what gets in the way of finding a good match, the patient pauses for a moment, looking at the therapist, and then replies "racism."

Dr. C pauses the video at this moment and muses, "That response may be a bit of a red flag."

Her comment triggers Dr. X to flinch with surprise. "What do you mean?" he asks.

Noticing his response, Dr. C realizes she has entered very important terrain without giving it sufficient thought. She can see that Dr. X is upset by her comment, though she is uncertain about the exact nature of his frustration. She tries to clarify the intention behind her comment: "I'm trying to point out that she's a high-powered executive with great insurance coverage; there are plenty of excellent therapists in this area. So, it's worth noting that she can't seem to find a good therapy match after 3 years of trying. We may be dealing with a patient who externalizes interpersonal issues."

"Oh," says Dr. X, "I guess that makes sense. I mean, I see what you're trying to say." Feeling frustrated, he stops himself from speaking up, due to respect for Dr. C as his superior—and due to his belief that disagreeing with her clinical opinion would be inappropriate and unprofessional.

Mindful that Dr. X was having a negative response to her comment and uncertain of how to move the conversation forward, Dr. C offers, "I think this topic is really important for us to explore, but we are out of time for today. Let's finish this conversation next week, okay?"

The following week, Dr. X arrives at supervision more anxious than usual but eager to have a follow-up conversation about what had transpired the previous week. He felt a strong working alliance with Dr. C and was curious to understand her perspective on this issue. On the way to supervision, Dr. X wonders what it will be like for Dr. C, who is a white female, to talk about these issues with a biracial male such as himself. He was eager to learn more about how to navigate the nuances of these topics with his therapy patients.

However, upon entering Dr. C's office, Dr. X suddenly feels awkward and uncertain about how to begin the conversation. He worries that Dr. C will think he is calling her racist if he returns to her "red flag" comment, so he instead starts the supervision session by asking about a clinical issue with a different patient. His comment diverts their attention from the previous session. Of note, neither Dr. C nor Dr. X returns to the patient's comment about racism from the previous week, or Dr. X's reaction.

In the vignette above, a critical breakdown of communication has occurred, resulting in discomfort and avoidance around deeply important and vulnerable issues. Aware that her comment upset Dr. X, the supervisor felt uncertain as to how to proceed without being judged as racist. Meanwhile, the supervisee felt protective of the patient but also unable to speak up because of the power differential between him and his supervisor.

It is important to note that the *power differential* within the supervisory relationship plays a significant role in this communication breakdown. In a traditional supervisory relationship, the power differential is well defined. Supervisors are, by definition, more knowledgeable and experienced than their supervisees. This asymmetry is crucial: maintaining a power differential helps create a sense of safety for the

14

beginning trainee, who will, at times, need to lean upon someone who they view as more powerful, knowledgeable, and skilled in order to navigate new clinical scenarios. However, when navigating issues of diversity and inclusion, a trainee may find themselves in the awkward position of having more lived experience or knowledge than the supervisor. In fact, given recent demographic shifts and the increasing value placed upon diversity within academic programs, many supervisory dyads in the United States today consist of a senior supervisor from a historically dominant culture or community (white, Christian, straight, male, etc.), paired with a trainee from a historically marginalized or exploited culture or community (eg, black, Latinx, Muslim, gay, female, etc.). In addition, due to cohort-related training requirements across generations, current supervisees may be imbued with the importance of cultural diversity training as a necessary and integral part of all good patient care training, whereas their supervisors may have only received mandatory "cultural diversity" training long after completing postgraduate education (if at all!). As a result, supervisors may find themselves in the unusual position of working with a trainee who holds more cross-cultural knowledge or expertise than themselves.

As demonstrated in this vignette, the demographic realities of the supervisory pair may shift the power differential in unique ways, creating a challenging scenario that may elicit feelings of anxiety, self-consciousness, and/or defensiveness within *both* the supervisor and supervisee. Supervisees may hesitate to bring up issues that are particularly relevant or vulnerable to them (sexuality, race, gender, religion, and other categories of identity and belonging). At the same time, supervisors may avoid talking about issues related to cultural identity and diversity, particularly if they feel criticized or judged by the trainee. The avoidance (and/or confrontation) that commonly results in these situations may have a negative impact on the supervisory relationship as well as the therapy.

Case Study—Diversity Issues in Supervision, Part II

The following week, Dr. X reflected on this avoidance in his trainee process group. Talking through the supervision session in a safe space with his colleagues, he came to understand that his frustration stemmed from the fact that he identified with the patient. Dr. X had experienced significant challenges trying to find a therapist who was well attuned to the psychological impact of racism. In fact, he had gone through three different therapists before finding someone who he felt understood his own lived experience as a biracial individual raised within a highly segregated society. While the content of his life story was very different from that of his patient, he nonetheless empathized with her struggle to find a mental health professional who understood her experience with race. In an attempt to help create a space and opportunity for him and his supervisor to return to the discussion of race and culture, Dr. X decided to send Dr. C an article about addressing issues of culture and race in supervision.

At the subsequent session, Dr. C starts the session by thanking Dr. X for sending the article. Reflecting on her initial "red flag" comment, she notes it was lacking in an appreciation for the racial issues at hand and no doubt impeded their communication. She recognizes that Dr. X's lived experience is different from hers. She was aware he was uncomfortable when they discussed the patient a few weeks ago, yet she also felt a bit judged and was uncertain how to proceed without becoming more defensive or upsetting him further. She makes it clear that she values his perspective and the supervisory alliance. She states that, unlike most moments in supervision, he may in fact have something to teach her about this clinical situation. She then invites him to share his thoughts about the article, his interpretation about the patient's comment, and/or any of the comments she has just made.

In response, Dr. X comments on a few sections from the academic article that resonated with him. He discloses that he felt a deep bond and empathy with the patient from the first moment, and that he was therefore offended by Dr. C's "red flag" comment, which felt dismissive to him. He goes on to describe some of his own experiences dealing with discrimination and racism as a child, which were deeply painful for him. Dr. X also notes that his own strong identification with the patient's experience in relation to race may have gotten in the way of him recognizing and appreciating other clinical nuances.

The previous vignette demonstrates several key themes and "best practices" that we have been outlining in this section. First, when confronted with rupture in the supervisory relationship, Dr. X seeks consultation from his peers in process group. Peer consultation allows him to recognize his own avoidance of an affectively charged topic with his supervisor. He then proactively addresses the avoidance by emailing his supervisor an academic article about race in the supervisory experience. Reading the article allows Dr. C to better understand the trainee's perspective in a less charged manner. By better understanding his perspective and being able to reflect on her own defensiveness, Dr. C was able to explicitly address what she felt was happening in the supervisory session and intentionally shift the traditional supervisory power differential by acknowledging the value of Dr. X's cultural expertise and lived experience. Once that power differential was reduced, Dr. X felt safer discussing his feelings more openly. Ultimately, Dr. C invites Dr. X to share about his experiences, and the two were able to have a valuable and deeper conversation that allowed them both to process and learn from one another.

The previous clinical example highlights the importance of *intentionally* breaking down (or at least reducing) power differentials between the supervisor and trainee when trying to engage in a meaningful discussion about cultural diversity. This strategy is particularly useful when the power differential between the supervisor and supervisee echoes historical patterns of oppression—such as a white male supervisor paired with a female from a historically marginalized or exploited minority group. Reducing power differentials in the context of such difficult issues can lead to a sense of shared vulnerability, facilitating a safer, more exploratory space for the trainee in relation to issues of culture and diversity. This is not to say that the power differential should *always* be intentionally reduced but, rather, knowing *when to reduce* the power differential and *when to maintain* it is an important task for your supervisor.

14

Sharing about such deeply personal and vulnerable issues in supervision can be difficult for both the supervisee and supervisor. The complexities of the supervisory relationship may not be straightforward or clearly appreciated by either party, so it is important to approach these topics with humility and a willingness to learn from one another. As in all other domains of supervision and clinical learning, you *will* make mistakes when addressing issues of diversity and inclusion. And, you *will* learn from them—regardless of your own background. Recognizing that different situations require different approaches, the text box below outlines concrete suggestions to help trainees and supervisors find ways to navigate challenging moments of tension related to questions of diversity.

Strategies to Navigate Issues of Diversity and Inclusion in Supervision

1. Establish mutual trust with your supervisor before trying to discuss these issues, as talking about culture carries a high degree of affective potency

2. Be prepared to reflect upon any interpersonal dynamics related to power differentials, race, ethnicity, gender, religion, sexuality, socioeconomic status, or other issues of diversity if and when those issues arise

3. Recognize that the typical power differential of the supervisor and trainee may become inverted in these scenarios

4. Pay attention to your own feelings and countertransference, and do not be afraid to discuss them with your supervisor

5. Recognize that we all bring our own unique culture, assumptions, and lived experiences into the supervisory space

6. Be ready and willing to examine the idea that both you and your supervisor may have unconscious biases, regardless of your cultural background

7. Listen actively—sometimes this is the most important intervention

8. Begin with open inquiry and humility when in doubt about how to proceed

9. Avoid following the initial instinct to defend and clarify your own position

10. Address perceived differences in interpretation between you and your supervisor with curiosity, rather than judgment. Use phrases like "I wonder" or "I'm curious about…," rather than "I know" or "It's obvious that…"

11. Ask for feedback in real time: "What is it like for you and me to talk about these issues?"

12. Seek outside perspective and consultation from peers

13. Although this is usually the responsibility of the supervisor, attempt to reduce the power differential to enhance a solid working alliance and allow for more open communication around these issues. What is the meaning of the power differential for you in this context? What is the meaning for your supervisor? This communication can happen through mutual self-disclosure, acknowledging limits of knowledge, and sharing vulnerabilities

14. Share articles related to diversity and inclusion with your supervisor as a prompt for discussion. Consider using this book chapter to serve as a prompt for discussion around issues of culture and diversity in supervision

15. Ask for articles to read that are related to the psychological impact of collective trauma, structural violence, and other topics important to integrating cultural factors into treatment (*see Chapter 8 for further reference*)

16. Consider obtaining a cultural consultation to help move through any roadblocks in the supervisory relationship

Evaluate and Provide Feedback

In addition to teaching how to do therapy, your supervisor will also be evaluating you and, hopefully, providing frequent, clear, and specific feedback. We encourage you to ask your supervisor for frequent and *specific* feedback. This will help you continually improve your skills on the path to becoming a competent therapist.

When it comes to feedback, an interactive approach has been shown to be particularly effective[26-29] compared to a more unidirectional approach. For example, the supervisor might ask you to first self-assess your performance, then offer one or two constructive and/or positive comments about the performance. Ideally, the feedback will be based on the initial goals set in the supervision. Before ending the feedback session, the supervisor might ask if you have any questions about the feedback, what it was like to receive the feedback, and/or suggest you and the supervisor develop an action plan together to tackle the areas for improvement. This is in contrast to a more unidirectional approach, such as the "feedback sandwich," where the supervisor would provide some positive comments about your performance followed by one or two constructive comments and end with another positive comment, without necessarily engaging you in a dialogue about the feedback. With a more collaborative approach to feedback, not only does your supervisor have the opportunity to learn more about you, but the process may lead to decreasing the power differential in the supervisory relationship and, in turn, allow for more effective learning. It is important that you be able to hear and try to integrate the feedback.

As a novice therapist, you also need encouragement! You are in a vulnerable position and are practicing a modality in which you have little experience. Positive feedback provides reassurance and a platform from which to integrate more corrective feedback. However, it is the corrective feedback that will allow you to grow and develop.[29] Try your best not to be defensive, but rather to listen with an open mind to any feedback your supervisor gives, even if you disagree. If you do not understand a part of the feedback, ask for clarification. If the feedback is vague (*"Great job!"*), ask for details. You will find that different supervisors will focus on different aspects of your skills and/or knowledge. Take whatever you can from *each* supervisor.

14

Mentor

Finally, mentorship, another feature of the working phase, weaves in and out of supervisory sessions. Mentorship within supervision can result in valuable opportunities for career growth and development and can enhance your identity as a psychotherapist and/or mental health provider. Your supervisor may provide mentorship in a variety of ways. First, your supervisor models professionalism and identity as a therapist, educator, and/or a parent or spouse. Supervisors also model clinical reasoning and skills, self-care, and how to process and deliver other content that is brought up in supervision. Beyond modeling, the supervisor may actively engage you around personal and professional growth and guidance. However, because of the evaluative role of a supervisor, you should be mindful to make purposeful choices of what you feel comfortable sharing in supervision. Such mentoring topics might include helping you identify your values as they relate to your career, how to develop your career, what organizations or national committees you might consider joining, how to balance your personal life with professional ambitions, and even how to engage in scholarship. The supervisor might also help you navigate some complicated administrative or political issues within your department.

Finally, depending on your supervisor's style, they might advocate on your behalf. Your supervisor might recommend you for a committee of an organization they are involved in, introduce you to colleagues to facilitate networking, invite you to coauthor a manuscript, or ask you to join a research project. Although these behaviors may appear as boundary crossings, if your supervisor has your best interests in mind, then they are appropriate. Should you feel uncomfortable in the least or confused about whether the boundary has been inappropriately crossed, it is important to reflect on the behavior, discuss this with your supervisor, seek advice from a trusted colleague, and/or check it out with your training director.

THE TERMINATION PHASE

This phase refers to the ending phase of the supervisory relationship—which does not necessarily correspond to the termination of a patient from therapy. Termination of supervision, like in therapy, involves a deliberate winding down of the relationship—often within the last month of supervision—depending on the length of the relationship. This phase involves reflection on the supervisory process and achievements, summative evaluation of you (and your supervisor), as well as your transition to a new supervisor.

During this period, you and your supervisor reflect on the supervisory experience. Supervisors may guide you in reflecting on what aspects of the supervisory experience have been helpful and not so helpful. If you are able to provide your supervisor with clear and constructive feedback directly, your supervisor might benefit from a powerful learning experience. However, this is often difficult given the inherent power differential in the relationship. At a minimum, it is important to provide anonymous feedback about your supervisor to the training program. This can be complicated, particularly if a supervisor only has one supervisee for the entire year. In some programs, supervisors would not receive feedback until at least three supervisee evaluations are available for anonymous collation. As a result, it might take 3 years before a supervisor receives any formalized feedback from the training program! Ideally, feedback helps the supervisor reconsider supervisory approaches and techniques and appropriateness of their use, in order to become an even more effective supervisor. If you are not comfortable providing direct feedback and your program is structured in such a way that your supervisor might not receive anonymous feedback for quite a while, it may be useful to meet with your training director or clinic chief to provide confidential feedback about the supervisory experience.

It is also important to consider those areas of your own development that may need ongoing attention. Once you have synthesized your progress and identified specific learning goals for the future, you might consider discussing how best to move forward with this work in your next supervisory relationship. Remember, supervision is a space for potentially deep learning and growth. It is also a place where you have the opportunity to develop life-long learning behaviors that will be critical once you leave the protected learning environment of your training program.

Case Study—Termination

About a month prior to Drs. C and X's last supervision session, Dr. C encourages Dr. X to start reflecting on what aspects of the supervision have been particularly helpful to him and what aspects have not been so helpful. She also will want him to develop some goals moving forward that may be useful within his next supervisory experience. Dr. C explains that she, too, will be considering her experience within the supervision with Dr. X, what she has seen in terms of his progress, and how he might continue to improve moving forward. She will also reflect on which supervisory behaviors of hers she has found useful and perhaps not so useful in terms of helping him develop and work together. She suggests that, at each of the subsequent four sessions, they carve out some time to attend to feedback and termination. If left to the last session where there may be limited time due to patient needs, she is concerned there would not be adequate time to process and respond to each other's comments. Dr. X agrees with the approach and suggests that he start as of next week to describe how he has evolved within supervision.

Conclusion

In this chapter, we have sought to define the important relationship-based activity where trainees learn to become psychotherapists, regardless of modality. We have broken down the supervisory experience into four key phases: Preparatory, Introductory, Working, and Termination. These have been illustrated through example vignettes. Through demystifying the supervisory process, we hope that trainees are able to make better use of the supervisory experience in order to provide the best care to patients and to develop their skills and identity as a psychotherapist.

14

Self-Study Questions

1. What are the overarching four stages of supervision?

2. Based on the research, what foundational element is at the basis for a successful supervision?

3. What are four key roles of a supervisor?

4. What jeopardizes confidentiality within supervision?

5. What are the three goals of supervision?

6. What three factors should you consider when selecting a supervisor?

7. How might you come prepared for supervision?

8. What are some of the steps to consider when navigating issues of diversity and inclusion in supervision?

9. What are the three components of termination?

RESOURCES FOR FURTHER LEARNING

Books

Bernard JM, Goodyear RK. *Fundamentals of Clinical Supervision.* 6th ed. Upper Saddle River, NJ: Merrill; 2019.

De Golia SG, Corcoran KM, eds. *Supervision in Psychiatric Practice: Practical Approaches Across Venues and Providers.* Washington, DC: American Psychiatric Association Publishing; 2019.

Falender CA, Shafranske EP. *Supervision Essentials for the Practice of Competency-Based Supervision (Clinical Supervision Essentials).* Washington, DC, American Psychological Association; 2016.

Hook JN, Watkins CE, Davis DE, Owen J, Van Tongeren DR, Ramos MJ. Cultural humility in psychotherapy supervision. *Am J Psychother* 2016;70(2):149-166.

Johnson EA. *Working Together in Clinical Supervision.* New York, NY: Momentum Press; 2017.

REFERENCES

1. De Golia SG. Elements of supervision. In: De Golia SG, Corcoran KM, eds. *Supervision in Psychiatric Practice: Practical Approaches Across Venues and Providers.* Washington, DC: American Psychiatric Association Publishing; 2019.

2. Wampold BE. How important are the common factors in psychotherapy? An update. *World Psychiatry.* 2015;14:270-277.

3. Hubregsen JJ, Brenner AM. How to select an individual psychotherapy supervisor: a practical guide. In: De Golia SG, Corcoran KM, eds. *Supervision in Psychiatric Practice: Practical Approaches Across Venues and Providers.* Washington, DC: American Psychiatric Association Publishing; 2019.

4. Watkins CE Jr. The supervisory alliance: a half century of theory, practice, and research in critical perspective. *Am J Psychother.* 2014;68:19-55.

5. Carifio MS, Hess AK. Who is the ideal supervisor? *Prof Psychol.* 1987;18:244-250.

6. Ratliff DA, Wampler KS, Morris GH. Lack of consensus in supervision. *J Marital Fam Ther.* 2000;26:373-384.

7. Shanfield SB, Matthews KL, Hetherly V. What do excellent psychotherapy supervisors do? *Am J Psychiatry.* 1993;150:1081-1084.

8. Ladany N, Friedlander ML, Nelson ML. *Supervision Essentials for the Critical Events in Psychotherapy Supervision Model.* Washington, DC: American Psychological Association; 2016.

9. Watkins CE Jr. The alliance in reflective supervision: a commentary on Tomlin, Weatherston, and Pavkov's critical components of reflective supervision. *Infant Ment Health J.* 2015;36:141-145.

10. Watkins CE, Callahan JL. Psychotherapy Supervision Research: a status report & proposed model. In: De Golia SG, Corcoran KM, eds. *Supervision in Psychiatric Practice: Practical Approaches Across Venues and Providers.* Washington, DC: American Psychiatric Association Publishing; 2019.

11. Mehr KE, Ladany N, Caskie GIL. Trainee nondisclosure in supervision: what are they not telling you? *Couns Psychother Res.* 2010;10:103-113.

12. Webb A, Wheeler S. How honest do counsellors dare to be in the supervisory relationship? An exploratory study. *Br J Guid Counc.* 1998;26:509-524.

13. Son EJ, Ellis MV. Clinical supervision in South Korea and the United States: a comparative descriptive study. *Couns Psychol.* 2013;41:48-65.

14. Tsong Y, Goodyear RK. Assessing supervision's clinical and multicultural impacts: the supervision outcome scale's psychometric properties. *Train Educ Prof Psychol.* 2014;8:189-195.

15. Livni D, Crowe TP, Gonsalvez CJ. Effects of supervision modality and intensity on alliance and outcomes for the supervisee. *Rehabil Psychol.* 2012;57:178-186.

16. Patton MJ, Kivlighan DM. Relevance of the supervisory alliance to the counseling alliance and the treatment adherence in counselor training. *J Couns Psychol.* 1997;44:108-115.

17. Kaufman J, Schwartz T. Models of supervision. *Clin Superv.* 2004;22(1):143-158.

18. Mazor KM, Holtman MC, Shchukin Y, Mee J, Katsufrakis PJ. The relationship between direct observation, knowledge, and feedback: results of a national survey. *Acad Med.* 2011;86(10):S63-S68.

19. Gottlieb MC, Robinson K, Younggren JN. Multiple relations in supervision: guidance for administrators, supervisors, and students. *Prof Psychol Res Pr.* 2007;38:241-247.

20. Wimmers P, Schmidt H, Splinter T. Influence of clerkship experiences on clinical competence. *Med Educ.* 2006;40:450-458.

21. Miller WR, Yahne CE, Moyers TB, Martinez J, Pirritano M. A randomized trial of methods to help clinicians learn motivational interviewing. *J Consult Clin Psychol.* 2004;72:1050-1062.

22. De Golia SG, Williams KE, Safer D. Working with transcripts: an underutilized supervisory approach. In: De Golia SG, Corcoran KM, eds. *Supervision in Psychiatric Practice: Practical Approaches Across Venues and Providers.* Washington, DC: American Psychiatric Association Publishing; 2019.

23. McGaghie WC, Issenberg SB, Cohen ER, Barsuk JH, Wayne DB. Medical education featuring mastery learning with deliberate practice can lead to better health for individuals and populations. *Acad Med.* 2011;86(11):e8-e9.

24. Bandstra B, Shah R, Tan M. Cultural issues within the supervisory relationship. In: De Golia SG, Corcoran KM, eds. *Supervision in Psychiatric Practice: Practical Approaches Across Venues and Providers.* Washington, DC: American Psychiatric Association Publishing; 2019.

25. Schen CR, Greenlee A. Race in supervision: let's talk about it. *Psychodyn Psychiatry.* 2018;46(1):1-21.

26. Sargeant J, Eva KW, Armson H, et al. Features of assessment learners use to make informed self-assessments of clinical performance. *Med Educ.* 2011;45:636-647.

14

27. Telio S, Ajjawi R, Regehr G. The "educational alliance" as a framework for reconceptualizing feedback in medical education. *Acad Med.* 2015;90(5):609-614.
28. Watling CJ, Kenyon CF, Zibrowski EM, et al. Rules of engagement: residents' perceptions of the in-training evaluation process. *Acad Med.* 2008;83(10 suppl):S97-S100.
29. Boehler ML, Rogers DA, Schwind CJ, et al. An investigation of medical student reactions to feedback: a randomized controlled trial. *Med Educ.* 2006;40:746-749.

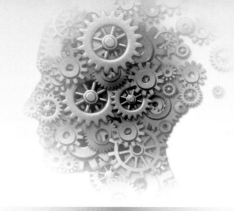

Acknowledgments

I am more grateful than I can say to all my patients who have shared their stories and struggles with me. It has been a great privilege to work with them, and they have taught me so much about how to actually be helpful.

Mentoring is essential to an academic career, and I was very lucky to have Bill Greenberg and Jon Borus. Bill showed me what it means to be a psychiatry residency director, and Jon made me into a scholarly writer. My work in psychiatry education is built on their examples.

As we make clear throughout the book, supervision is a critical part of becoming a therapist. I have had many wonderful supervisors, but Humphrey Morris and Philip Freeman deserve special mention as residency teachers who I later returned to for supervision during analytic training. They were models of both analytic attitude and kindness. Over the years, I have also relied on peer supervision and am thankful to many colleagues who have provided guidance, especially John Cain, whose generosity and acumen remain invaluable.

Finally, thank you to my parents, Sol and Gloria Brenner, who first set me on this path. And to my sons, Max and Caden, who have been very patient during this book process and have taught me so much about both development and play.

And the most heartfelt appreciation to my coauthor, peer-mentor, peer-supervisor, editor, and spouse, Amy Brenner. She is the wisest person and keenest clinician I know and has made my work and this book better in every possible way.

Adam Brenner, MD

First, I want to thank all of my students—past, present, *and* future. You are the reason I am in academic medicine, and you forever push me to be a better teacher, supervisor, and psychologist. I have also learned from many incredible patients—there are not enough words for all you have taught me. Thank you to the many colleagues and mentors within the APA and the UT Southwestern Medical Center Department of Psychiatry, who helped raise me professionally for the past 10 years and continue to nurture my growth.

Inspiration to teach and write starts with having good teachers. So many teachers have indelibly imprinted their lessons on me—Ms. Holloway and Ms. Herbert (discipline and tenacity), Ms. Watkins (a love of writing), Mr. Bodine (creating safe spaces), and Ms. Hall (always finding potential). Later, I had many graduate school mentors who provided their own lessons—Dr. Sharon Jenkins (how to edit, with her fierce, blue, felt-tipped pen), Dr. Randall Cox (immense and unwavering support), and Dr. Amy Murrell (the art of Mattering).

I am fortunate to have an extremely "deep bench" of personal support and encouragement. First, endless thanks to my parents (Jeanie and Roger), who expected a boy, got a baby woman, and taught me the values of integrity, faith, and compassion. And much love to the rest of my bench—my best friend (Urmi), sister-friend (Michelle), aunt (Sukie), brothers (Josh and Aaron), and in-laws (Susan and Mike).

To my three children, who were (mostly) patient during evenings and weekends while "mommy worked on the book"—hopefully you will understand someday!

Finally, I want to express limitless gratitude and affection for my husband. He shows up for his family, supports academic pursuits such as this one, engages in spirited debates that challenge my perspective, and is witty beyond measure.

Laura Howe-Martin

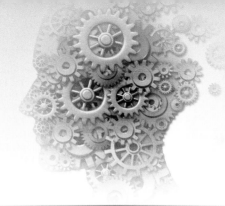

Index

Note: Page numbers followed by "f" indicate figures, "t" indicate tables and "b" indicate boxes.